RADIOLOGY

CASE REVIEW SERIES | Thoracic Imaging

RADIOLOGY
CASE REVIEW SERIES | Thoracic Imaging

Amr M. Ajlan, MD

Consultant Radiologist and Assistant Professor
Radiology Department
King Abdulaziz University Hospital
King Abdulaziz University
Jeddah, Saudi Arabia

Alexandre Semionov, MD

Assistant Professor
Department of Diagnostic Radiology
McGill University
Montreal, Quebec, Canada

SERIES EDITOR

Roland Talanow, MD, PhD

Consultant Radiologist
Department of Radiology
Chrissie Tomlinson Memorial Hospital
George Town, Cayman Islands
Affiliate Professor
University of Bern
Bern, Switzerland

Mc
Graw
Hill
Education

New York   Chicago   San Francisco   Athens   London
Madrid   Mexico City   Milan   New Delhi   Singapore
Sydney   Toronto

Radiology Case Review Series: Thoracic Imaging

3 4 5 6 7 8   QVS/QVS   24 23 22 21 20

ISBN 978-0-07-181808-7
MHID 0-07-181808-1

This book was set in Times LT Std. by Thomson Digital.
The editors were Michael Weitz and Robert Pancotti.
The production supervisor was Richard Ruzycka.
Project management was provided by Sarita Yadav, Thomson Digital.
The text designer was Elise Lansdon.
Quad/Graphics was the printer and binder.

Library of Congress Cataloging-in-Publication Data

Ajlan, Amr M., author.
  Thoracic imaging / Amr M. Ajlan, Alexandre Semionov.
    p. ; cm. — (Radiology case review series)
  Includes bibliographical references.
  ISBN 978-0-07-181808-7 (softcover : alk. paper) — ISBN 0-07-181808-1 (alk. paper)
  I. Semionov, Alexandre, author. II. Title. III. Series: Radiology case review series.
  [DNLM: 1. Thoracic Diseases—diagnosis—Case Reports. 2. Thoracic Diseases—diagnosis—Problems and Exercises. 3. Diagnostic Imaging—Case Reports. 4. Diagnostic Imaging—Problems and Exercises. WF 18.2]
  RC941
  617.5'40754—dc23
                                                                                2015015571

McGraw-Hill Education books are available at special quantity discounts to use as premiums and sales promotions or for use in corporate training programs. To contact a representative, please visit the Contact Us pages at www.mhprofessional.com.

I am grateful to Dr. Roland Talanow for giving me the opportunity to author this book. I am especially thankful that my dear friend Dr. Alexandre Semionov kindly agreed to co-author this project, adding his touch of expected excellence. I had the help of many friends and colleagues along the way. Drs. Jonathon Leipsic, Cameron Hague, and Jennifer Ellis provided me with unlimited support during my fellowship. I am also thankful to Drs. Nestor Muller, John Mayo, Patrick Vos, Joseph Casullo, John Kosiuk and Ida Khalili. No words of thanks can express my appreciation for the boundless help provided by my mother, wife, and kids. In the end, I would like to dedicate this effort to the memory of my father, God bless his soul. His love for teaching has always inspired me in ways that are immeasurable.

— Amr M. Ajlan, MD

I would like to dedicate this book to Dr. Max Palayew, an outstanding chest radiologist, a great mentor, a true scholar, and a genuine gentleman.
To Dr. John Kosiuk, who unostentatiously has taught me to become some of the above.
And to my family, without whom none of this would be possible or meaningful.
Special thanks to my brother-in-arms, Dr. Amr Ajlan, for soliciting me for this project and for seeing it through.

— Alexandre Semionov, MD

Contents

Series Preface

Maybe I have an obsession for cases, but when I was a radiology resident I loved to learn especially from cases, not only because they are short, exciting, and fun—similar to a detective story in which the aim is to get to "the bottom" of the case—but also because, in the end, that's what radiologists are faced with during their daily work. Since medical school, I have been fascinated with learning, not only for my own benefit but also for the sake of teaching others, and I have enjoyed combining my IT skills with my growing knowledge to develop programs that help others in their learning process. Later, during my radiology residency, my passion for case-based learning grew to a level where the idea was born to create a case-based journal: integrating new concepts and technologies that aid in the traditional learning process. Only a few years later, the *Journal of Radiology Case Reports* became an internationally popular and PubMed indexed radiology journal—popular not only because of the interactive features but also because of the case-based approach. This led me to the next step: why not tackle something that I especially admired during my residency but that could be improved: creating a new interactive case-based review series. I imagined a book series that would take into account new developments in teaching and technology and changes in the examination process.

As did most other radiology residents, I loved the traditional case review books, especially for preparation for the boards. These books are quick and fun to read and focus in a condensed way on material that will be examined in the final boards. However, nothing is perfect and these traditional case review books had their own intrinsic flaws. The authors and I have tried to learn from our experience by putting the good things into this new book series but omitting the bad parts and exchanging them with innovative features.

What are the features that distinguish this series from traditional series of review books?

To save space, traditional review books provide two cases on one page. This requires the reader to turn the page to read the answer for the first case but could lead to unintentional "cheating" by seeing also the answer of the second case. Doesn't this defeat the purpose of a review book? From my own authoring experience on the *USMLE Help* book series, it was well appreciated that we avoided such accidental cheating by separating one case from the other. Taking the positive experience from that book series, we decided that each case in this series should consist of two pages: page 1 with images and questions and page 2 with the answers and explanations. This approach avoids unintentional peeking at the answers before deciding on the correct answers yourself. We keep it strict: one case per page! This way it remains up to your own knowledge to figure out the right answer.

Another example that residents (including me) did miss in traditional case review books is that these books did not highlight the pertinent findings on the images: sometimes, even looking at the images as a group of residents, we could not find the abnormality. This is not only frustrating but also time-consuming. When you prepare for the boards, you want to use your time as effectively as possible. Why not show annotated images? We tackled that challenge by providing, on the second page of each case, the same images with annotations or additional images that highlight the findings.

When you are preparing for the boards and managing your clinical duties, time is a luxury that becomes even more precious. Does the resident preparing for the boards truly need lengthy discussions as in a typical textbook? Or does the resident rather want a "rapid fire" mode in which he or she can "fly" through as many cases as possible in the shortest possible time? This is the reality when you start your work after the boards! Part of our concept with the new series is in providing short "pearls" instead of lengthy discussions. The reader can easily read and memorize these "pearls."

Another challenge in traditional books is that questions are asked on the first page and no direct answer is provided, only a lengthy block of discussion. Again, this might become time-consuming to find the right spot where the answer is located if you have doubts about one of several answer choices. Remember: time is money—and life! Therefore, we decided to provide explanations to *each* individual question, so that the reader knows exactly where to find the right answer to the right question. Questions are phrased in an intuitive way so that they fit not only the print version but also the multiple-choice questions for that particular case in our online version. This system enables you to move back and forth between the print version and the online version.

In addition, we have provided up to three references for each case. This case review is not intended to replace traditional textbooks. Instead, it is intended to reiterate and strengthen your already existing knowledge (from your training) and to fill potential gaps in your knowledge.

However, in a collaborative effort with the *Journal of Radiology Case Reports* and the international radiology community Radiolopolis, we have developed an online repository with more comprehensive information for each case, such as demographics, discussions, more image examples, interactive image stacks with scroll, a window/level feature, and other interactive features that almost resemble a workstation. In addition, we are planning ahead toward the new Radiology Boards format and are providing rapid-fire online sessions and mock examinations that use the cases in the print version.

I am particularly proud of such a symbiotic endeavor of print and interactive online education and I am grateful to McGraw-Hill for giving me and the authors the opportunity to provide such a unique and innovative method of radiology education, which, in my opinion, may be a trendsetter.

The primary audience of this book series is the radiology resident, particularly the resident in the final year who is preparing for the radiology boards. However, each book in this series is structured on difficulty levels so that the series also becomes useful to an audience with limited experience in radiology (nonradiologist physicians or medical students) up to subspecialty-trained radiologists who are preparing for their CAQs or who just want to refresh their knowledge and use this series as a reference.

I am delighted to have such an excellent team of US and international educators as authors on this innovative book series. These authors have been thoroughly evaluated and selected based on their excellent contributions to the *Journal of Radiology Case Reports*, the Radiolopolis community, and other academic and scientific accomplishments.

It brings especially personal satisfaction to me that this project has enabled each author to be involved in the overall decision-making process and improvements regarding the print and online content. This makes each participant not only an author but also part of a great radiology product that will appeal to many readers.

Finally, I hope you will experience this case review book as it is intended to be: a quick, pertinent, "come to the point" radiology case review that provides essential information for the radiology boards in the shortest time available, which in the end is crucial for preparation for the boards.

Roland Talanow, MD, PhD

Preface

As radiology residents, we used to rely heavily on case review books for our studying, especially during the preparation for the American Board of Radiology and Royal College of Physicians and Surgeons of Canada certification examinations. Although great case review resources were available for most radiology subspecialties, such as neuroradiology and musculoskeletal imaging, their counterparts for thoracic imaging were scarce.

This work is our attempt to rectify this situation. We hope that we have created a textbook in which judiciously selected images illustrate a wide range of typical thoracic pathologies and their less typical presentations. We provide short and concise text, which yet contains all necessary information. Questions and answers, which accompany each case, are geared toward better understanding and memorization of the relevant material. Many of these questions are the very same ones we, as radiology residents and fellows, have been asked by our mentors and examiners. Knowing these answers and understanding them is what makes one a competent chest radiologist and a useful consultant.

The cases included in this book range in scope from radiography basics to unusual thoracic pathologies. Thus, this book can be used as a study guide for junior and senior residents and fellows alike. The online version of the book includes more extensive discussions and additional images, for those who might be interested in deepening their knowledge of certain thoracic pathologies.

Although geared primarily toward those who study radiology and prepare for accreditation exams in diagnostic imaging, this book can also serve as a useful and easy-to-use reference for any radiologist and clinician.

Amr M. Ajlan, MD
Alexandre Semionov, MD

Acute fever and productive cough

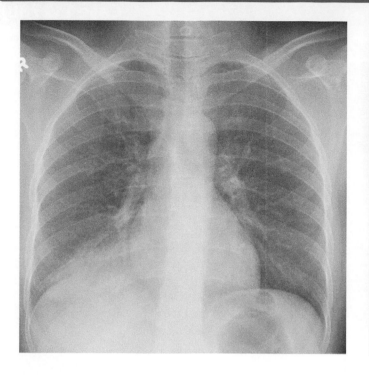 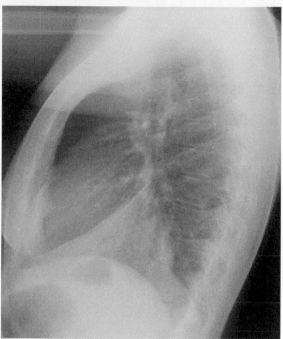

1. What are the findings?

2. What is the favored diagnosis?

3. What allows localization of the abnormality to the right lower lobe on the frontal view?

4. What is the name of the sign resulting from obliteration of the diaphragm by a consolidation?

5. What is the most common pathogen of community-acquired pneumonia?

Case ranking/difficulty: 🐾

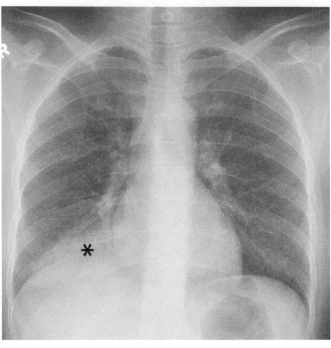

Frontal chest radiograph shows a right lung base consolidation (*asterisk*) obliterating the medial aspect of the right hemidiaphragm ("silhouette sign").

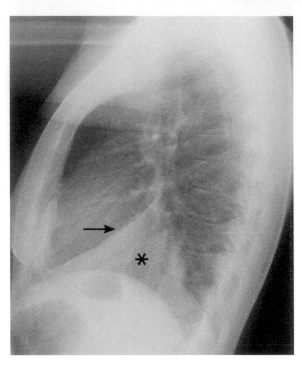

Lateral chest radiograph shows the right lower lobe consolidation (*asterisk*), bordered by the right major fissure anteriorly (*arrow*), obscuring the right hemidiaphragm ("silhouette sign").

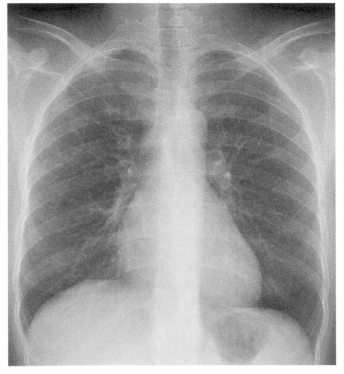

Follow-up frontal chest radiograph, done 3 weeks after the original study, shows complete resolution of the right lung base consolidation.

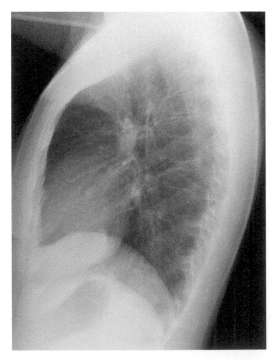

Follow-up lateral chest radiograph, done 3 weeks after the original study, shows complete resolution of the right lower lobe consolidation. The right hemidiaphragm is now sharply outlined by the normally aerated lung.

Answers

1. There is a large right lower lobe consolidation.

2. Patient's age and clinical history favor pneumonia.

3. Obliteration of the medial aspect of the right hemidiaphragm and concomitant preservation of the right heart border allow confident localization of the abnormality to the right lower lobe on the frontal view.

4. Obliteration of the contour of an anatomical structure (eg, mediastinal, cardiac or diaphragmatic border) by a lesion in the adjacent lung parenchyma, is known as "silhouette sign."

5. *Streptococcus pneumoniae* is the most common pathogen of community-acquired pneumonia.

Pearls

- Pneumonia should be the first diagnostic consideration of a consolidation on chest radiography in a febrile patient.
- Lobar pneumonia is an infection that only involves a single lobe or segment, whereas bronchopneumonia affects the lungs in patches around the airways.
- In cases of pneumonia, the radiological response lags behind the clinical response by several days.
- "Silhouette sign" is useful in localizing lung lesions, as all structures forming the cardiac, mediastinal and diaphragmatic silhouettes are in contact with a specific portion of the lung.

Suggested Readings

Becker-Dreps S, Amaya E, Liu L, Rocha J, Briceño R, Moreno G, Alemán J, Hudgens MG, Woods CW, Weber DJ. Impact of a combined pediatric and adult pneumococcal immunization program on adult pneumonia incidence and mortality in Nicaragua. *Vaccine*. January 2015;33(1):222-227.

Felson B, Felson H. Localization of intrathoracic lesions by means of the postero-anterior roentgenogram; the silhouette sign. *Radiology*. September 1950;55(3):363-374.

Franquet T. Imaging of pneumonia: trends and algorithms. *Eur Respir J*. July 2001;18(1):196-208.

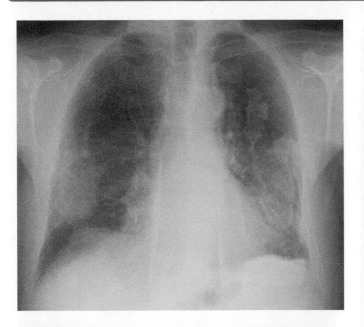
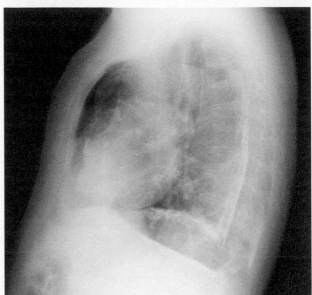
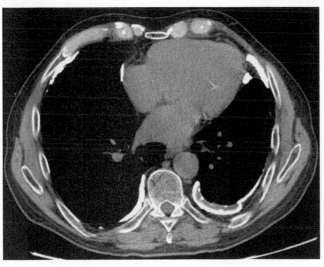
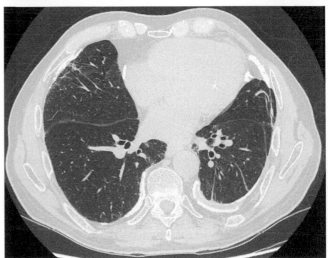

1. What are the radiographic findings?

2. What is the likely diagnosis?

3. What are the CT findings?

4. What is the difference between asbestosis and asbestos-related pleural disease?

5. List a few imaging manifestations of asbestos exposure.

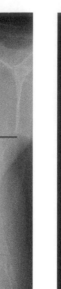

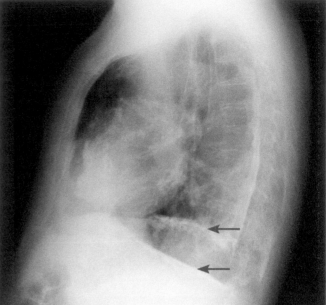

Bilateral irregular calcific densities project over both hemithoraces, in keeping with pleural plaques. The plaques have a partially well-defined lateral "rolled edge" (*red arrows*). The plaques also show an ill-defined inner border (*blue arrow*), suggesting pleural location. The smoothly lobulated configuration of the plaques resembles that of a "holly leaf." Note the presence of mediastinal and diaphragmatic plaques (*green arrows*). Diaphragmatic plaques are highly suggestive of asbestos-related pleural disease.

Some plaques have a different configuration on this lateral view, while others are less conspicuous on this view, when compared to the frontal radiograph. This feature is supportive of pleural location of the lesions. Note the presence of the diaphragmatic plaques (*arrows*).

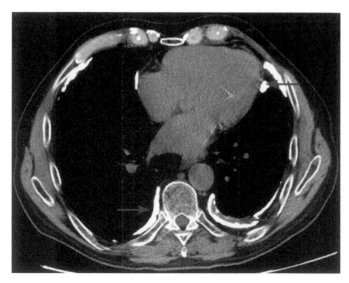

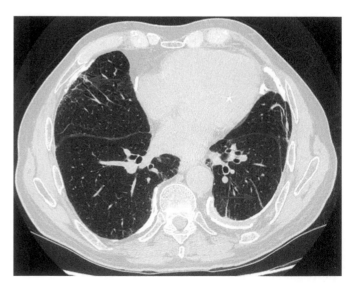

Multiple bilateral densely calcified pleural plaques are seen (*arrows*).

There are multiple areas of bilateral lung parenchymal scarring (*arrows*), which represent reaction to the adjacent pleural disease (so-called "hairy plaque" appearance). No obvious fibrosis is seen on this selected image.

Answers

1. The radiographs show bilateral irregular calcific densities, with lateral "rolled edges" and ill-defined inner borders, suggesting their pleural location. The smoothly lobulated configuration of the plaques resembles that of a "holly leaf." Note the presence of mediastinal and diaphragmatic plaques.

2. Asbestos-related pleural plaques are the likely diagnosis.

3. Multiple bilateral densely calcified pleural plaques are seen on CT, with areas of pleuroparenchymal lung scarring.

4. The term *asbestosis* should be strictly used to describe lung fibrosis secondary to asbestos exposure and should not be used to describe pleural changes.

5. Asbestos exposure can manifest as pleural effusions, pleural plaques, pleural thickening, pleural calcifications, round atelectasis, mesothelioma, asbestosis, and lung cancer.

Pearls

- Asbestos exposure can lead to different processes: asbestos-related pleural diseases (which include pleural effusions, pleural plaques, pleural thickening, pleural calcifications, round atelectasis, and mesothelioma), asbestosis (which is secondary pulmonary fibrosis), and lung cancer.
- Diaphragmatic and mediastinal pleural plaques are highly suggestive of asbestos-related pleural disease.
- Pleural plaques and thickening are commonly associated with adjacent parenchymal scarring, which should not be confused for asbestosis.

Suggested Readings

Kim KI, Kim CW, Lee MK, Lee KS, Park CK, Choi SJ, Kim JG. Imaging of occupational lung disease. *Radiographics.* November-December 2001;21(6):1371-1391.

Roach HD, Davies GJ, Attanoos R, Crane M, Adams H, Phillips S. Asbestos: when the dust settles an imaging review of asbestos-related disease. *Radiographics.* October 2002;22 Spec No:S167-S184.

Yang HY, Wang JD, Chen PC, Lee JJ. Pleural plaque related to asbestos mining in Taiwan. *J Formos Med Assoc.* December 2010;109(12):928-933.

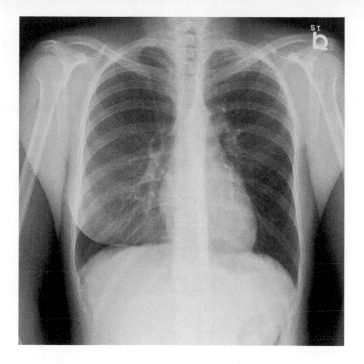

1. What is the reason for the patient's hyperlucent left hemithorax?

2. What is the eponym used to describe hyperlucent hemithorax secondary to massive pulmonary embolism?

3. What is the most common reason for a hyperlucent hemithorax?

4. How do you determine that a frontal chest radiograph is well centered?

5. What eponym describes congenital absence of the pectoralis muscle?

Case ranking/difficulty: 🐾

Category: Chest wall/Extrapleural

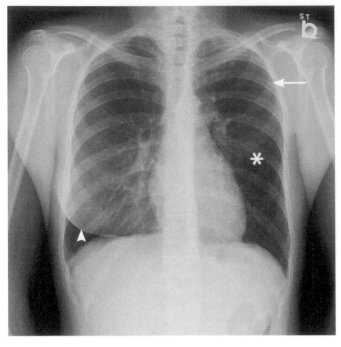

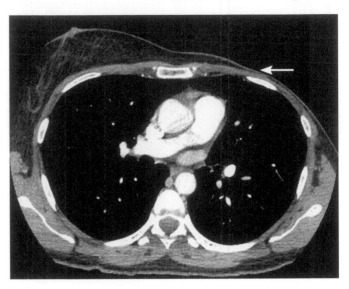

CT confirms absent left breast (*arrow*).

Chest radiograph demonstrates a hyperlucent left hemithorax (*asterisk*), absent left breast shadow, and left chest wall surgical clips (*arrow*). Note the normal right breast shadow (*arrowhead*).

Answers

1. The left hemithorax hyperlucency is due to previous left mastectomy.

2. Hyperlucent hemithorax secondary to massive pulmonary embolism is known as "Westermark sign." The sign (and hyperlucent hemithorax) is secondary to oligemia distal to the pulmonary embolism (PE). The Westermark sign is seen in 2% of patients with PE.

3. Rotation is the most common cause of a hyperlucent hemithorax on chest radiography.

4. The spinous processes of the thoracic vertebrae are in the midline of the chest. They should form a vertical line that lies equidistant from the medial margins of the clavicles. Rotation of the patient will lead to offsetting of the spinous processes so they would lie nearer one clavicular head than the other.

5. Poland syndrome is a congenital abnormality characterized by unilateral underdevelopment or absence of pectoral muscles. It is often associated with cutaneous syndactyly of the ipsilateral hand.

Pearl

- The differential diagnosis for a hyperlucent hemithorax on radiography can be remembered with the CRAWLS mnemonic: C—contralateral lung increased density, for example, supine pleural effusion; R—radiograph rotation; A—air, for example, pneumothorax; W—wall, for example, chest wall mass, mastectomy, poliomyelitis, Poland syndrome; L—lungs, for example, airway obstruction, emphysema, Swyer-James syndrome, pulmonary atresia, unilateral large bullae, large pulmonary embolus; S—scoliosis.

Suggested Reading

Altinsoy B, Altintas N. Diagnostic approach to unilateral hyperlucent lung. *JRSM Short Rep.* December 2011;2(12):95.

Rule out pneumonia

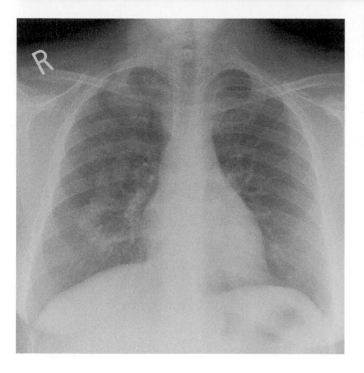 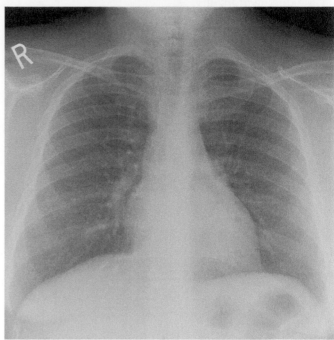

1. What are the findings on the two chest radiographs of the same patient done 15 minutes apart?

2. What is the most likely diagnosis?

3. What might have happened between the initial and follow-up radiographs?

4. Why is it important to recognize such an artifact?

5. Why is it important to repeat the chest radiograph after removing the presumed artifact?

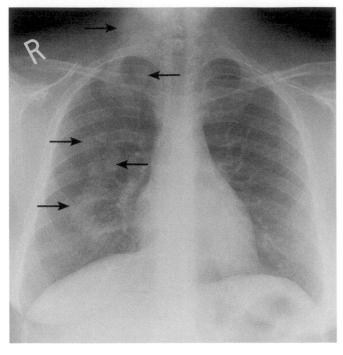

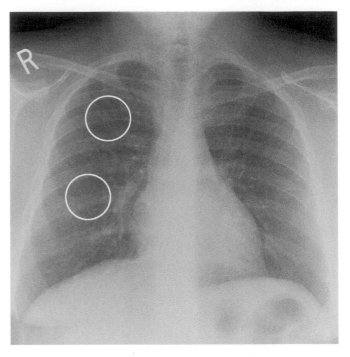

The initial chest radiograph shows a long, wavy, lobulated band opacity in the right hemithorax, extending to the supraclavicular region (*arrows*).

Repeat chest radiograph done on the same day demonstrates complete resolution of the right hemithorax abnormality. Only normal structures are present in the areas, where the abnormality was previously seen (*circles*).

Answers

1. The initial radiograph shows a right hemithoracic long, wavy, lobulated band opacity, extending to the supraclavicular region. The abnormality is absent on the repeat chest radiograph.

2. The finding is classical for a hair braid artifact.

3. On the follow-up radiograph, care was taken to remove the braid from the thoracic area.

4. Prompt recognition of the artifact might avoid unnecessary additional investigations, treatment and stress to the patient, and embarrassment and potential legal issues to the radiologist.

5. A repeat chest radiograph is indicated in order to confirm the artifactual nature of the abnormalities and to ensure that no pathology was obscured by the artifact.

Pearls

- Radiologists should be familiar with the possibility of hairstyles creating perplex radiographic artifacts.
- Radiology technologists should make every effort to remove patients' hair and any foreign objects (jewelry, garments, electronic devices) from the field of imaging.
- After removing the presumed cause of artifact, repeat imaging should be performed in order to confirm the artifactual nature of the abnormalities and to ensure that no pathology was obscured by the artifact.

Suggested Reading

Scheifele C, Lemke AJ, Reichart PA. Hair artifacts in the head and neck region. *Dentomaxillofac Radiol.* July 2003;32(4):255-257.

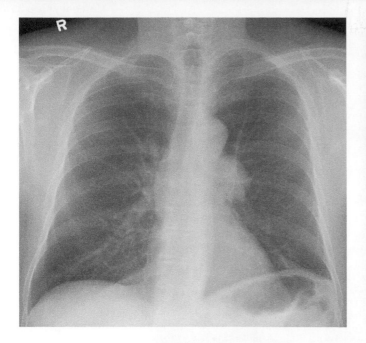 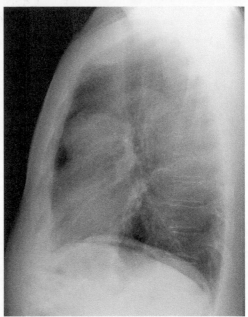

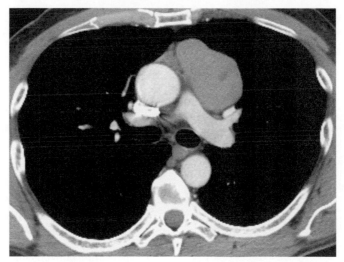

1. What are the radiographic findings?

2. What is the "hilum overlay sign?"

3. What is the "hilum convergence sign?"

4. What are the CT findings?

5. What is the differential diagnosis?

Case ranking/difficulty: 🎋

Category: Mediastinum

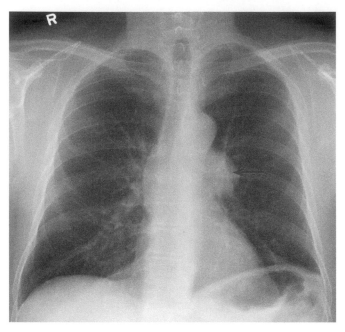

A well-defined round opacity projects over the left hilar region (*arrow*). Note that the pulmonary arterial branches can be clearly seen through the abnormal opacity, representing a "hilum overlay sign."

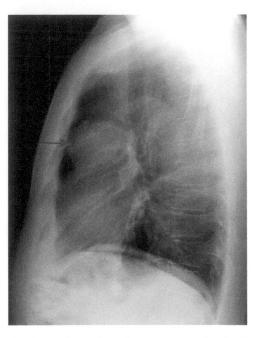

The lateral radiograph confirms the anterior mediastinal location of the abnormal opacity (*arrow*).

Answers

1. A well-defined round opacity projects over the left hilar region, with a "hilum overlay sign." The lateral radiograph confirms the anterior mediastinal location of the abnormal opacity.

2. The "hilum overlay sign" refers to visualization of the right or left main pulmonary arteries 1 cm or more within the lateral edge of an abnormal radiographic opacity. It implies that the lesion is not contacting the hilum, and is therefore either anterior or posterior to it.

3. The "hilum convergence sign" refers to visualization of the pulmonary arterial branches in continuity with an abnormal central hilar opacity, so that the arterial branches appear "converging" toward the abnormality. This denotes that the hilar abnormality is pulmonary arterial in nature and is not due to other mediastinal pathologies.

4. There is a large anterior mediastinal mass of soft tissue attenuation with a small cystic area, but no internal calcification or fat. The abnormality shows a well-defined and slightly lobulated margin. The adjacent fat planes are preserved.

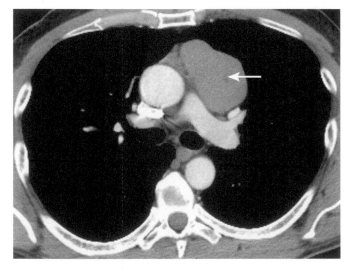

There is a large anterior mediastinal mass of soft tissue attenuation with a small internal cystic area (*arrow*), but no internal calcification or fat. The abnormality shows a well-defined and slightly lobulated margin. The adjacent fat planes are preserved.

5. The classic 4Ts of the anterior mediastinal mass differential diagnosis are thymic lesions, thyroid lesions, teratoma, and terrible lymphoma. However, many other lesions can involve the anterior mediastinum (such as seminoma, nerve sheath tumors, aneurysms, parathyroid lesions, and several other entities). This differential diagnostic list can be shortened by considering the patient's age.

Pearls

- Pathological evaluation of the entire thymic capsule is absolutely required in order to rule out invasiveness of the thymoma since microinvasion can be missed on imaging modalities alone.
- Look carefully for any pleural thickening, nodularity, irregularity, or effusion, since thymoma might be associated with occult pleural drop metastases.
- Thymoma spread does not usually involve lymph nodes.

Suggested Readings

Inaoka T, Takahashi K, Mineta M, et al. Thymic hyperplasia and thymus gland tumors: differentiation with chemical shift MR imaging. *Radiology*. June 2007;243(3):869-876.

Nasseri F, Eftekhari F. Clinical and radiologic review of the normal and abnormal thymus: pearls and pitfalls. *Radiographics*. March 2010;30(2):413-428.

Nishino M, Ashiku SK, Kocher ON, Thurer RL, Boiselle PM, Hatabu H. The thymus: a comprehensive review. *Radiographics*. March-April 2006;26(2):335-348.

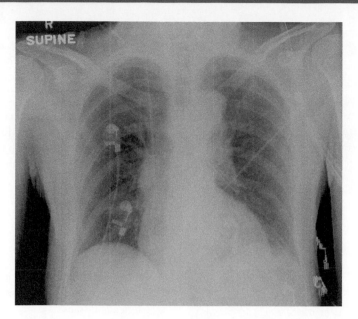

1. What is the most important finding on this radiograph?

2. What are the risk factors for malpositioning an enteric tube?

3. What are the complications of a malpositioned enteric tube?

4. What would be your actions in daily practice, if faced with such an abnormality?

5. What should the treating physician do when notified about an enteric tube that is malpositioned into an airway?

Case ranking/difficulty:

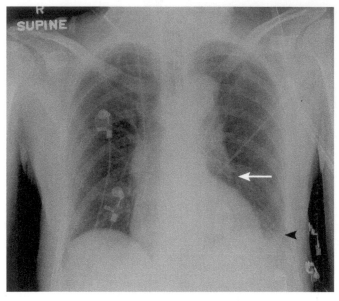

Median sternotomy wires and support equipment are noted, but the most important finding is that the enteric tube has an abnormal course with its tip residing in the left lower lobe bronchus (*arrow*). Note the subtle ill definition of the left hemidiaphragm (*arrowhead*), likely denoting aspiration pneumonitis or atelectasis.

Answers

1. The most important finding on this radiograph is that the enteric tube has an abnormal course with its tip in the left lower lobe bronchus.

2. Dysfunctional swallowing and gag reflex in neurologically impaired or sedated patients are known risks for enteric tube abnormal positioning.

3. A malpositioned enteric tube may be complicated by atelectasis, aspiration pneumonitis, superadded pneumonia, pneumothorax, hydropneumothorax, and empyema.

4. When faced with such an abnormality in practice, you should verbally inform the person or team responsible for taking care of the patient about the malpositioned enteric tube and then mention the finding in your report.

5. When notified about a malpositioned enteric tube, the treating physician should remove the tube and obtain a repeat chest radiograph (ie, to exclude associated complications, such as an iatrogenic pneumothorax).

Pearls

- Always start by checking the course and tip location of tubes and lines on chest radiographs.
- Given the usually low quality of ICU films, always adjust your image contrast to optimally visualize the tubes and lines.
- Note that an abnormally positioned enteric tube tip in the posterior costophrenic sulcus might falsely show an infradiaphragmatic location on frontal chest radiographs.

Suggested Readings

Agha R, Siddiqui MR. Pneumothorax after nasogastric tube insertion. *JRSM Short Rep.* 2011;2(4):28.

Hunter TB, Taljanovic MS. Medical devices of the abdomen and pelvis. *Radiographics.* October 2011;25(2):503-523.

McLean GK, Meranze SG, Burke DR. Inadvertent tracheobronchial placement of feeding tubes. *Radiology.* January 1989;170(1 pt 1):278.

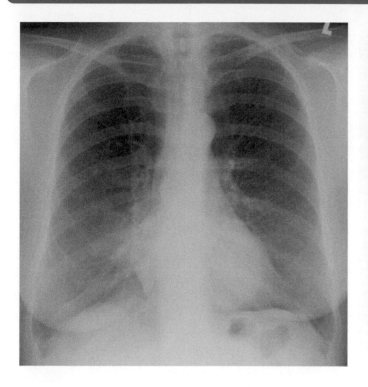
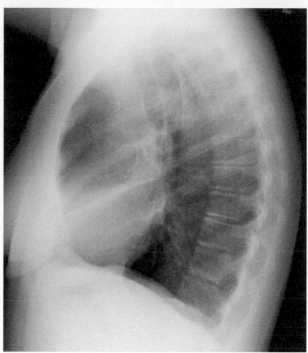

1. What is the most important finding on the frontal chest radiograph?

2. What is your differential diagnosis based on the frontal radiographic appearance?

3. What is the most important finding on the lateral chest radiograph?

4. What is the final diagnosis?

5. How would this abnormality appear on a lordotic chest radiograph?

Case ranking/difficulty: 🔥

Category: Airways

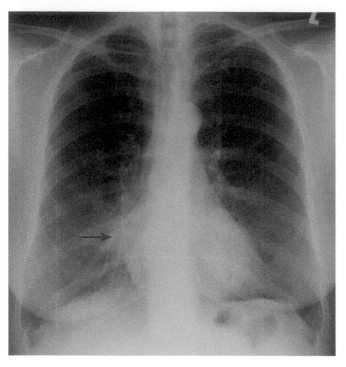

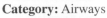

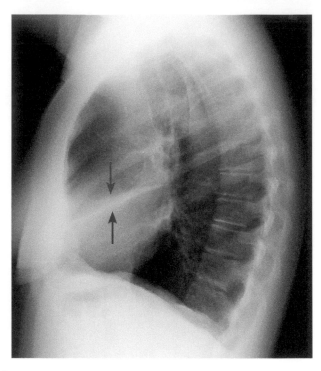

There is subtle ill-defined opacification of the medial lower right lung with partial obscuration of the right cardiac border (*arrow*). Note that the minor fissure is not seen, which may be normal or related to fissural displacement. Also note that the right hemithorax is of normal size, and that there is no obvious hilar displacement, mediastinal shift, or diaphragmatic elevation.

There is an obvious thin triangular opacity, with its apex at the hilum and its base at the lower retrosternal region. On this lateral radiograph, the minor (*red arrow*) and major (*blue arrow*) fissures are clearly displaced and apposed.

Answers

1. The most important finding on the frontal radiograph is an ill-defined opacity that partially obscures the right cardiac border.

2. Since the abnormality obscures the right cardiac border, it is located in the right middle lobe (RML). Thus, this can represent RML collapse or pneumonia. A classic mimicker would be pectus excavatum.

3. There is a thin triangular opacity on the lateral radiograph, with its apex at the hilum and its base at the lower retrosternal region. The opacity is outlined by the displaced and apposed minor and major fissures.

4. The diagnosis is that of RML collapse.

5. On a frontal lordotic view, the opacity might appear as a triangular abnormality with the base at the hilum.

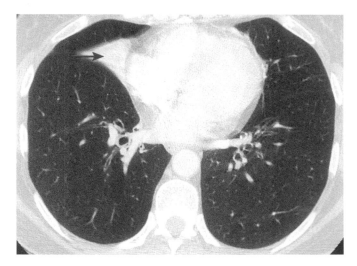

The collapsed right middle lobe is clearly identified on this selected CT image (*arrow*).

Pearls

- The usual features of lobar collapse may be absent on a frontal chest radiograph of RML atelectasis.
- The cardiac borders should always be sharply defined on a normal frontal chest radiograph.
- RML collapse is better visualized on lateral chest radiographs as a triangular opacity with the apex pointing to the hilum.

Suggested Readings

Ajlan AM, Belley G, Kosiuk J. "V V O I": a swift hand motion in detecting atelectasis on frontal chest radiographs. *Can Assoc Radiol J*. May 2011;62(2):146-150.

Ashizawa K, Hayashi K, Aso N, Minami K. Lobar atelectasis: diagnostic pitfalls on chest radiography. *Br J Radiol*. January 2001;74(877):89-97.

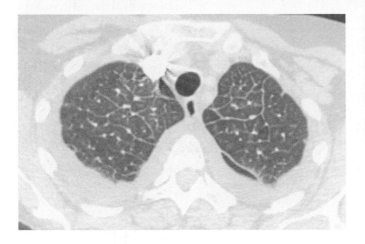 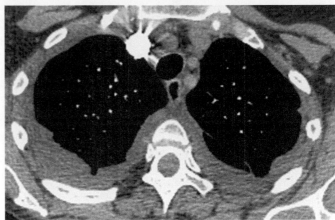

1. What are the findings?

2. What radiographic finding is equivalent to interlobular septal thickening on CT?

3. What is the differential diagnosis of smooth interlobular septal thickening?

4. What is the differential diagnosis of nodular interlobular septal thickening?

5. What is the most likely diagnosis for the CT findings above?

Case ranking/difficulty: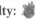

Category: Basic interpretation

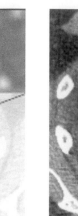

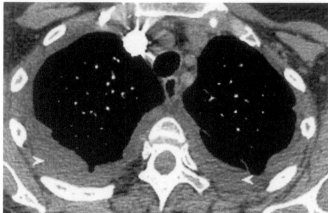

Lung window: Bilateral diffuses smooth interlobular septal thickening (*arrowheads*) and bilateral pleural effusions.

Mediastinal window: Bilateral pleural effusions (*arrowheads*).

Answers

1. CT chest demonstrates diffuse bilateral smooth interlobular septal thickening and bilateral pleural effusions.

2. Radiographic equivalent of interlobular septal thickening seen on CT are Kerley B lines.

3. Differential diagnoses of smooth interlobular septal thickening include the following. Common: pulmonary edema, lymphangitic carcinomatosis, lymphoproliferative disorders, interstitial pneumonia (viral, *Mycoplasma*), pulmonary hemorrhage. Less common: amyloidosis, pulmonary venoocclusive disease, Erdheim-Chester disease acute eosinophilic pneumonia.

4. Differential diagnoses of nodular interlobular septal thickening include sarcoidosis, lymphangitic carcinomatosis, lymphoproliferative disorders, silicosis, and amyloidosis.

5. Combination of smooth interlobular septal thickening and pleural effusions argues in favor of pulmonary edema due to heart failure.

Pearls

- Primary differential diagnosis of smooth septal thickening: pulmonary edema, lymphangitic carcinomatosis, lymphoproliferative disorders.
- Primary differential diagnosis of nodular septal thickening: sarcoidosis, lymphangitic carcinomatosis, lymphoproliferative disorders, occupational lung diseases.

Suggested Readings

Collins J. CT signs and patterns of lung disease. *Radiol Clin North Am*. November 2001;39(6):1115-1135.

Storto ML, Kee ST, Golden JA, Webb WR. Hydrostatic pulmonary edema: high-resolution CT findings. *AJR Am J Roentgenol*. October 1995;165(4):817-820.

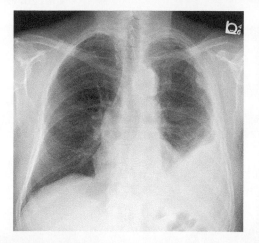
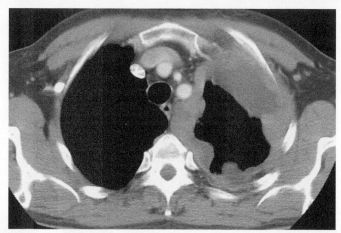
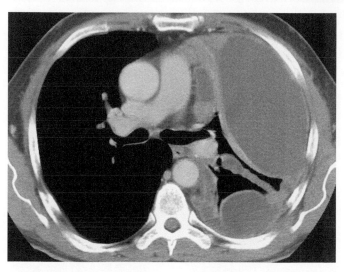
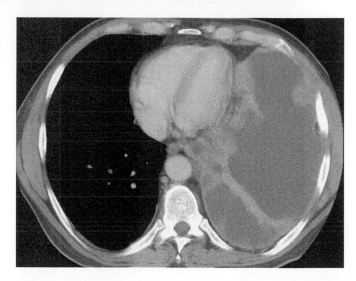

1. What are the radiographic findings?

2. What are the CT findings?

3. What is the differential diagnosis based on the CT findings?

4. What is the most common primary pleural neoplasm?

5. Is fine needle aspiration sufficient to diagnose mesothelioma?

Case ranking/difficulty: 🔥   **Category:** Pleura

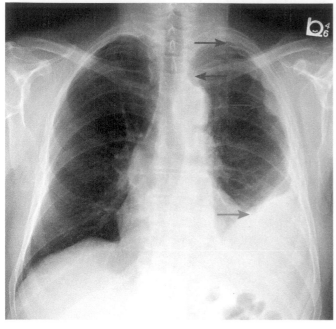

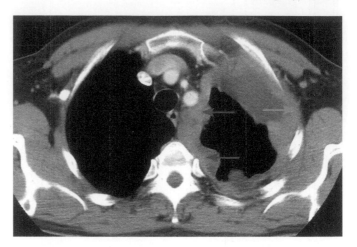

There is circumferential nodular left pleural thickening, with involvement of the mediastinum (*red arrows*) and invasion of the subpleural fat (*green arrow*).

There are smooth, pleural-based, lobular opacities along the lateral, apical, and mediastinal borders of the left hemithorax (*red arrows*). The homogenous and well-defined opacification of the left hemithoracic base is likely due to a loculated pleural effusion, but an underlying soft tissue component is also possible (*green arrow*).

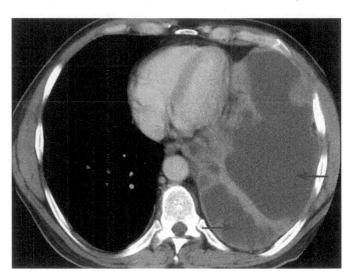

There are multiple large pleural loculations at the lower hemithorax (*red arrows*).

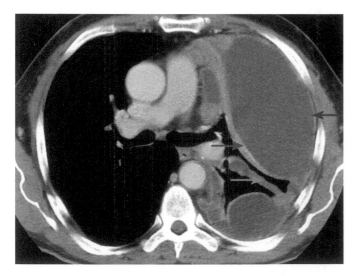

The left visceral (*red arrow*) and parietal (*blue arrow*) pleura are involved. The process extends into the left major fissure (*green arrow*) and is associated with a loculated pleural effusion.

Answers

1. There are smooth, pleural-based, lobular opacities along the lateral, apical, and mediastinal borders of the left hemithorax. The opacification of the left hemithoracic base may be due to a loculated pleural effusion, but a soft tissue component is also possible.

2. There is marked circumferential nodular thickening of the left visceral and parietal pleura, with a multiloculated pleural effusion. The process extends into the left major fissure and there are several areas where soft tissue nodules extend to the subpleural fat and chest wall.

3. The differential diagnosis of malignant pleural thickening is mesothelioma, metastases (particularly from thymic neoplasms), and lymphoma.

4. Mesothelioma is the most common primary pleural neoplasm.

5. Fine needle aspiration is not sufficient to diagnose mesothelioma.

Pearls

- Pleural thickening can be benign (ie, tuberculosis, empyema, hemothorax, radiation, pleurodesis, prior surgery, and asbestos exposure) or malignant (mesothelioma, metastases, and lymphoma).
- Features of malignant pleural thickening are thickening of more than 1 cm, nodular thickening, circumferential thickening, or involvement of the mediastinal pleura.
- The surgical approach may be modified if there is transdiaphragmatic extension of mesothelioma. Careful assessment of the coronal and sagittal CT reformats is helpful in evaluation of the integrity of the diaphragm.

Suggested Readings

Gill RR, Umeoka S, Mamata H, et al. Diffusion-weighted MRI of malignant pleural mesothelioma: preliminary assessment of apparent diffusion coefficient in histologic subtypes. *AJR Am J Roentgenol*. August 2010;195(2):W125-W130.

Tyszko SM, Marano GD, Tallaksen RJ, Gyure KA. Best cases from the AFIP: Malignant mesothelioma. *Radiographics*. January-February 2007;27(1):259-264.

Wang ZJ, Reddy GP, Gotway MB, et al. Malignant pleural mesothelioma: evaluation with CT, MR imaging, and PET. *Radiographics*. January-February 2004;24(1):105-119.

Immigration radiograph in asymptomatic female

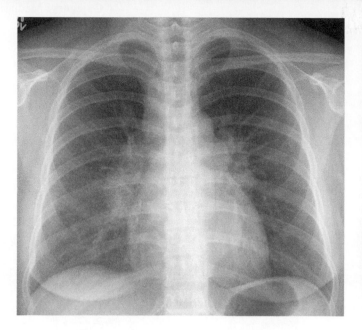 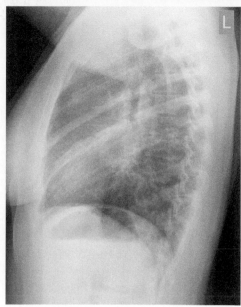

1. What are the radiographic imaging findings?

2. What is the differential diagnosis based on the imaging findings?

3. What is the most common imaging presentation of sarcoidosis?

4. Is hilar lymphadenopathy in sarcoidosis more commonly unilateral, bilateral symmetric, or bilateral asymmetric?

5. What is the most characteristic histopathological feature of sarcoidosis?

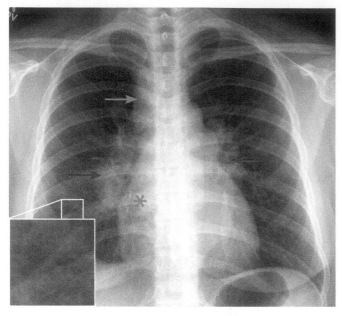

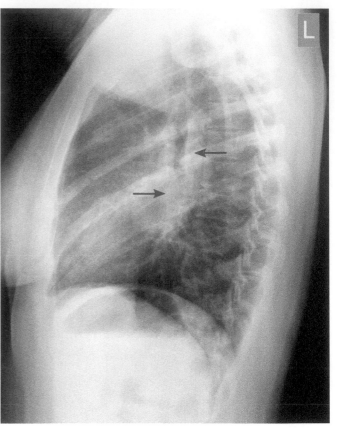

There is bilateral symmetric hilar enlargement (*red arrows*). There is thickening of the right paratracheal stripe, which should normally measure <4 mm (*green arrow*). There is a subcarinal opacity that displaces the azygoesophageal recess laterally (*green asterisk*). The overall picture is that of lymphadenopathy. Subtle nodularity is questioned in the right mid and lower lung zones (*magnification*).

Well-defined lobulated opacities circumferentially surround the hilar structures (*arrows*), consistent with lymphadenopathy. Subtle lung nodularity is questioned (*arrowhead*).

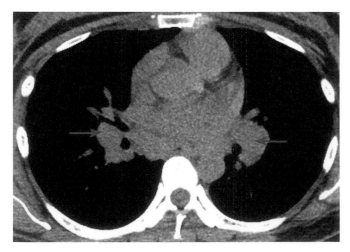

There is bilateral symmetric hilar lymph node enlargement (*arrows*).

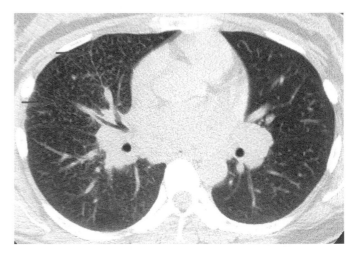

Minimal right lung nodular septal thickening is seen (*arrows*).

Answers

1. There is bilateral symmetric hilar enlargement, thickening of the right paratracheal stripe, subcarinal opacity, and subtle nodularity in the right mid and lower lung zones.

2. The differential for bilateral symmetric hilar lymphadenopathy is sarcoidosis, infections (ie, mainly viral, but could be due to mycobacterial, fungal, or bacterial causes), and neoplasms (eg, metastases and lymphoma).

3. The most common imaging manifestation of sarcoidosis is intrathoracic lymphadenopathy.

4. Hilar lymphadenopathy in sarcoidosis is more commonly bilateral symmetric, but less commonly may present as bilateral asymmetric or unilateral hilar involvement.

5. The most characteristic histopathological feature of sarcoidosis is the presence of noncaseating granulomas.

Suggested Readings

Criado E, Sánchez M, Ramírez J, et al. Pulmonary sarcoidosis: typical and atypical manifestations at high-resolution CT with pathologic correlation. *Radiographics*. October 2010;30(6):1567-1586.

Kanne JP, Yandow DR, Haemel AK, Meyer CA. Beyond skin deep: thoracic manifestations of systemic disorders affecting the skin. *Radiographics*. October 2011;31(6):1651-1668.

Park HJ, Jung JI, Chung MH, et al. Typical and atypical manifestations of intrathoracic sarcoidosis. *Korean J Radiol*. November-December 2009;10(6):623-631.

Pearls

- Bilateral hilar lymphadenopathy is caused in general by inflammatory, infectious, and neoplastic etiologies.
- When bilateral hilar lymphadenopathy is symmetric, sarcoidosis should be considered first, followed by viral infections.
- When bilateral hilar lymphadenopathy is asymmetric or unilateral, infectious and neoplastic etiologies are favored.
- Garland triad, also known as 1-2-3 sign, results from enlargement of the right paratracheal, right hilar, and left hilar lymph nodes on frontal radiographs in cases of sarcoidosis.
- The "donut sign," denoting lymphadenopathy on lateral radiographs, refers to soft tissue density surrounding a lucent hilar bronchus.

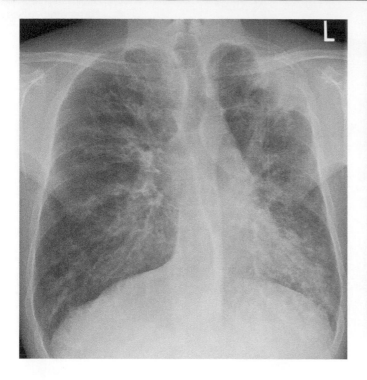 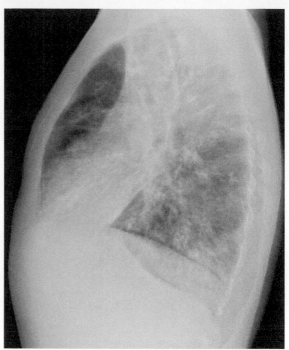

1. What are the radiographic abnormalities?

2. What is the differential diagnosis?

3. What is the mode of inheritance of cystic fibrosis?

4. Mention three organisms that typically infect cystic fibrosis patients.

5. What are the pancreatic changes that can be seen in cystic fibrosis?

Case ranking/difficulty:

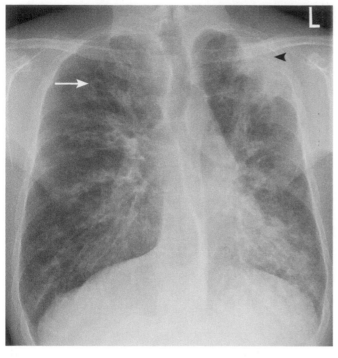

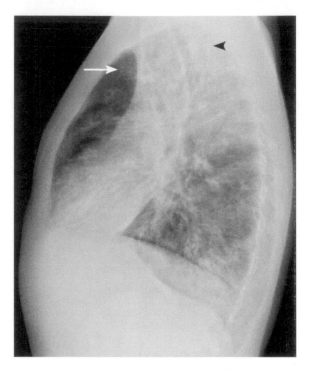

There are bilateral diffuse rounded and linear opacities with central lucencies, in keeping with bronchiectasis (*arrow*). There is lung hyperinflation. There are scattered consolidations, the largest located in the left upper lobe (*arrowhead*).

Bronchiectasis (*arrow*), hyperinflation and upper lung consolidation (*arrowhead*) are demonstrated on the lateral radiograph.

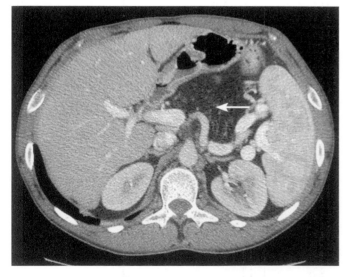

Note the complete fatty pancreatic replacement (*arrow*), a sign which could clinch the diagnosis of cystic fibrosis when seen in combination with classic lung features!

Answers

1. The radiographs show bilateral diffuse bronchiectasis, hyperinflation, and scattered consolidations.

2. The differential diagnosis of bronchiectasis includes congenital causes (eg, cystic fibrosis primary ciliary dyskinesia, hypogammaglobulinemia, Williams-Campbell syndrome, Mounier-Kuhn syndrome, and Swyer-James syndrome) and acquired causes (eg, allergic bronchopulmonary aspergillosis, atypical mycobacterial infection, other infections, and severe bronchiolitis obliterans of any etiology).

3. Cystic fibrosis is an autosomal recessive disease, with mutations located on chromosome 7. The mutation affects the gene coding for cystic fibrosis transmembrane conductance regulator (CFTR) protein, which is essential for normal function of chloride ion channels.

4. *Pseudomonas aeruginosa*, *Staphylococcus aureus*, *Burkholderia cepacia*, and other bacteria can infect cystic fibrosis patients.

5. The pancreas in cystic fibrosis can undergo fatty replacement, atrophy, fibrosis, and cystic changes.

Pearls

- Bronchiectasis in cystic fibrosis is usually upper lung predominant.
- When faced with a chest CT showing diffuse bronchiectasis, check the pancreas for possible fatty replacement.
- Other abdominal findings of cystic fibrosis include a small gallbladder and bowel obstruction secondary to meconium ileus equivalent.

Suggested Readings

Hartman TE, Primack SL, Lee KS, Swensen SJ, Müller NL. CT of bronchial and bronchiolar diseases. *Radiographics.* September 1994;14(5):991-1003.

King LJ, Scurr ED, Murugan N, Williams SG, Westaby D, Healy JC. Hepatobiliary and pancreatic manifestations of cystic fibrosis: MR imaging appearances. *Radiographics.* May-June 200;20(3):767-777.

Robertson MB, Choe KA, Joseph PM. Review of the abdominal manifestations of cystic fibrosis in the adult patient. *Radiographics.* May-June 2006;26(3):679-690.

Recurrent pneumonia in a 37-year-old female

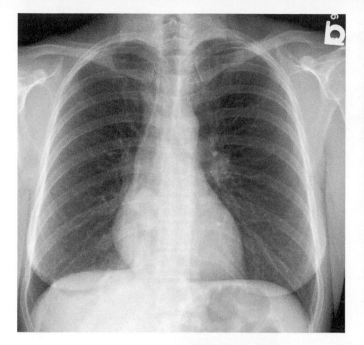

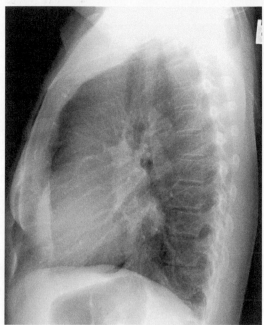

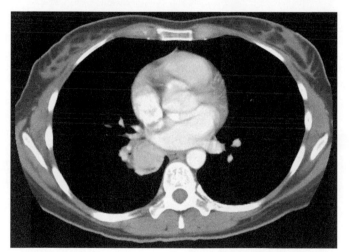

1. What are the radiographic findings?

2. What are the CT findings?

3. What is the differential diagnosis?

4. What are the types of bronchopulmonary neuroendocrine tumors?

5. Are all carcinoid tumors sporadic?

Case ranking/difficulty: 🐾

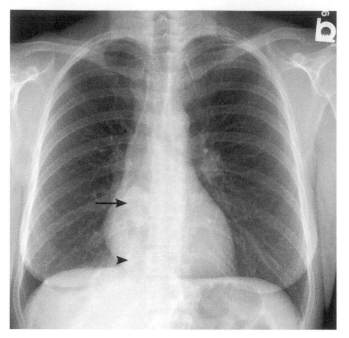

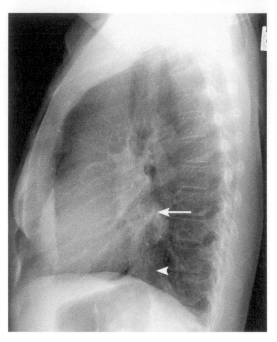

The frontal chest radiograph shows a well-defined, ovoid right retrocardiac opacity (*arrow*). A right lower lobar opacity is seen, secondary to postobstructive changes (*arrowhead*). This is a nice example of a radiographic abnormality in a hidden area. Always make sure the cardiac density is equal on both sides of the midline!

The abnormality is clearly depicted on this lateral radiograph and localizes to the hilar/infrahilar region (*arrow*). It obscures the infrahilar clear window. Hilar lymphadenopathy is suspected. Right lower lobar postobstructive changes are also seen (*arrowhead*).

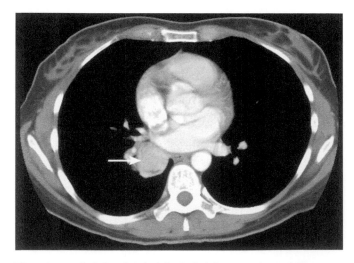

There is a well-defined right hilar/infrahilar mass (*arrow*). The lesion is homogenous (the surrounding crescents of low density are due to mucus-filled and compressed airway). The mass has high density on this contrast-enhanced CT, suggesting high vascularity.

Answers

1. There is a well-defined, ovoid right retrocardiac opacity, with postobstructive changes and possible right hilar lymph node enlargement.

2. There is a well-defined right hilar/infrahilar mass. The mass has high attenuation on this contrast-enhanced CT, suggesting high vascularity.

3. Typical or atypical carcinoid is the major consideration given the patient's age, presentation, and imaging appearance. However, other neoplasms such as squamous cell carcinoma (SCC), metastasis, and hamartoma are among the possible considerations.

4. Bronchopulmonary neuroendocrine tumors are divided into typical carcinoid (low-grade malignancy), atypical carcinoid (medium-grade malignancy), large cell neuroendocrine carcinoma (high-grade malignancy), and small cell lung cancer (highest-grade malignancy).

5. Although most carcinoids are sporadic, a small proportion arises in the context of multiple endocrine neoplasia and neurofibromatosis type 1.

Pearls

- The retrocardiac area is one of the 'blind spots' on chest radiography.
- On a normal chest radiograph, the retrocardiac density should be equal on each side of the midline.
- Unless liver metastases are present, carcinoid syndrome does not develop with pulmonary carcinoid.
- Carcinoid tumors are typically negative on PET scanning. However, low PET activity may be seen with atypical carcinoid.
- Octreotide scintigraphy may be of value in detecting occult primary carcinoid or distant carcinoid metastasis.

Suggested Readings

Jeung MY, Gasser B, Gangi A, et al. Bronchial carcinoid tumors of the thorax: spectrum of radiologic findings. *Radiographics*. March-April 2002;22(2):351-365.

Park CM, Goo JM, Lee HJ, Kim MA, Lee CH, Kang MJ. Tumors in the tracheobronchial tree: CT and FDG PET features. *Radiographics*. January-February 2009;29(1): 55-71.

Scarsbrook AF, Ganeshan A, Statham J, et al. Anatomic and functional imaging of metastatic carcinoid tumors. *Radiographics*. March-April 2007;27(2):455-477.

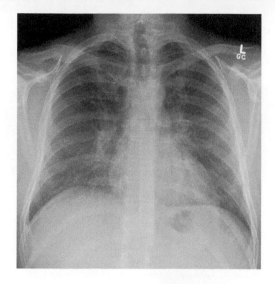
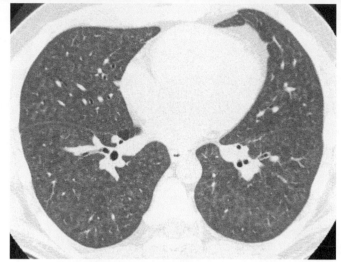
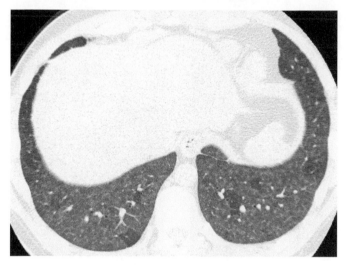

1. What are the radiographic findings?

2. What are the CT findings?

3. What is the differential diagnosis based on the
   CT findings?

4. What substances are implicated in causing the
   presented entity?

5. What would you expect in the bronchoalveolar
   lavage of this patient?

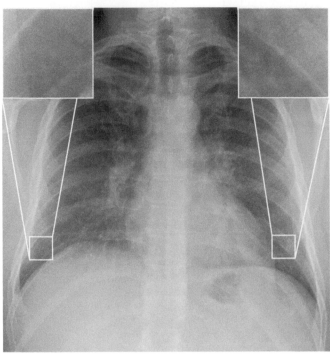

Bilateral and diffuse, subtle, small, nodular opacities are seen (*magnification*).

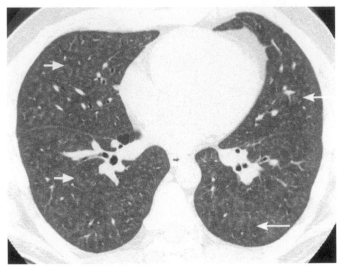

There are bilateral, diffuse, ill-defined, parenchymal ground-glass nodules (*arrows*). Note that these nodular opacities are sparing the pleural and fissural surfaces, denoting a centrilobular location.

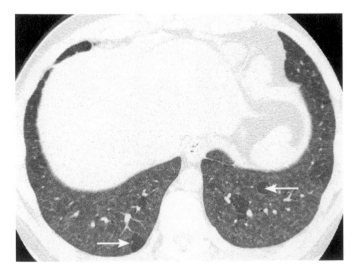

There are multifocal areas of lobular hypoattenuation (*arrows*), where paucity of pulmonary vasculature is noted.

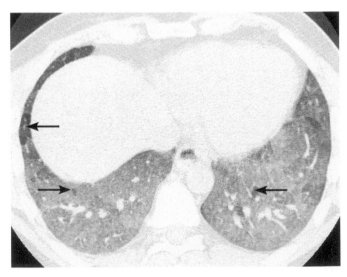

This expiratory image shows persistent focal areas of hypoattenuation (*arrows*), demonstrating no change in density or volume when compared to the inspiratory acquisition. This is in keeping with air trapping.

Answers

1. There are bilateral and diffuse, subtle, small, nodular opacities.

2. There are bilateral, diffuse, ill-defined, centrilobular ground-glass nodules and multifocal areas of lobular hypoattenuation, where paucity of pulmonary vasculature is noted. The expiratory image confirms the presence of lobular areas of air trapping.

3. The differential diagnosis for bilateral centrilobular ground-glass nodularity mainly includes hypersensitivity pneumonitis (HP), respiratory bronchiolitis (associated with smoking), and infectious bronchiolitis (viral and atypical pneumonias).

4. HP is an allergic airway reaction due to exposure to various organic or nonorganic materials (eg, bacteria, fungi, protozoa, bird excreta, mold, grain, and many others).

5. Bronchoalveolar lavage in cases of HP typically shows a high white blood cell count, with more than 30% lymphocytosis.

Pearls

- Fever and leukocytosis in HP can lead to erroneous diagnosis of pneumonia.
- Entities that present on CT as ground-glass opacities (eg, *Pneumocystis* or viral pneumonias), small airway disease (eg, HP or respiratory bronchiolitis), or vascular abnormalities (eg, pulmonary embolism or vasculitis) may appear normal or near normal on chest radiography.
- Some of the HP-related 'buzzword' centrilobular ground-glass nodularity, mosaic attenuation, headcheese sign, and air trapping.
- Mosaic attenuation (due to air trapping) + ground-glass opacities (due to infiltrative lung disease) = headcheese sign.

Suggested Readings

Hirschmann JV, Pipavath SN, Godwin JD. Hypersensitivity pneumonitis: a historical, clinical, and radiologic review. *Radiographics*. November 2009;29(7):1921-1938.

Olson AL, Huie TJ, Groshong SD, et al. Acute exacerbations of fibrotic hypersensitivity pneumonitis: a case series. *Chest*. October 2008;134(4):844-850.

Trahan S, Hanak V, Ryu JH, Myers JL. Role of surgical lung biopsy in separating chronic hypersensitivity pneumonia from usual interstitial pneumonia/idiopathic pulmonary fibrosis: analysis of 31 biopsies from 15 patients. *Chest*. July 2008;134(1):126-132.

Right-sided pleuritic chest pain

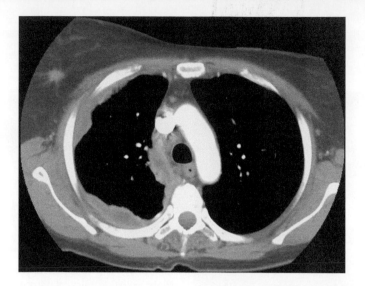

1. What are the CT findings?

2. What is the differential diagnosis based on the CT findings?

3. What is the likely diagnosis?

4. What are the expected features of malignant pleural involvement?

5. List a few malignancies which are associated with pleural metastases.

Case ranking/difficulty: 🌑   **Category:** Pleura

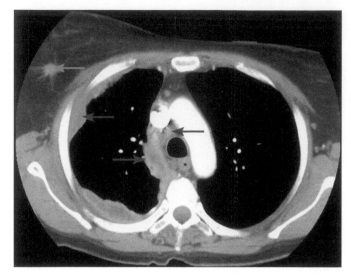

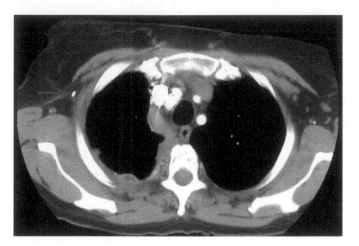

This image shows the same abnormality, in addition to a right axillary surgical clip from a prior lymph node dissection procedure (*arrow*).

There is near-circumferential right hemithoracic pleural involvement by soft tissue-attenuated lesions (*red arrows*). The right mediastinal pleura is involved. The lesions show areas of internal hypodensity, denoting necrosis. Some of the lesions appear nodular and exceed 1 cm in thickness. There is mediastinal lymphadenopathy (*blue arrow*). Note the irregular and spiculated right breast lesion (*green arrow*).

Answers

1. There is near-circumferential right hemithoracic pleural involvement by soft tissue-attenuated lesions. The right mediastinal pleura is involved. The lesions show areas of internal hypodensity, denoting necrosis. Some of the lesions appear nodular and exceed 1 cm in thickness. There is mediastinal lymphadenopathy. An irregular and spiculated right breast lesion is seen.

2. The differential diagnosis based on the CT findings is that of metastases, mesothelioma, and lymphoma.

3. Given the right breast abnormality, metastases from breast carcinoma should be favored.

4. The expected features of malignant pleural thickening are thickening of more than 1 cm, nodular thickening, circumferential thickening, or involvement of the mediastinal pleura.

5. Pleural metastases can be due to thymoma, adenocarcinomas (from lung, breast, colon, and stomach), and a variety of other tumors.

Pearls

- Always check the periphery of any provided image, since a peripheral or "hidden" finding might be the diagnosis "clincher" in a board examination setting!
- Features of malignant pleural thickening are thickening of more than 1 cm, nodular thickening, circumferential thickening, or involvement of the mediastinal pleura.
- Although pleural effusion very commonly accompanies metastatic pleural diseases, some cases will have no associated pleural effusion.

Suggested Readings

Gill RR, Umeoka S, Mamata H, et al. Diffusion-weighted MRI of malignant pleural mesothelioma: preliminary assessment of apparent diffusion coefficient in histologic subtypes. *AJR Am J Roentgenol.* August 2010;195(2):W125-W130.

Tyszko SM, Marano GD, Tallaksen RJ, Gyure KA. Best cases from the AFIP: Malignant mesothelioma. *Radiographics.* January-February 2007;27(1):259-264.

Wang ZJ, Reddy GP, Gotway MB, et al. Malignant pleural mesothelioma: evaluation with CT, MR imaging, and PET. *Radiographics.* January-February 2004;24(1):105-119.

Febrile neutropenia after recent bone marrow transplantation for myelofibrosis

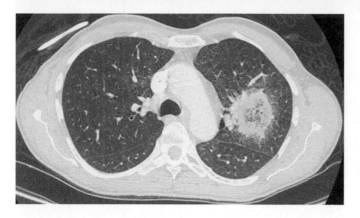 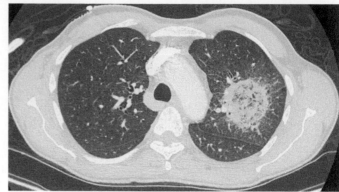

1. What are the CT findings?

2. What is the main diagnostic possibility in this patient with recent bone marrow transplantation?

3. What are the types of *Aspergillus* lung involvement?

4. What is semi-invasive aspergillosis?

5. What is the "halo sign?"

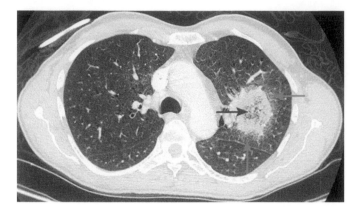

There is a large, rounded, heterogeneous consolidation in the left upper lobe (*red arrow*), with a subtle surrounding ground-glass halo (*green arrows*).

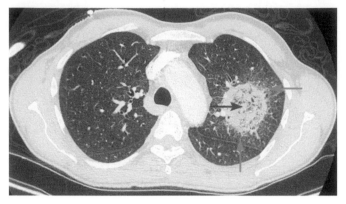

The lesion is redemonstrated on this image (*red arrow*), with more obvious surrounding ground-glass attenuation and minimal interlobular septal thickening (*green arrows*).

those on steroids). In addition, the disease is indolent, with slow progression over weeks to months.

5. The "halo sign" represents a central consolidative nodular opacity that is surrounded by a rim of ground-glass attenuation. The halo is commonly due to surrounding hemorrhage, but can appear due to other causes (eg, inflammation, tissue compression, or neoplastic invasion).

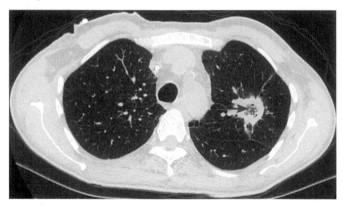

The lesion shows a substantial decrease in size on this posttreatment follow-up image. Note that the abnormality now has a more confined central area of heterogeneous ground-glass attenuation (*red arrow*) and a thick consolidative rim (*blue arrow*).

Answers

1. There is a large, rounded, heterogeneous consolidation in the left upper lobe, with a surrounding halo of ground-glass attenuation and minimal interlobular septal thickening.

2. Invasive pulmonary aspergillosis (IPA) is the main diagnosis.

3. The main types of *Aspergillus* lung diseases are aspergilloma (ie, fungal ball), allergic bronchopulmonary aspergillosis, semi-invasive aspergillosis, and invasive aspergillosis (ie, angio- and/or airway-invasive forms).

4. Semi-invasive aspergillosis (also called chronic necrotizing *Aspergillus* infection) may have a very similar imaging appearance to invasive pulmonary aspergillosis, but the clinical picture is different. Patients at risk for semi-invasive aspergillosis have only mild immunity impairment (ie, patients with diabetes, alcoholism, malnutrition, chronic obstructive airway diseases, and

Pearls

- Any new lung opacity in a patient with recent bone marrow transplantation (BMT) should be considered invasive pulmonary aspergillosis (IPA) until proven otherwise.
- The "halo sign" is highly suggestive of IPA in the correct clinical context, but can be seen with many other pathologies.
- Cavitation can be seen in BMT patients with IPA in cases of disease worsening, but can also develop as neutropenia resolves.

Suggested Readings

Franquet T, Müller NL, Giménez A, Guembe P, de La Torre J, Bagué S. Spectrum of pulmonary aspergillosis: histologic, clinical, and radiologic findings. *Radiographics*. July-August 2001;21(4):825-837.

Kenney HH, Agrons GA, Shin JS; Armed Forces Institute of Pathology. Best cases from the AFIP. Invasive pulmonary aspergillosis: radiologic and pathologic findings. *Radiographics*. November-December 2002;22(6):1507-1510.

Worthy SA, Flint JD, Müller NL. Pulmonary complications after bone marrow transplantation: high-resolution CT and pathologic findings. *Radiographics*. November-December 1997;17(6):1359-1371.

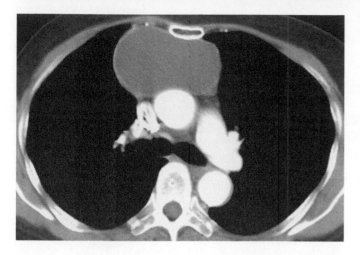 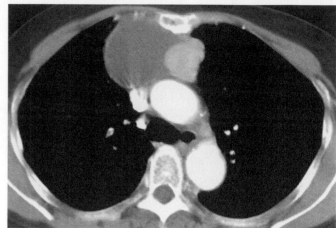

1. What are the CT findings?

2. Given the patient's age, what is the most likely diagnosis?

3. List the differential diagnosis for a thymic lesion.

4. What are the types of thymic hyperplasia?

5. What are the two epithelial thymic neoplasms?

Case ranking/difficulty:

Category: Mediastinum

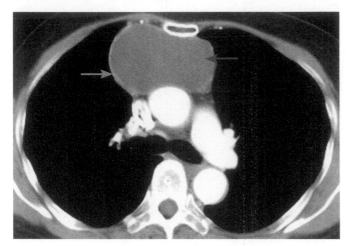

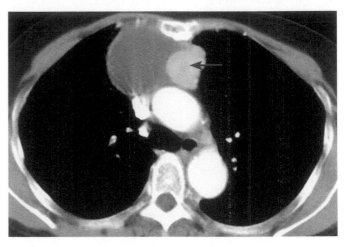

There is a large anterior mediastinal lesion, showing a predominant cystic component (*red arrow*). The abnormality is well circumscribed by a thin capsule (*green arrow*). The lesion shows close contact with the retrosternal chest wall and major mediastinal vasculature.

The anterior mediastinal lesion has a sizable peripheral nodular soft tissue component (*arrow*).

Answers

1. There is a large anterior mediastinal lesion, showing a predominant cystic component. The abnormality is well circumscribed by a thin capsule and has a sizable peripheral nodular soft tissue component. The lesion shows close contact with the retrosternal chest wall and major mediastinal vasculature.

2. The most likely diagnosis, given the patient's age, is cystic thymoma.

3. The differential diagnosis of a thymic lesion includes thymic hyperplasia, cyst, thymoma, carcinoma, carcinoid, lymphoma, and thymolipoma.

4. Thymic hyperplasia is divided into true hyperplasia and lymphoid hyperplasia.

5. The epithelial thymic neoplasms are thymomas and thymic carcinomas.

Pearls

- Thymoma can be predominantly cystic.
- Assess for the possibility of any enhancing components in cystic mediastinal lesions.
- The differential diagnosis of a cystic or predominantly cystic anterior mediastinal lesion includes cystic thymoma, thymic cyst, teratoma, necrotic lymph node (from metastases or lymphoma), cystic changes in a thyroid lesion, foregut duplication cyst, pericardial cyst, lymphangioma, hydatid cyst, and abscess.

Suggested Readings

Nasseri F, Eftekhari F. Clinical and radiologic review of the normal and abnormal thymus: pearls and pitfalls. *Radiographics*. March 2010;30(2):413-428.

Nishino M, Ashiku SK, Kocher ON, Thurer RL, Boiselle PM, Hatabu H. The thymus: a comprehensive review. *Radiographics*. March-April 2006;26(2):335-348.

Parker MS, Chasen MH, Paul N. Radiologic signs in thoracic imaging: case-based review and self-assessment module. *AJR Am J Roentgenol*. March 2009;192(3 suppl):S34-S48.

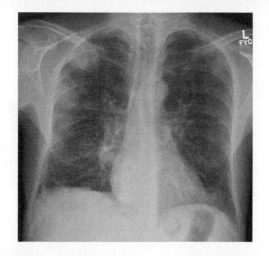
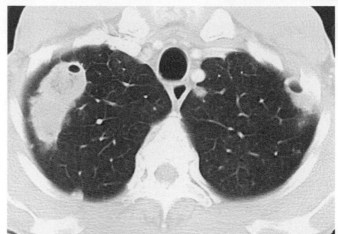
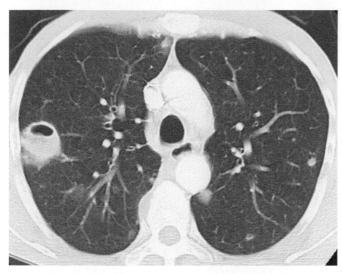
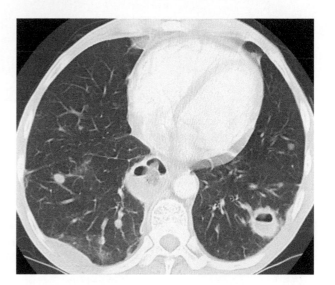

1. What are the radiographic abnormalities?

2. What are the CT abnormalities?

3. What is the differential diagnosis?

4. What is Lemierre syndrome?

5. What is the "feeding vessel sign?"

Case ranking/difficulty: 🔥

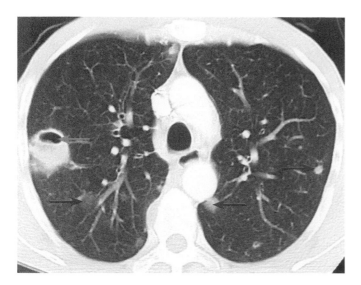

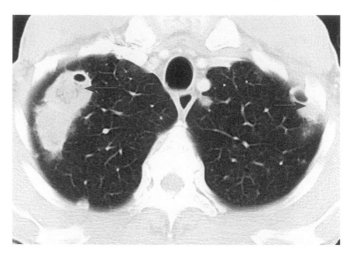

Bilateral, peripheral, and well-defined lung opacities are present (*arrows*), with internal debris and air-fluid levels due to cavitations.

There are multifocal, bilateral, peripheral, well-defined, and rounded lung opacities of variable size. Some lesions show internal air-fluid levels, suggesting cavitations (*red arrows*). Blunting of the right costophrenic angle denotes a small pleural effusion (*blue arrow*). There is a right-sided peripherally inserted central catheter.

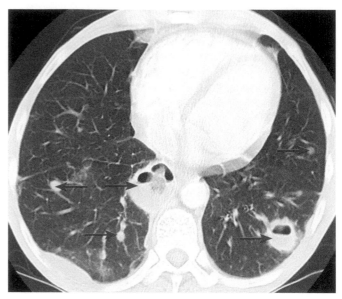

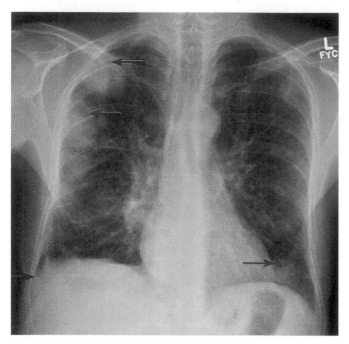

Similar lesions are identified in both lower lung lobes (*arrows*).

Answers

1. The radiograph shows bilateral, multifocal, peripheral, well-defined, rounded lung opacities of variable size. Some lesions show internal air-fluid levels, suggesting cavitations. Blunting of the right costophrenic angle denotes a small pleural effusion.

2. The CT shows bilateral, scattered, peripheral, well-defined lung opacities, with internal debris and air-fluid levels due to cavitations.

Bilateral and scattered lung parenchymal lesions are seen (*red arrows*). Note the larger cavitary lesion of the right lung (*green arrow*).

3. The differential diagnosis of multiple, bilateral, cavitary lesions includes metastases (most often from squamous cell carcinoma, sarcoma, and transitional cell carcinoma), connective tissue disorders (eg, rheumatoid arthritis), vasculitis (eg, Wegener granulomatosis), infections (eg, *S aureus*, anaerobes, gram-negative organisms, tuberculosis, and fungi), septic emboli, and posttraumatic lung contusions/lacerations.

4. Lemierre syndrome is an otolaryngeal infection, which is complicated by internal jugular venous thrombosis and secondary septic emboli (typically involving the lung).

5. The "feeding vessel sign" has been classically described as a pulmonary artery fading into a pulmonary opacity related to septic embolism.

Pearls

- Imaging features of septic pulmonary emboli can be seen even before the diagnosis is clinically suspected.
- If septic emboli are suspected due to bilateral multifocal lung opacities, a short-term radiographic or CT follow-up (about 24 hours) would classically show rapid development or progression in the cavitary component of the lesions.
- The differential diagnosis for end-of-vessel lesions: septic emboli, hematogenous infection, vasculitis (eg, Wegener granulomatosis), metastases, and pulmonary infarcts.

Suggested Readings

Cook RJ, Ashton RW, Aughenbaugh GL, Ryu JH. Septic pulmonary embolism: presenting features and clinical course of 14 patients. *Chest*. July 2005;128(1):162-166.

Gadkowski LB, Stout JE. Cavitary pulmonary disease. *Clin Microbiol Rev*. April 2008;21(2):305-333, table of contents.

Han D, Lee KS, Franquet T, et al. Thrombotic and nonthrombotic pulmonary arterial embolism: spectrum of imaging findings. *Radiographics*. November-December 2003;23(6):1521-1539.

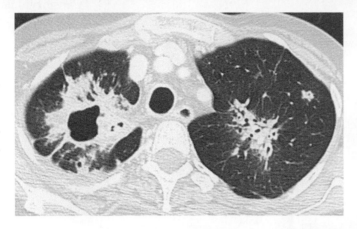
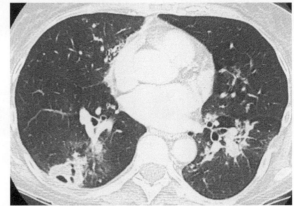

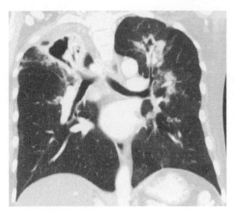
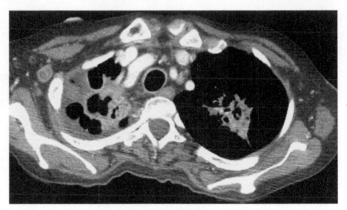

1. What are the CT findings?

2. What is the differential diagnosis?

3. What are the imaging findings of active tuberculosis?

4. What is the hallmark of postprimary tuberculosis?

5. List a few risk factors for developing tuberculosis.

Case ranking/difficulty:

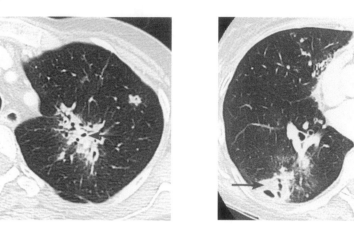

Bilateral, multifocal, irregular cavitary lung parenchymal opacities are seen (*arrows*).

Additional cavities are seen in the lower lungs (*arrows*). Note the sparing of the middle lobe and lingula.

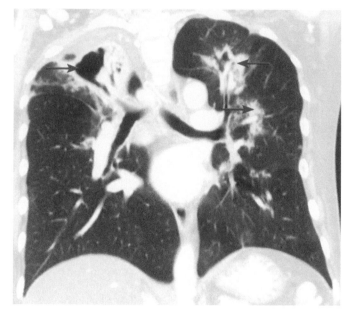

This coronal image shows an upper lung predominance of the abnormalities (*arrows*).

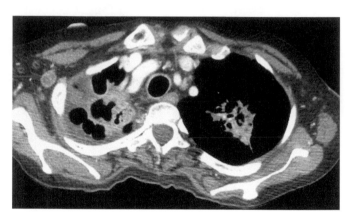

There are a few enlarged right axillary lymph nodes, with the largest showing hypodense central necrosis (*arrow*).

4. Cavitation is the hallmark of postprimary tuberculosis.

5. Risk factors for developing tuberculosis include human immunodeficiency virus (HIV) infection, extremes of age, malnutrition, diabetes, chemotherapy, chronic renal failure, and living in endemic countries.

Answers

1. The CT shows bilateral, multifocal, irregular cavitary lesions, with upper lung predominance. There are a few enlarged right axillary lymph nodes, with the largest showing central necrosis.

2. The differential diagnosis is mainly that of infections (ie, tuberculous and nontuberculous mycobacterial infection or fungal pneumonia) and neoplasms (ie, cavitary metastases).

3. Imaging findings of active tuberculosis include cavitations, necrotic lymph nodes, tree-in-bud pattern, miliary pattern and change from prior imaging.

Pearls

• When active tuberculosis (TB) is suspected on imaging, the radiologist should recommend isolating the patient till appropriate workup and treatment are implemented.

• A unilateral pleural effusion in an adult has several etiologies, but the *two Ts* should always be considered: TB and Tumor (ie, lung cancer or metastases).

- Lymphadenopathy is the most common extrapulmonary TB manifestation. This can appear as cervical, axillary, or upper abdominal lymphadenopathy on chest CT examinations.
- In immunocompromised patients, reactivation TB may appear similar to primary TB, since these patients may not mount an adequate immune response to form cavities.
- The classic classification of TB into primary and post-primary (also known as secondary or reactivation) types is based on older literature and has been recently challenged. The current direction is to interrupt the clinical and imaging findings of TB in the context of the patient's immune status.

Suggested Readings

Burrill J, Williams CJ, Bain G, Conder G, Hine AL, Misra RR. Tuberculosis: a radiologic review. *Radiographics*. September-October 2007;27(5):1255-1273.

Jeong YJ, Lee KS. Pulmonary tuberculosis: up-to-date imaging and management. *AJR Am J Roentgenol*. September 2008;191(3):834-844.

Rossi SE, Franquet T, Volpacchio M, Giménez A, Aguilar G. Tree-in-bud pattern at thin-section CT of the lungs: radiologic-pathologic overview. *Radiographics*. May-June 2005;25(3):789-801.

Rozenshtein A, Hao F, Starc MT, Pearson GD. Radiographic appearance of pulmonary tuberculosis: dogma disproved. *AJR Am J Roentgenol*. May 2015;204(5):974-978.

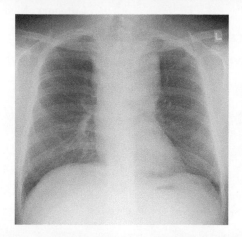
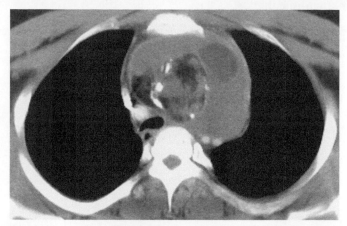
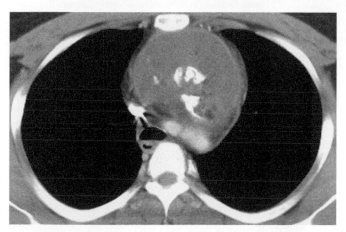
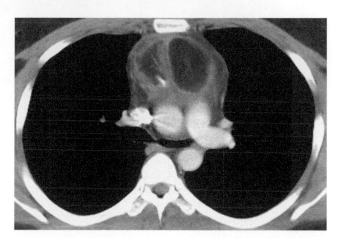

1. What are the radiographic findings?

2. What is the differential diagnosis based on the radiographic findings?

3. What are the CT findings?

4. What is the diagnosis based on the CT findings?

5. How are germ cell tumors (GCT) classified?

Case ranking/difficulty: 　　　　　　　　　　　　　　　　**Category:** Mediastinum

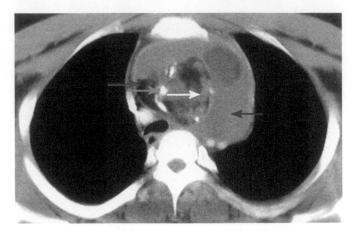

There is a large and well-defined central anterior mediastinal mass, containing areas of fat (*red arrow*), dense calcifications (*green arrow*), cystic regions (*blue arrow*), and soft tissue components (*white arrow*). The lesion displaces the vascular structures and airway, with no obvious invasive features.

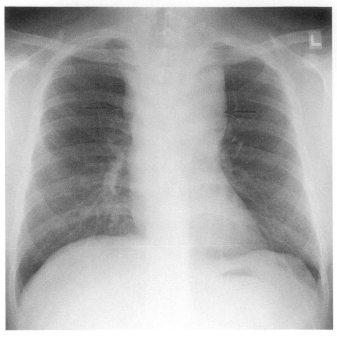

Widening of the mediastinum is seen, with no obscuration of the aortic border or the hilar structures, denoting that the abnormality is in the anterior mediastinum (*arrows*). The lesion shows a homogenous opacity with no obvious calcifications.

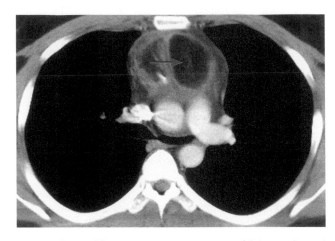

Large intralesional fat components are seen on this image (*arrow*).

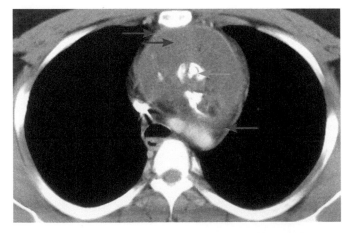

A lower level slice through the lesion shows tooth-like calcifications (*green arrow*), a large cystic portion (*blue arrow*), and a thin enhancing capsule (*red arrows*).

Answers

1. There are findings consistent with an anterior mediastinal lesion.

2. The typical anterior mediastinal lesions are germ cell tumors (GCT), lymphoma, thyroid-related masses, and thymic lesions. The young age of the patient favors GCT or lymphoma. Although less favored, vascular aneurysms should be also considered, whenever a mediastinal mass is seen.

3. There is a large and well-defined central anterior mediastinal mass, containing areas of fat, dense calcifications, cystic regions, and soft tissue components. The lesion displaces the vascular structures and airway.

4. Teratoma is the diagnosis of choice in this case.

5. GCTs are divided into seminomas and nonseminomas. Nonseminomatous types are teratomas (mature, immature, and with malignant transformation), yolk sac tumors, embryonal cell carcinomas, choriocarcinomas, and mixed type GCTs.

Pearls

- An anterior mediastinal mass with fat, cystic, and calcific components is characteristic of teratoma.
- Teratomas, followed by seminomas, are the most common mediastinal germ cell tumors.
- Teratomas are not hormonally active, unless they are malignant or contain other types of nonseminomatous components.

Suggested Readings

Gaerte SC, Meyer CA, Winer-Muram HT, Tarver RD, Conces DJ. Fat-containing lesions of the chest. *Radiographics*. October 2002;22 Spec No:S61-S78.

Jeung MY, Gasser B, Gangi A, et al. Imaging of cystic masses of the mediastinum. *Radiographics*. October 2002;22 Spec No:S79-S93.

Ueno T, Tanaka YO, Nagata M, et al. Spectrum of germ cell tumors: from head to toe. *Radiographics*. March-April 2004;24(2):387-404.

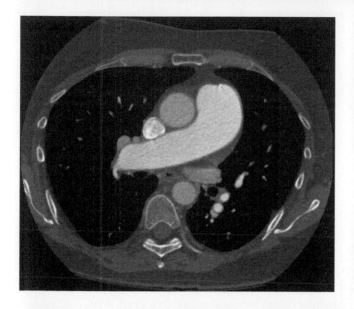
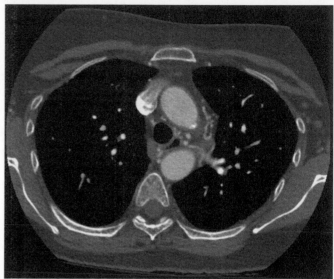
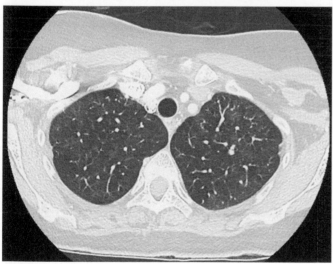
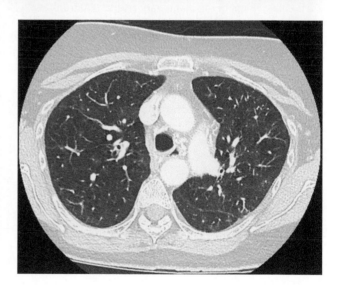

1. What are the pertinent CT findings?

2. What is the diagnosis?

3. What is the clinical definition of pulmonary arterial hypertension?

4. How should the pulmonary arterial (PA) trunk be measured on a chest CT?

5. How should the PA-to-aortic ratio be measured on a chest CT?

Case ranking/difficulty:

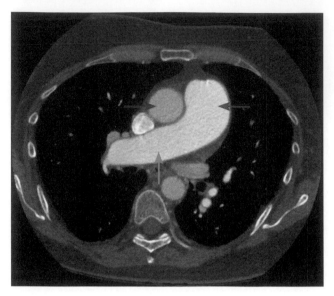

There is enlargement of the pulmonary arterial (PA) trunk (*red arrow*) and right main PA branch (*green arrow*). The PA shows a larger caliber when compared to the ascending aorta (*blue arrow*), resulting in a PA-to-aortic ratio >1.

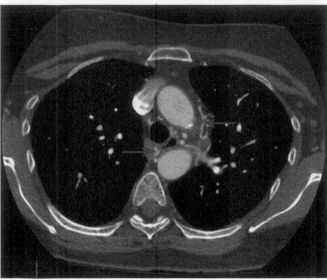

Markedly dilated bronchial collaterals are seen in the mediastinum (*arrows*).

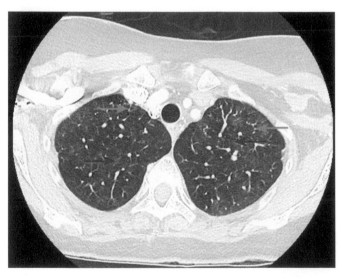

Bilateral, small, ill-defined, centrilobular ground-glass nodular-like opacities are seen (*red arrows*). There are also serpentine intraparenchymal vessels that do not follow the normal intraparenchymal pulmonary arterial branching pattern (*green arrows*).

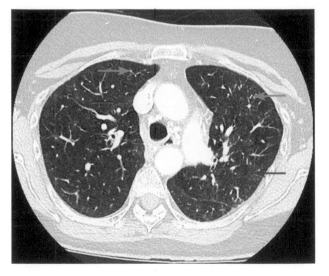

Subtle mosaic lung attenuation is noted (*red arrows* denoting areas of increased attenuation). Abnormal intraparenchymal pulmonary arterial vessels are reidentified (*green arrows*).

Answers

1. There is enlargement of the pulmonary arterial (PA) trunk and right PA branch. Markedly dilated systemic bronchial and nonbronchial collaterals are seen as well. In addition, bilateral, subtle, mosaic lung attenuation and small, ill-defined, centrilobular ground-glass nodular-like opacities are noted.

2. The diagnosis is that of pulmonary arterial hypertension (PAHTN).

3. PAHTN is clinically diagnosed when the mean PA pressure is >25 mm Hg at rest or >30 mm Hg during exercise, with an increased pulmonary vascular resistance.

4. The PA should be measured on axial CT images at the level of the pulmonary arterial bifurcation. A diameter of >28 mm is suggestive of PAHTN.

5. The maximal diameter of the PA trunk should be compared to maximum diameter of the ascending aorta on the same transverse image, at the level where the PA trunk sweeps to become the right main PA branch. A PA-to-aortic ratio >1 is a sign suggestive of PAHTN.

Pearls

• The direct pulmonary arterial trunk measurement and the PA-to-aortic ratio measurement are both performed on axial CT images, but at different levels (as described in the imaging findings section).

• Mosaic perfusion in the context of PAHTN may be mistaken for small airway disease, unless expiratory CT images are acquired.

• Centrilobular ground-glass nodules can be seen in cases of PAHTN and are postulated to be due to cholesterol granuloma formation. This should not be mistaken for hypersensitivity pneumonitis.

Suggested Readings

Devaraj A, Hansell DM. Computed tomography signs of pulmonary hypertension: old and new observations. *Clin Radiol.* August 2009;64(8):751-760.

Dupont MV, Drăgean CA, Coche EE. Right ventricle function assessment by MDCT. *AJR Am J Roentgenol.* January 2011;196(1):77-86.

Tsai IC, Tsai WL, Wang KY, et al. Comprehensive MDCT evaluation of patients with pulmonary hypertension: diagnosing underlying causes with the updated Dana Point 2008 classification. *AJR Am J Roentgenol.* September 2011;197(3):W471-W481.

Left-sided chest pain and hemoptysis

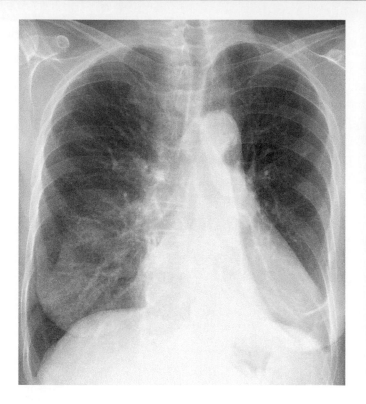 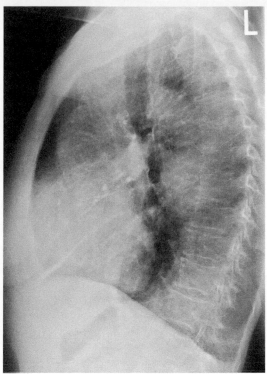

1. What are the radiographic findings?

2. What is the diagnosis?

3. List two signs of left lower lobe (LLL) collapse.

4. What is the "flat waist sign?"

5. What is the "spine sign?"

Case ranking/difficulty: 🦃

Category: Airways

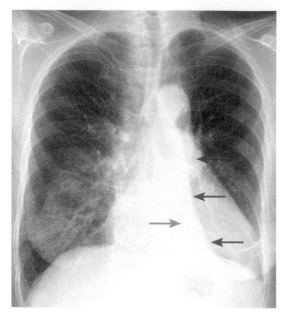

The left hemithorax appears smaller than expected and the left hilum is displaced inferiorly. The medial part of the left retrocardiac region shows increased opacification, creating the so-called "ivory heart sign" (*green arrow*). This area of opacification is well defined by the medially displaced fissure, which assumes an abnormal vertical orientation (*red arrows*). A well-defined convex opacity projects over the left hilum (*blue arrow*). The remainder of the left lung is more lucent than the right lung, suggesting compensatory left upper lobe hyperinflation. The left costophrenic angle is obliterated, in keeping with a small pleural effusion.

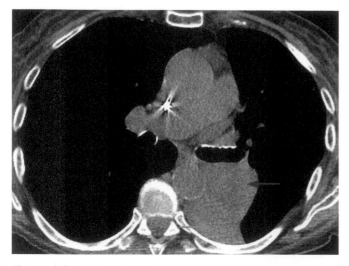

There is left lower lobe (LLL) collapse (*green arrow*). Note that the LLL bronchus is obliterated by a soft tissue density bulge (*blue arrow*), which is difficult to appreciate as it blends with the collapsed LLL on this unenhanced study. This finding suggests that the LLL collapse is actually caused by a neoplastic process (which turned out to be a squamous cell carcinoma).

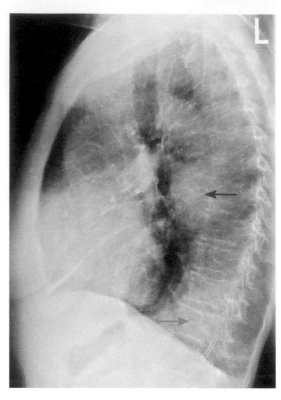

There is opacification of the left posterior hemithorax, in keeping with the so-called "spine sign" (*green arrow*). This opacity obscures the left hemidiaphragm. The left hilar mass–like opacity is also seen (*blue arrow*). Also note the increased anteroposterior chest diameter and slight flattening of the right hemidiaphragm, suggesting emphysema.

Answers

1. The left hemithorax appears smaller than expected and the left hilum is displaced inferiorly. The medial part of the left retrocardiac region shows increased opacification. This area of opacification is well defined by the medially displaced fissure, which assumes an abnormal vertical orientation. An additional convex opacity projects over the left hilar region. There is opacification of the left posterior hemithorax on the lateral radiograph, with obscuration of the left hemidiaphragm. Features suggesting emphysema are also seen.

2. Left lower lobe (LLL) collapse is the diagnosis and a neoplastic process should be considered as a probable cause for the collapse.

3. Two signs of LLL collapse are the "flat waist sign" and the "ivory heart sign."

4. The "flat waist sign" represents flattening of the aortic arch and adjacent pulmonary arterial contours due to cardiac rotation secondary to LLL collapse.

5. On normal lateral chest radiographs, the posterior hemithoracic density should have a decreasing craniocaudal gradient. When this is not the case, due to a lower lung abnormality, it is termed the "spine sign."

Pearls

- On normal frontal chest radiographs, the cardiac density should be equal on either side of the midline.
- On normal lateral chest radiographs, the posterior hemithoracic density must decrease in a craniocaudal direction.
- When lobar collapse is detected on chest radiographs, a thorough search for a cause should be performed, with specific attention to the hilar region.

Suggested Readings

Ajlan AM, Belley G, Kosiuk J. "V V O I": a swift hand motion in detecting atelectasis on frontal chest radiographs. *Can Assoc Radiol J*. May 2011;62(2):146-150.

Ho ML, Gutierrez FR. Chest radiography in thoracic polytrauma. *AJR Am J Roentgenol*. March 2009;192(3): 599-612.

Kattan KR, Wlot JF. Cardiac rotation in left lower lobe collapse. "The flat waist sign". *Radiology*. February 1976;118(2):275-279.

Parker MS, Chasen MH, Paul N. Radiologic signs in thoracic imaging: case-based review and self-assessment module. *AJR Am J Roentgenol*. March 2009;192(3 suppl):S34-S48.

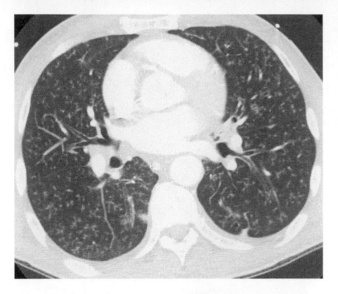
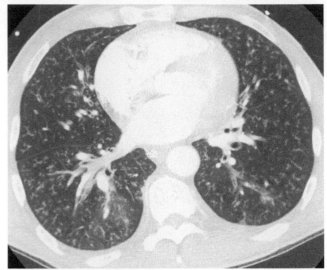
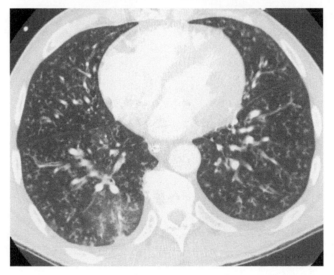

1. What are the CT findings?

2. How can centrilobular nodules be further characterized based on their CT appearance?

3. What is "tree-in-bud" pattern?

4. With which type of tuberculosis is "tree-in-bud" pattern seen: primary or postprimary?

5. In the context of tuberculosis, what does "tree-in-bud" pattern imply?

Case ranking/difficulty: 🐾

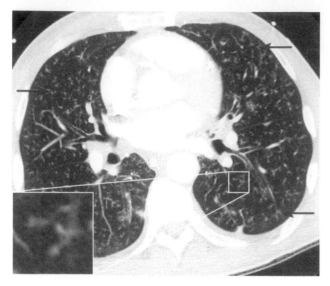

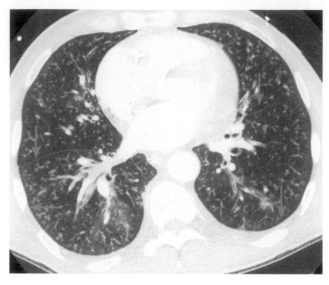

There are bilateral diffuse, tiny, branching centrilobular nodular, and linear opacities (*arrows* and *magnification*), in keeping with a "tree-in-bud" pattern.

Note the sparing of the pleura, septa, and fissures (*arrows*), which implies that the nodular distribution is neither perilymphatic nor random.

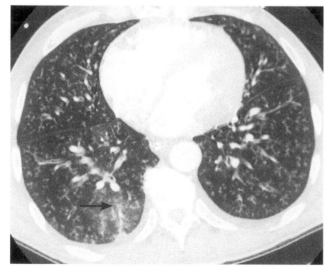

"Tree-in-bud" nodules are also seen in this more caudal image, along with right lower lobe ground-glass and consolidative opacities (*arrow*).

Answers

1. The CT shows bilateral diffuse, tiny, branching centrilobular nodular, and linear opacities, in keeping with a "tree-in-bud" pattern. There are right lower lobar ground-glass and consolidative opacities as well.

2. Centrilobular nodules can be generally divided into those which are of soft-tissue attenuation (where the nodules

are well-defined) and those of ground-glass attenuation (where the nodules are ill defined).

3. "Tree-in-bud" pattern is a chest CT sign, where centrilobular nodules have a branching and linear appearance, following the pathway of the involved small airways.

4. "Tree-in-bud" pattern is more commonly seen with primary tuberculosis (TB), but is also seen with the postprimary type.

5. "Tree-in-bud" pattern is a sign of active TB. Thus, the patient should be isolated and treated accordingly.

Pearls

- Features of active TB include cavitations, necrotic lymph nodes, "tree-in-bud" pattern, miliary spread change from prior imaging, chest wall invasion, and suggestive symptomatology.
- "Tree-in-bud" pattern can be seen with various infectious (eg, TB, atypical mycobacteria bacteria, fungi, and viruses) and noninfectious (aspiration, cystic fibrosis, primary ciliary dyskinesia, connective tissue disease, diffuse panbronchiolitis, and allergic bronchopulmonary aspergillosis) causes.
- "Tree-in-bud" pattern was originally thought to be pathognomonic of TB, but turned out to be nonspecific, and only implies small airway involvement.
- Peripheral pulmonary vascular metastases is a rare mimicker of the airway-related "tree-in-bud" pattern.

Suggested Readings

Burrill J, Williams CJ, Bain G, Conder G, Hine AL, Misra RR. Tuberculosis: a radiologic review. *Radiographics*. September-October 2007;27(5):1255-1273.

Jeong YJ, Lee KS. Pulmonary tuberculosis: up-to-date imaging and management. *AJR Am J Roentgenol*. September 2008;191(3):834-844.

Rossi SE, Franquet T, Volpacchio M, Giménez A, Aguilar G. Tree-in-bud pattern at thin-section CT of the lungs: radiologic-pathologic overview. *Radiographics*. May-June 2005;25(3):789-801.

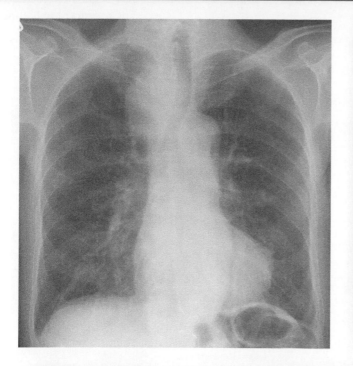
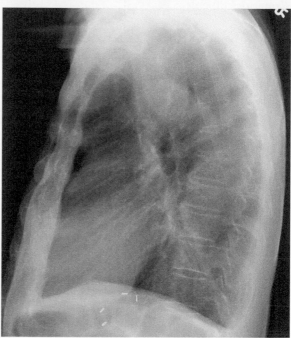
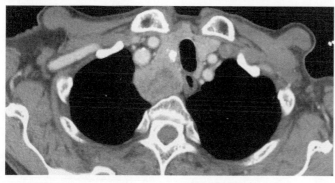
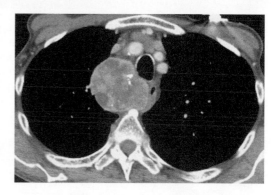

1. What are the radiographic abnormalities?

2. What are the CT abnormalities?

3. What is the "cervicothoracic sign?"

4. What is Raider triangle?

5. List a few abnormalities that can occur in Raider triangle.

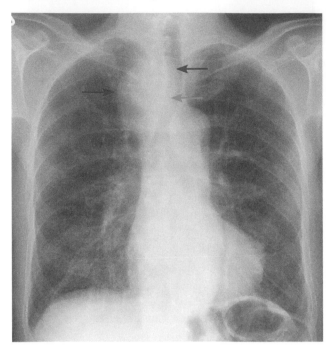

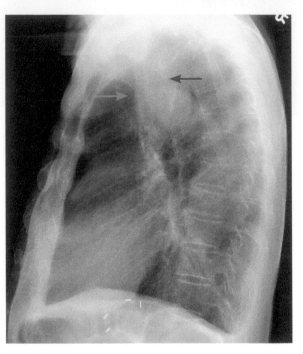

There is a large, homogenous, smoothly marginated right-sided, paratracheal opacity that shows partial projection over the tracheal air column (*red arrows*). The lesion displaces the tracheal air column, with no substantial airway narrowing (*green arrow*). The remainder of the mediastinal and hilar structures appear unremarkable.

The mediastinal abnormality occupies the retrotracheal space (*red arrow*) and displaces the trachea anteriorly (*green arrow*). Flattening of the diaphragms secondary to emphysema and upper abdominal surgical clips are additional unrelated findings.

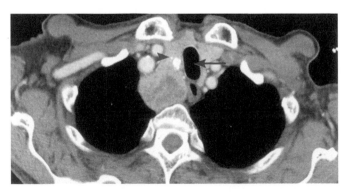

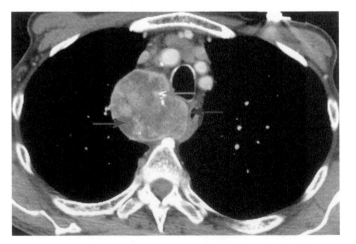

There is a right paratracheal, heterogeneous, soft tissue mass which is continuous with the thyroid gland (*red arrowhead*). The abnormality displaces the trachea to the left (*blue arrow*), but does not compromise the airway.

The lesion shows cystic changes (*red arrow*) and scattered foci of calcification (*green arrow*). The abnormality extends into the retrotracheal triangle and displaces a partially compressed esophagus to the left side (*blue arrow*).

Answers

1. The radiographs show a large, homogenous, smoothly marginated, right-sided paratracheal opacity that extends into the retrotracheal space. The lesion displaces the tracheal air column anteriorly and to the left, with no substantial airway narrowing.

2. The CT shows a right paratracheal, heterogeneous, soft tissue mass that is in continuity with the thyroid gland and has internal cystic and calcific components. The abnormality displaces the trachea to the left, but does not compromise the airway. The abnormality extends into the retrotracheal triangle and displaces a partially compressed esophagus to the left.

3. While the posterior lung extends up to the apex, the anterior lung terminates at the clavicles. Thus, if a mediastinal mass extends above the clavicle, the lateral border of the supraclavicular extension can be used to further localize the lesion. If the supraclavicular component has a well-defined lateral border, the lesion should be in the posterior mediastinum. If the supraclavicular part has an ill-defined lateral margin, it is anterior, since it is in contact with neck soft tissues and not the lung, constituting the "cervicothoracic sign."

4. Raider triangle is another name for the retrotracheal space, which is a mediastinal compartment defined by the posterior tracheal wall, the anterior spinal border, the aortic arch, and the thoracic inlet.

5. Thyroid goiter, esophageal Zenker diverticulum, right or left aberrant subclavian artery, lymphoma, foregut duplication cyst, and descending neck abscess are examples of abnormalities that can reside in or extend into the retrotracheal space.

Pearls

- Whereas a left-sided tracheal impression might be normal (ie, secondary to the aortic arch), a right-sided tracheal impression is never normal (ie, thyroid goiters are a common cause).
- Although retrosternal goiters commonly extend into the anterior mediastinum, they may also assume middle or posterior mediastinal locations or even completely encircle the trachea.
- Airway compromise is the main clinical concern with large thyroid goiters and should always be addressed in the radiology report.

Suggested Readings

Franquet T, Erasmus JJ, Giménez A, Rossi S, Prats R. The retrotracheal space: normal anatomic and pathologic appearances. *Radiographics*. October 2002;22 Spec No:S231-S246.

Vanderpump MP, Tunbridge WM, French JM, et al. The incidence of thyroid disorders in the community: a twenty-year follow-up of the Whickham Survey. *Clin Endocrinol (Oxf)*. July 1995;43(1):55-68.

Whitten CR, Khan S, Munneke GJ, Grubnic S. A diagnostic approach to mediastinal abnormalities. *Radiographics*. May-June 2007;27(3):657-671.

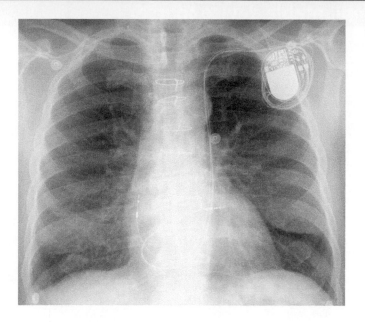

1. What is the most pertinent radiographic finding?

2. What would be your differential diagnosis based on this radiographic finding?

3. Why is the word *persistent* used to describe a left-sided SVC?

4. On imaging, how can you differentiate this entity from partial anomalous pulmonary venous return (PAPVR)?

5. What is the "ligament of Marshall?"

Case ranking/difficulty:

Category: Mediastinum

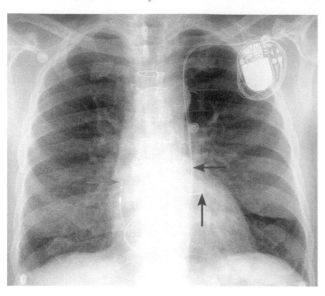

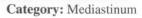

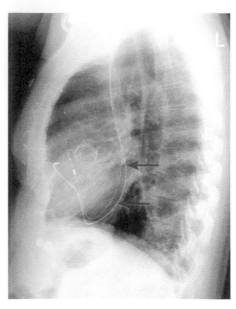

The leads of the cardiovascular implantable electronic device (CIED) have an abnormal course along the left mediastinal border, instead of crossing to the right of the mediastinal midline (*red arrows*). The atrial lead tip projects over the right atrial area (*green arrow*). The ventricular lead tip projects in a high position over the left paramedian cardiac shadow, suggesting a right ventricular outflow tract (RVOT) location (*blue arrow*). Features of prior aortic valve replacement are noted. There is minimal blunting of the costophrenic angles, due to small pleural effusions or mild pleural thickening.

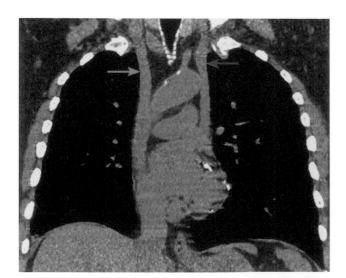

This is a selected coronal CT image before placement of the CIED. There is a tubular structure at the left lateral mediastinal border, representing a persistent left superior vena cava (PLSVC) (*red arrow*). On evaluation of the axial data set, this structure was tubular and connected the left brachiocephalic vein with coronary sinus. A right SVC is present (*green arrow*).

The lateral radiograph shows a posterior course of both CIED leads (*arrows*), likely within the coronary sinus, before projecting over the cardiac shadow.

Answers

1. The leads of the cardiovascular implantable electronic device (CIED) have an abnormal course along the left mediastinal border, instead of showing the expected midline crossing to the right side.

2. The abnormal course of the CIED leads raises the possibility of an arterial location, placement within a persistent left superior vena cava (PLSVC), placement within a dilated venous collateral, internal mammary vein or hemiazygos veins, abnormal course in a partial anomalous pulmonary venous return (PAPVR), or even perforation with an extravascular position.

3. Since a PLSVC results from failure of the normal regression of a left superior cardinal vein, the word *persistent* is used to describe left-sided SVC.

4. PLSVC drains deoxygenated systemic venous blood into the coronary sinus or right atrium, while PAPVR drains oxygenated pulmonary venous blood (from the lung parenchyma) into a systemic vein (eg, brachiocephalic or subclavian vein). Thus, the origin of these two conditions is not the same, despite the fact that both might present as a tubular structure running along the left mediastinal border.

5. The left superior cardinal vein normally regresses to become a noncanalized fibrous ligament called the "ligament of Marshall" or the "ligament of the left vena cava."

Pearls

- Central venous catheter or CIED leads inserted via the left-sided venous system should cross the mediastinal midline to the right, along the expected normal venous course.
- PLSVC can present as an unusual central venous catheter or CIED course on chest radiographs.
- PLSVC most commonly drains into the coronary sinus.
- PLSVC is only one of the causes of coronary sinus dilatation; elevation of the right atrial pressure being the most common cause. Other causes include coronary arteriovenous fistula and PAPVR into the coronary sinus.

Suggested Readings

Goyal SK, Punnam SR, Verma G, Ruberg FL. Persistent left superior vena cava: a case report and review of literature. *Cardiovasc Ultrasound*. 2008;6(6):50.

Lanzman RS, Winter J, Blondin D, et al. Where does it lead? Imaging features of cardiovascular implantable electronic devices on chest radiograph and CT. *Korean J Radiol*. September-October 2011;12(5):611-619.

Paval J, Nayak S. A persistent left superior vena cava. *Singapore Med J*. March 2007;48(3):e90-e93.

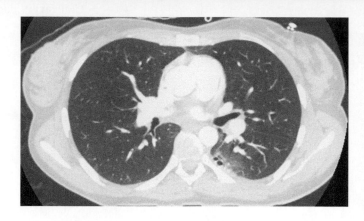 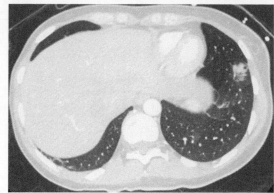

1. What are the findings?

2. What is the differential diagnosis of small cavitary lung nodules?

3. What are the differential diagnostic considerations of lung opacities in the setting of trauma?

4. What is the treatment for pulmonary contusions and lacerations?

5. What is the natural evolution of pulmonary contusions on imaging?

Case ranking/difficulty:

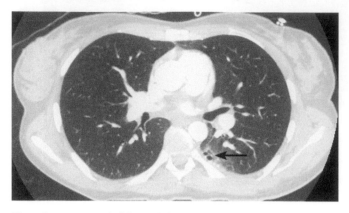

There is a posterior left lower lobe subpleural, heterogenous, nodular density with internal lucencies (*arrow*).

Answers

1. The CT findings include left lung peripheral heterogenous nodular densities with internal lucencies.

2. The differential diagnosis of the small cavitary lung nodules includes bronchogenic carcinoma, tuberculosis, septic emboli, pulmonary abscesses, cavitary metastases such as squamous or transitional cell carcinoma metastases, pulmonary lacerations, rheumatoid nodules, and Wegener granulomatosis.

3. The differential diagnostic considerations of lung opacities in a setting of trauma include pulmonary contusions, pulmonary lacerations, fat emboli, aspiration, atelectasis, pulmonary edema from fluid overload, and neurogenic pulmonary edema.

4. Pulmonary contusions and lacerations are self-limiting and require no treatment.

5. Pulmonary contusions resolve within days.

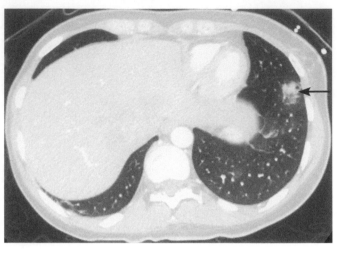

A more caudal image shows a peripheral, lingular, heterogenous, nodular density with internal lucency (*arrow*).

Pearls

- Pulmonary contusions appear at the time of injury and resolve within days.
- Pulmonary lacerations heal more slowly than contusions and may last up to several months.
- Pulmonary contusions and laceration require no treatment.

Suggested Reading

Kaewlai R, Avery LL, Asrani AV, Novelline RA. Multidetector CT of blunt thoracic trauma. *Radiographics*. October 2008;28(6):1555-1570.

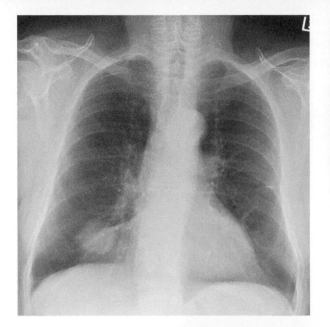
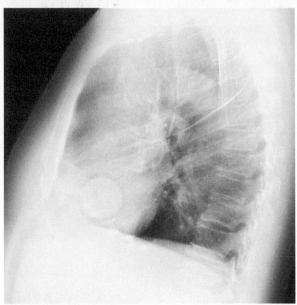
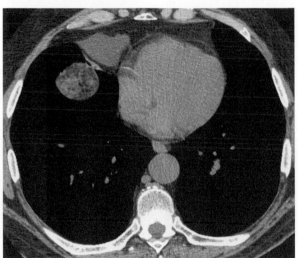

1. What is the salient radiographic finding?

2. What is the differential diagnosis based on the radiographic findings?

3. What are the CT findings?

4. What is the differential diagnosis based on the CT findings?

5. What is "Carney triad?"

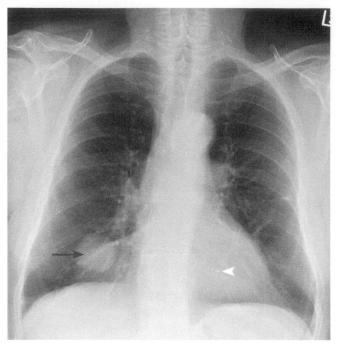

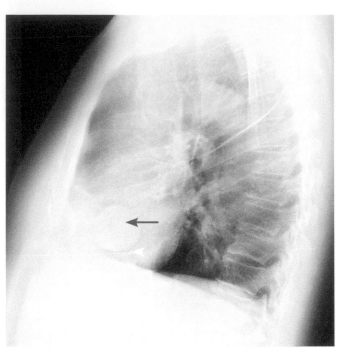

A well-defined, round, homogenous opacity involves the right middle lobe (*arrow*). Unrelated scattered calcified granulomata and an intracardiac metallic density from prior pacemaker lead placement (*arrowhead*) are also seen.

The right middle lobar opacity is identified on this lateral radiograph (*arrow*). Unrelated scattered calcified granulomata and an intracardiac metallic density from prior pacemaker lead placement (*arrowhead*) are also seen.

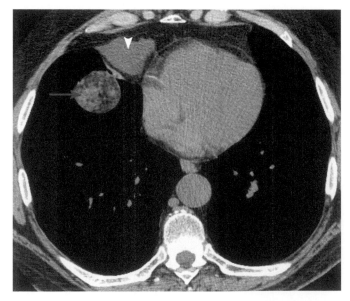

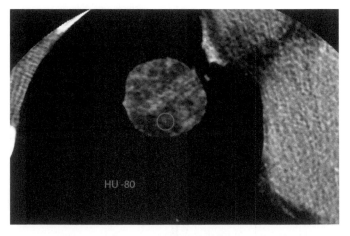

The right lung mass has both soft tissue and fat attenuations (*arrow*). An incidental right pericardial cyst is also present (*arrowhead*).

This magnified image shows the lesion with internal attenuation of −80 Hounsfield units, consistent with fat.

Answers

1. A single well-defined right middle lobe mass is seen.

2. The differential diagnosis of a solitary pulmonary mass includes lung cancer, carcinoid, hamartoma, and solitary metastasis.

3. There is a right middle lobe lung mass with both soft tissue and fat attenuations.

4. The differential diagnosis of a fat-containing lung parenchymal lesion includes hamartoma, metastatic liposarcoma, and lipoid pneumonia.

5. Carney triad is a syndrome of multiple pulmonary hamartomas/chondromas, gastrointestinal stromal tumors, and extraadrenal paragangliomas. Carney triad is different from Carney complex, which is a syndrome of endocrine overactivity, skin pigmentation, myxomas, and schwannomas.

Pearls

- Hamartomas are a common cause of benign solitary pulmonary nodule (SPN).
- Hamartomas can remain stable or slowly grow over time.
- Hamartomas will show calcifications in only about half of the cases.

Suggested Readings

Brandman S, Ko JP. Pulmonary nodule detection, characterization, and management with multidetector computed tomography. *J Thorac Imaging.* May 2011;26(2):90-105.

Meyer CA, White CS. Cartilaginous disorders of the chest. *Radiographics.* September-October 1998;18(5):1109-1123; quiz 1241-1242.

Molinari F, Bankier AA, Eisenberg RL. Fat-containing lesions in adult thoracic imaging. *AJR Am J Roentgenol.* November 2011;197(5):W795-W813.

Smoker with a few days of chest pain

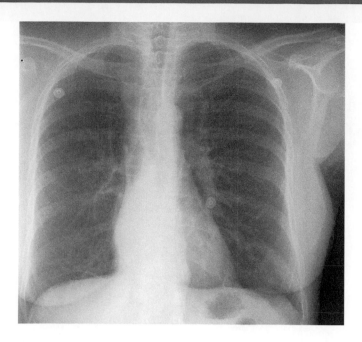

1. What major findings are seen on this radiograph?

2. On a normal chest radiograph, which hilum is usually higher than the other?

3. What is the working diagnosis?

4. What is the "upper triangle sign?"

5. Which bronchus is usually obstructed in cases of combined right middle and lower lobes collapse?

Case ranking/difficulty:

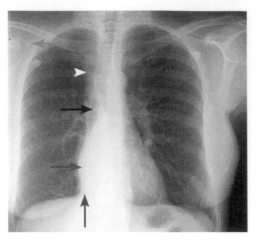

There is a homogenous increase in the right retrocardiac density (*red arrow*) when compared to the left retrocardiac region, with partial obscuration of the medial aspect of the right hemidiaphragm (*blue arrow*). The right hilum is depressed as denoted by a straighter than usual course of the right main stem bronchus (*black arrow*). In addition, the right interlobar pulmonary artery is not visualized in its expected location. Although there is hyperinflation due to smoking-induced emphysema, the right hemithorax appears relatively smaller than expected. There is apparent widening of the right superior mediastinum due to mediastinal displacement and rotation, leading to the "upper triangle sign" (*white arrowhead*). The right scapula is only partially seen (*green arrow*), in contrast to the clearly visualized left scapula.

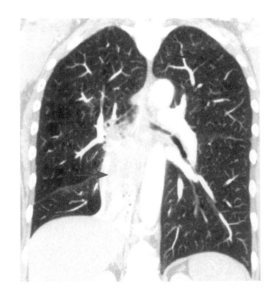

RLL collapse is also seen on this coronal image (*red arrow*), explaining the radiographically detected right retrocardiac density. Centrilobular emphysema is also noted (*blue arrows*).

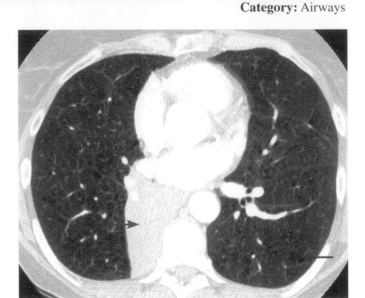

The collapsed right lower lobe (RLL) is seen on CT (*red arrow*) along with centrilobular emphysema (*blue arrows*).

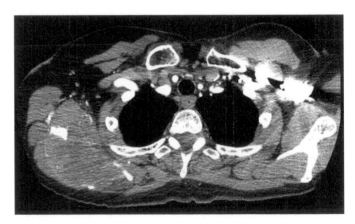

There is a large chest wall soft tissue mass destroying the right scapula (*arrow*), consistent with a metastatic bone lesion.

Answers

1. There is right retrocardiac opacification, with obscuration of the medial right hemidiaphragm, right hilar depression, and a relative decrease in the right hemithoracic size. Additionally, there is suspected destruction of the right scapula.

2. Normally, the left hilum is higher than the right in most individuals. In a minority of normal cases, the right hilum may be at the same level as the left. Importantly, the right hilum should never be higher than the left on normal radiographs.

3. Right lower lobe (RLL) collapse is the main diagnosis. In view of the right scapular lesion, this should raise the possibility of bronchial obstruction by lung cancer.

4. In the case of RLL collapse, apparent widening of the right superior mediastinum may be seen due to mediastinal displacement and rotation, resulting in the so-called "upper triangle sign."

5. Obstruction of the bronchus intermedius results in collapse of both the right middle and lower lobes.

Pearls

- The right interlobar pulmonary artery should be normally seen on all technically adequate frontal radiographs.
- The interlobar artery may be obscured in RLL collapse.
- RLL collapse causes mediastinal displacement and rotation that results in apparent widening of the superior mediastinum, resulting in the "upper triangle sign."
- All the osseous structures, including the scapula, should be assessed during routine reading of chest radiographs.
- Chest wall soft tissues should be routinely assessed on chest CT.

Suggested Readings

Ajlan AM, Belley G, Kosiuk J. "V V O I": a swift hand motion in detecting atelectasis on frontal chest radiographs. *Can Assoc Radiol J*. May 2011;62(2):146-150.

Ho ML, Gutierrez FR. Chest radiography in thoracic polytrauma. *AJR Am J Roentgenol*. March 2009;192(3): 599-612.

Parker MS, Chasen MH, Paul N. Radiologic signs in thoracic imaging: case-based review and self-assessment module. *AJR Am J Roentgenol*. March 2009;192(3 suppl):S34-S48.

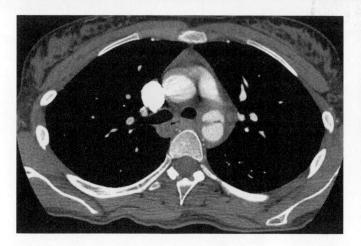
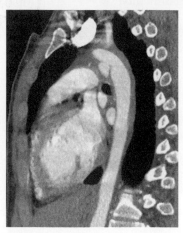

1. What are the findings?

2. What are differential diagnostic considerations of aortic pseudoaneurysm?

3. What is the most common type of injury resulting in aortic aneurysm?

4. What is the most frequent site of traumatic aortic injury in survivors?

5. What are potential diagnostic pitfalls simulating aortic injury on imaging?

Case ranking/difficulty: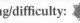

Category: Mediastinum

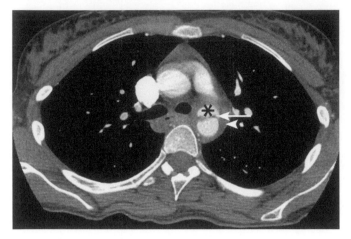

There is focal contour irregularity (*asterisk*) and linear filling defect (*arrow*) in the aortic isthmus, and a periaortic hematoma (*arrowhead*).

Answers

1. The CT shows outpouching/contour irregularity of the inferior wall at the aortic isthmus (ie, pseudoaneurysm), linear filling defect in the lumen of the aorta, and periaortic hematoma.

2. Differential diagnosis of aortic pseudoaneurysm includes traumatic aortic injury, mycotic aneurysm, penetrating atheromatous ulcer, and complication of connective-tissue diseases and of vasculitis.

3. Motor vehicle collision is the mechanism of injury most commonly associated with aortic injury resulting in aneurysm formation.

4. The most common location of traumatic aortic injury is at the root, but the victims usually do not survive to reach the hospital. Aortic isthmus is the most frequent site of acute traumatic aortic injury seen in survivors.

5. There are several potential diagnostic pitfalls simulating aortic injury. Takeoff of bronchial and intercostal arteries can have small infundibula that may give the impression of a small pseudoaneurysm. Enhancement of the collapsed lung adjacent to the aorta may simulate an intimal flap. Left superior intercostal and hemiazygos veins opacified with contrast can approximate the appearance of an intimal flap. Motion artifacts can simulate intimal flap. Finally, ductus diverticulum can simulate a traumatic pseudoaneurysm.

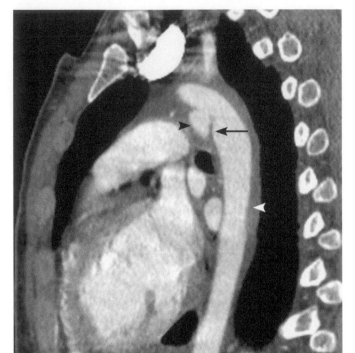

Sagittal reformation shows an outpouching of the inferior wall of the aortic isthmus (*black arrowhead*), linear filling defect in the lumen of the aorta (*arrow*), and periaortic hematoma (*white arrowhead*).

Pearls

- Acute traumatic aortic injuries are almost exclusively seen in setting of high-velocity deceleration trauma.
- Aortic isthmus is the most common site of injury in survivors reaching the hospital.
- Aortic contour irregularity should be viewed with high index of suspicion in the context of trauma.
- In addition to assessing the aorta on axial images, aortic contour evaluation on the sagittal and coronal reformats is extremely valuable.

Suggested Reading

Steenburg SD, Ravenel JG, Ikonomidis JS, Schönholz C, Reeves S. Acute traumatic aortic injury: imaging evaluation and management. *Radiology*. September 2008;248(3):748-762.

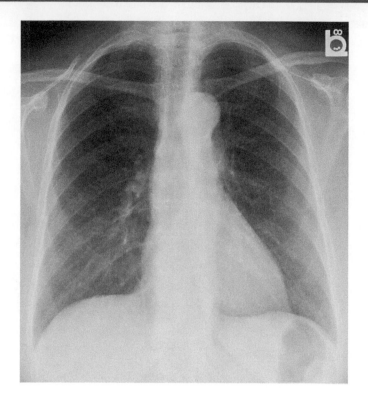

1. What line/stripe appears abnormal on the chest radiograph?

2. What is the normal configuration of the line that appears abnormal on the provided radiograph?

3. What are the boundaries of the recess that give rise to this line?

4. What is the differential diagnosis of the radiographic abnormality?

5. What is the most common etiology of this radiographic abnormality?

Case ranking/difficulty:

Category: Basic interpretation

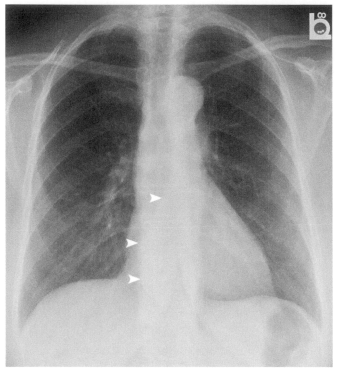

There is abnormal rightward bulging of the lower azygoesophageal line (*arrowheads*).

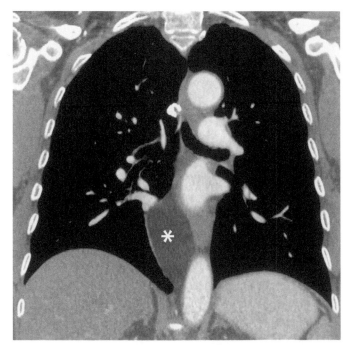

Coronal reformation of CT chest shows the craniocaudal extent of the right paraesophageal lipoma (*asterisk*).

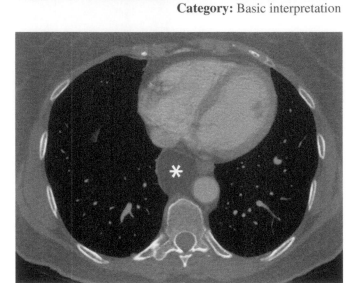

CT chest shows that the radiographic abnormality is due to a right paraesophageal fat-density lesion (*asterisk*), consistent with a lipoma.

Answers

1. There is abnormal rightward bulging of the azygoesophageal line.

2. A normal azygoesophageal line should be straight or mildly convex to the left.

3. Azygoesophageal recess represents a space lying lateral or posterior to the esophagus and anterior to the spine, extending from the level of the anterior turn of the azygos vein superiorly, to the level of the aortic hiatus inferiorly.

4. The differential diagnosis of a bulging azygoesophageal line includes lymphadenopathy, hiatal hernia, bronchopulmonary-foregut malformation, esophageal neoplasm, pleural abnormalities, and left atrial enlargement.

5. In clinical practice, the bulging azygoesophageal line is most commonly secondary to a hiatal hernia.

Pearls

- On a normal chest radiograph, the azygoesophageal line should be straight or slightly convex to the left.
- Rightward convexity of the azygoesophageal line could be due to lymphadenopathy, hiatal hernia, bronchopulmonary-foregut malformation, esophageal neoplasm, esophageal varices, pleural abnormalities, and left atrial enlargement.
- Systematic assessment of the azygoesophageal line should be part of the normal routine in chest radiograph interpretation.

Suggested Reading

Gibbs JM, Chandrasekhar CA, Ferguson EC, Oldham SA. Lines and stripes: where did they go?—From conventional radiography to CT. *Radiographics*. January-February 2007;27(1):33-48.

Right chest pain, fever, and productive cough

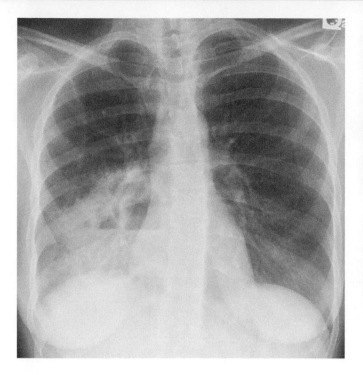
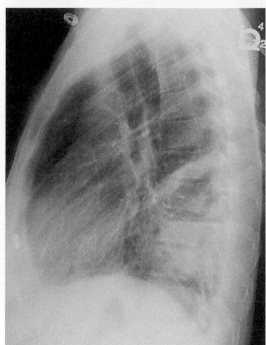

1. What are the findings?

2. What is the differential diagnosis?

3. What are the pathogens most commonly associated with this condition?

4. What are the recognized predisposing factors to this condition?

5. What is the standard treatment for this condition?

Case ranking/difficulty:

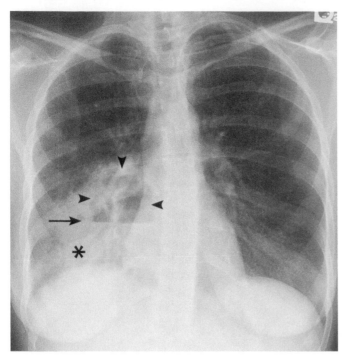

Frontal chest radiograph shows a large right lower lobe consolidation (*asterisk*) and cavity (*arrowheads*) with an air-fluid level (*arrow*).

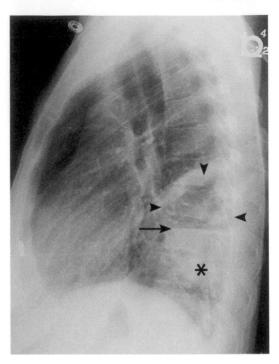

Lateral chest radiograph shows posterior right lower lobe consolidation (*asterisk*) and cavity (*arrowheads*) with an air-fluid level (*arrow*). The air-fluid level has similar length on the frontal and lateral views, confirming its intraparenchymal location.

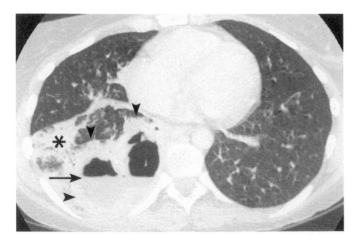

CT chest in lung window confirms a right lower lobe cavitary lesion with thick, irregular walls (*arrowheads*), an air-fluid level (*arrow*) and adjacent patchy consolidation (*asterisk*).

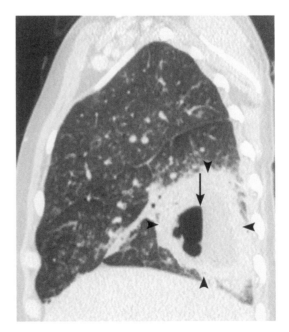

Sagittal reformation depicts the craniocaudal span of the posterior right lower lobe cavity with thick, irregular walls (*arrowheads*) and an air-fluid level (*arrow*).

Answers

1. Chest radiographs show an extensive consolidation and a large thick-walled cavity with an air-fluid level in the posterior aspect of the right lower lobe.

2. The differential diagnosis should include a pulmonary abscess, cavitating bronchogenic carcinoma, necrotic metastasis, infected bulla, and tuberculosis.

3. Microorganisms most commonly associated with lung abscesses are *Staphylococcus aureus*, *Klebsiella* species, *Pseudomonas* species, and *Proteus* species.

4. The recognized factors predisposing to pulmonary abscess are aspiration and chronic pneumonia.

5. Intravenous antibiotics are the recommended treatment for pulmonary abscess.

Pearls

- Pulmonary abscesses most often arise as a complication of aspiration pneumonitis, necrotizing pneumonia, or chronic pneumonia.
- Large pulmonary abscesses and aerobic bacteria are associated with a worse outcome.
- Most patients with a pulmonary abscess improve with antibiotics.
- Air-fluid level on chest radiography is not normal and should prompt a search for upper gastrointestinal abnormality (eg, esophageal diverticulum, hiatal hernia), hydropneumothorax, or pulmonary cavitary lesions.
- Intraparenchymal air-fluid level can be differentiated from that in the pleural space by comparing its length on frontal and lateral views, which should be nearly equal for an intraparenchymal collection and different for a pleural collection.

Suggested Reading

Hirshberg B, Sklair-Levi M, Nir-Paz R, Ben-Sira L, Krivoruk V, Kramer MR. Factors predicting mortality of patients with lung abscess. *Chest*. March 1999;115(3):746-750.

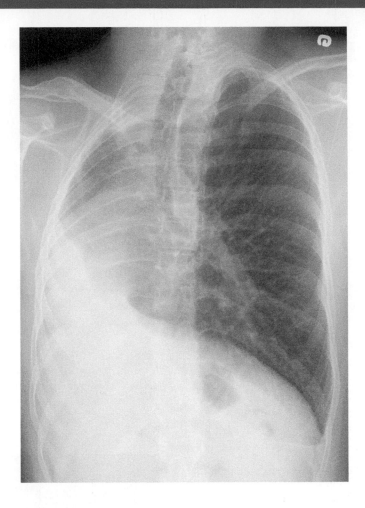

1. What are the radiographic findings?

2. What is the differential diagnosis based on the radiographic findings?

3. How is pulmonary aplasia different from pulmonary agenesis?

4. What additional abnormalities could be encountered in this patient?

5. What syndrome could be associated with pulmonary agenesis?

Case ranking/difficulty: 🐾

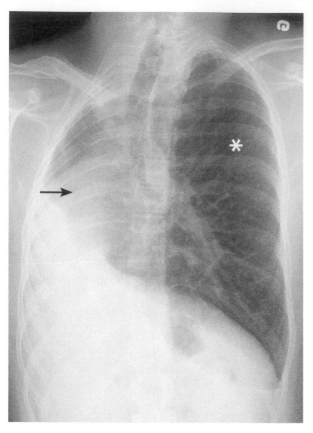

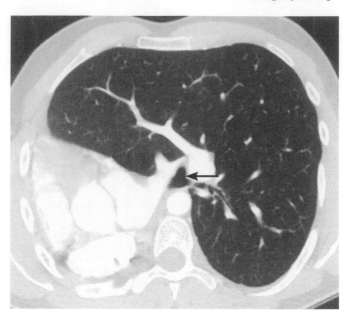

CT chest in lung window at the level of left main stem bronchus bifurcation (*arrow*) demonstrates complete absence of the right lung parenchyma and of the right bronchopulmonary structures, mediastinal shift to the right, and compensatory hyperinflation of the left lung.

Posteroanterior chest radiograph demonstrating marked right lung volume loss with mediastinal shift to the right (*arrow*) and left lung hyperinflation (*asterisk*). Note smaller right hemithorax.

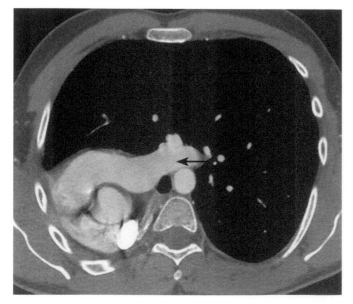

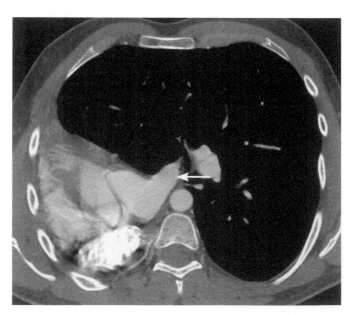

Note normal left superior pulmonary vein (*arrow*) and absence of the right pulmonary veins.

Note normal left main pulmonary artery (*arrow*) and absence of the right main pulmonary artery.

Answers

1. The chest radiograph demonstrates marked right lung volume loss, mediastinal shift to the right, smaller right hemithorax, and left lung hyperinflation.

2. The differential diagnosis of such extensive right lung volume loss should include right pneumonectomy, right pulmonary agenesis or aplasia, and complete right lung collapse.

3. Imaging findings in pulmonary aplasia and agenesis are similar, except for the presence of a short blind-ending bronchus in aplasia.

4. Pulmonary agenesis is frequently associated with additional congenital abnormalities of the cardiovascular, gastrointestinal, genitourinary, or skeletal systems.

5. Pulmonary agenesis has been reported in VACTERL, which is a syndrome of nonrandom co-occurrence of birth defects including Vertebral anomalies, Anal atresia, Cardiac defects, Tracheoesophageal fistula and/or Esophageal atresia, Renal anomalies, and Limb defects.

Pearls

- Pulmonary agenesis is a rare congenital abnormality.
- Pulmonary agenesis is different from pulmonary aplasia, in that the latter features a blind-ending bronchus.
- Pulmonary agenesis is often associated with other congenital abnormalities.
- Differential diagnosis of marked lung volume loss should include pneumonectomy, pulmonary agenesis, pulmonary aplasia, and complete lung collapse.

Suggested Reading

Biyyam DR, Chapman T, Ferguson MR, Deutsch G, Dighe MK. Congenital lung abnormalities: embryologic features, prenatal diagnosis, and postnatal radiologic-pathologic correlation. *Radiographics*. October 2010;30(6):1721-1738.

Remote thyroidectomy

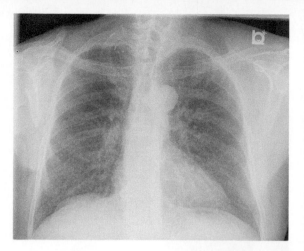
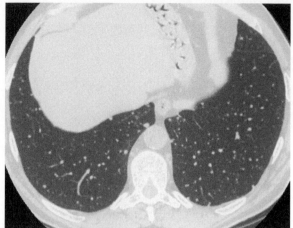
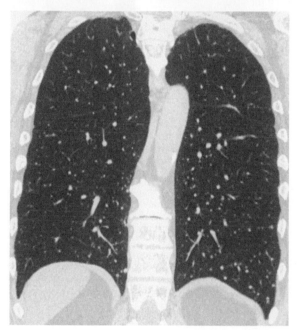

1. What are the findings?

2. What is the pattern of distribution of the nodules?

3. What is the differential diagnosis of miliary
   pattern of pulmonary nodules on CT?

4. What primary malignancies typically give
   miliary pattern of pulmonary metastases?

5. What kind of imaging should be avoided in
   patients with suspected metastatic thyroid
   cancer?

Case ranking/difficulty: 🍂

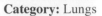

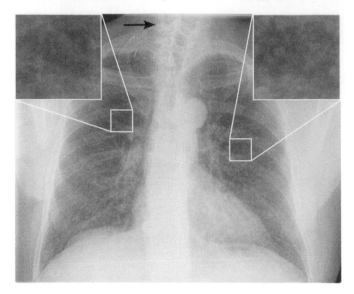

Posteroanterior chest radiograph shows diffuse bilateral micronodules (*magnifications*) and thyroidectomy clips (*arrow*).

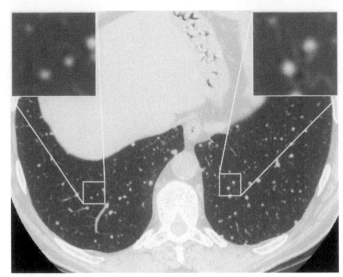

CT chest confirms diffuse bilateral micronodules in random distribution (*magnifications*).

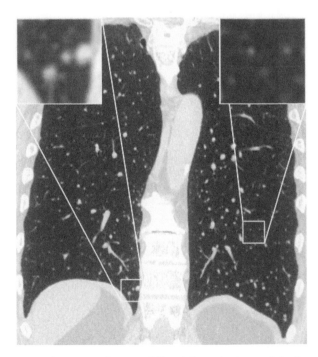

Coronal reformation showing diffuse bilateral micronodules in random distribution.

Answers

1. Both chest radiograph and CT demonstrate diffuse bilateral micronodules.

2. The pattern of distribution of the nodules is random. Since the nodules are less than 2-3 mm in size, the pattern is designated as 'miliary'.

3. Differential diagnosis of miliary nodules comprises hematogenous spread of infection (most commonly tuberculosis, fungal infections, and varicella) and metastases.

4. Malignancies commonly associated with miliary pulmonary metastases are malignant melanoma, osteosarcoma, renal cell carcinoma, thyroid carcinoma, and trophoblastic disease.

5. Imaging studies that require intravenous administration of iodine-containing contrast agents should be avoided, because the iodine in contrast will interfere with radioactive iodine treatment for up to 2 months.

Pearls

- The pattern of micronodular distribution cannot be reliably ascertained on chest radiography. However, in most cases, CT allows precise pattern identification, thus narrowing down the differential diagnosis.
- Miliary pattern of lung nodules is most commonly associated with hematogenous spread of infections (most commonly tuberculous or fungal) and of metastases (most commonly from thyroid cancer).
- Intravenous iodinated contrast should be avoided in patients with suspected metastatic thyroid cancer, as it will preclude radioactive-iodine therapy for 2 months.

Suggested Reading

Roche CJ, O'Keeffe DP, Lee WK, Duddalwar VA, Torreggiani WC, Curtis JM. Selections from the buffet of food signs in radiology. *Radiographics*. November-December 2002;22(6):1369-1384.

Routine follow-up in a heavy smoker

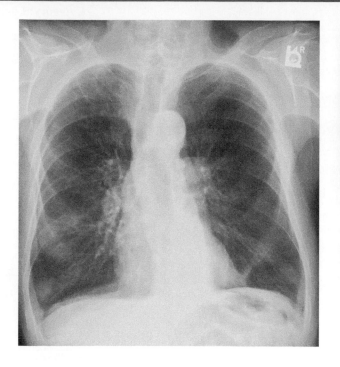 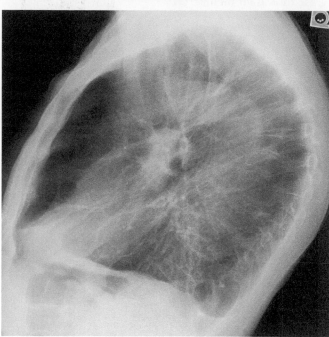

1. What are the findings on the frontal radiograph?

2. What are the findings on the lateral radiograph?

3. What are the recognized morphological types of pulmonary emphysema?

4. What type of pulmonary emphysema is strongly associated with cigarette smoking?

5. What CT finding allows to differentiate centrilobular emphysema from pulmonary cysts?

Case ranking/difficulty: 🌰

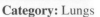

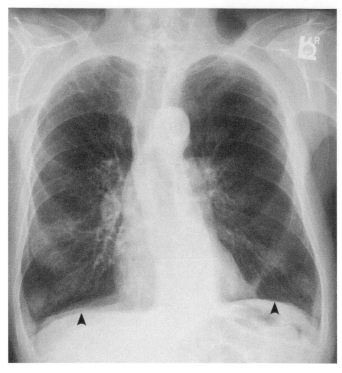

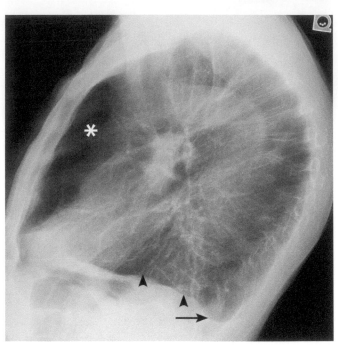

There is hyperinflation manifesting as hyperlucent lungs, overall increased lung volume, and flattened hemidiaphragms (*arrowheads*).

The lateral radiograph shows increased retrosternal space (*asterisk*), flattened diaphragm (*arrowheads*), resulting in blunted posterior costophrenic angles (*arrow*), and increased anteroposterior diameter of the chest.

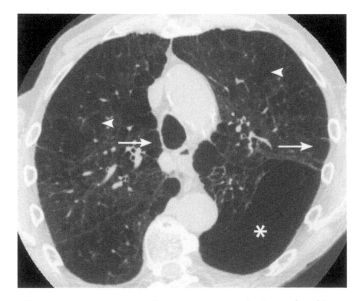

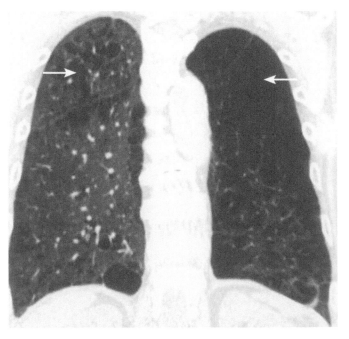

CT demonstrates severe pulmonary centrilobular (*arrowheads*) and paraseptal (*arrows*) emphysema with large bulla on the left (*asterisk*).

Coronal image shows that emphysema is more advanced in the upper lobes (*arrows*).

Answers

1. The frontal radiograph demonstrates classical findings of hyperinflation: hyperlucent lung parenchyma, increased pulmonary volume, and flattened diaphragm.

2. The lateral radiograph shows additional findings related to hyperinflation: increased anteroposterior diameter of the chest ("barrel chest"), increased retrosternal space, and flattened hemidiaphragms, resulting in costophrenic angles blunting.

3. The recognized morphological types of pulmonary emphysema are panacinar (ie, panlobular), centrilobular (ie, centriacinar), and paraseptal (ie, distal acinar or distal lobular).

4. Centrilobular emphysema is strongly associated with cigarette smoking.

5. Two features that allow confident differentiation of centrilobular emphysema from pulmonary cysts: imperceptible wall in emphysema; presence of the central dot within the lucent area of emphysema, corresponding to the bronchovascular bundle.

Pearls

- Pulmonary emphysema is defined as abnormal permanent enlargement of the air spaces distal to the terminal bronchioles, accompanied by destruction of the alveolar walls, without fibrosis.
- There are three recognized types of pulmonary emphysema: panlobular, centrilobular, and paraseptal.
- Centrilobular emphysema is the most common type of emphysema and is strongly associated with cigarette smoking.
- Smoking-related emphysema is typically upper lung predominant, as opposed to panlobular emphysema of alpha-1-antitrypsin deficiency, which shows basilar predominance.

Suggested Readings

Stern EJ, Frank MS. CT of the lung in patients with pulmonary emphysema: diagnosis, quantification, and correlation with pathologic and physiologic findings. *AJR Am J Roentgenol*. April 1994;162(4):791-798.

Takahashi M, Fukuoka J, Nitta N, et al. Imaging of pulmonary emphysema: a pictorial review. *Int J Chron Obstruct Pulmon Dis*. 2008;3(2):193-204.

Progressive exertional shortness of breath

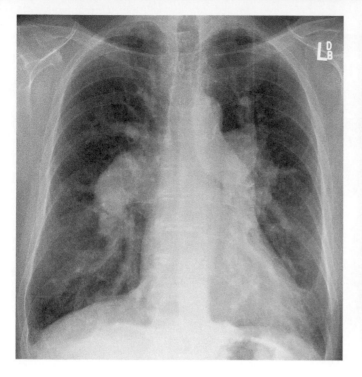 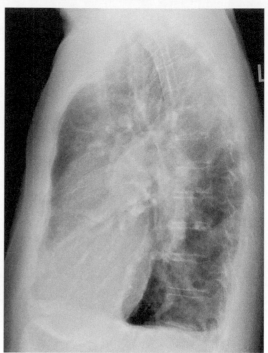

1. What are the radiographic findings?

2. What is the overall diagnosis?

3. What does "pruning" mean in the context of pulmonary arterial hypertension?

4. What is the 2008 Dana Point Classification?

5. What are the categories that are included in the 2008 Dana Point Classification?

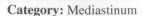

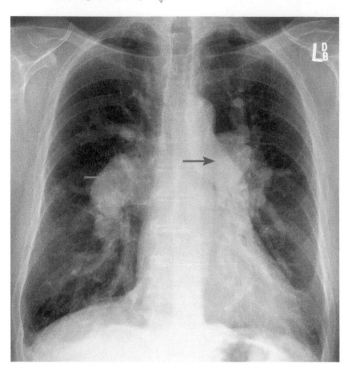

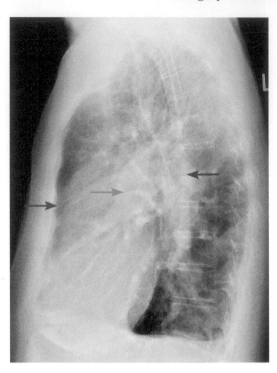

There is enlargement of the pulmonary arterial trunk (*red arrow*), right pulmonary artery (*green arrow*), and left pulmonary artery (*blue arrow*). Note the relative paucity of peripheral lung markings bilaterally, consistent with peripheral pruning. There is cardiomegaly, with no features to suggest pulmonary edema. Unrelated minimal biapical pleuroparenchymal scarring, costophrenic angle blunting from chronic pleural thickening, and aortic atherosclerotic calcifications are seen.

There is enlargement of the right (*green arrow*) and left (*blue arrow*) pulmonary arteries. Note that the right ventricle abuts more than half of the sternum (*red arrow*), denoting RV enlargement. There is costophrenic angle blunting from chronic pleural thickening.

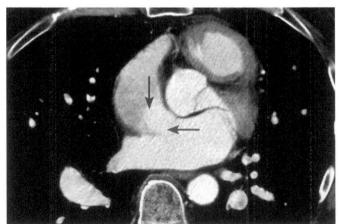

There is a large secundum atrial septal defect (*red arrow*) and high-density contrast appears to pass from the left to the right atrium (*blue arrow*).

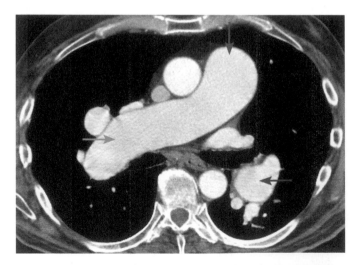

The pulmonary arterial trunk (*red arrow*), right pulmonary artery (*green arrow*), and left pulmonary artery (*blue arrow*) are all larger than the ascending aorta.

Answers

1. There is enlargement of the central pulmonary arteries and relative paucity of peripheral lung markings bilaterally.

2. The diagnosis is that of pulmonary arterial hypertension (PAHTN).

3. "Pruning" is a term that describes peripheral pulmonary arterial attenuation as a result of long-standing PAHTN that appears as peripheral paucity of lung markings on chest radiographs.

4. The 2008 Dana Point Classification is the newest PAHTN classification system and incorporates five major categories, according to the etiology of PAHTN.

5. The 2008 categories included in the 2008 Dana Point Classification are idiopathic PAHTN, PAHTN from left heart disease, PAHTN from lung diseases or hypoxia, chronic thromboembolic PAHTN, and PAHTN from miscellaneous causes.

Pearls

- PAHTN can be classified according to the 2008 Dana Point Classification.
- The pulmonary artery (PA) can be of normal caliber in cases of PAHTN and can be enlarged in patients without PAHTN. Thus, a thoughtful multidisciplinary approach is needed when increased PA diameter is found on imaging.
- It is important to carefully assess the cardiac structures on IV-enhanced chest CTs, since abnormalities are commonly seen even on non-ECG-synchronized exams.

Suggested Readings

Devaraj A, Hansell DM. Computed tomography signs of pulmonary hypertension: old and new observations. *Clin Radiol.* August 2009;64(8):751-760.

Dupont MV, Drăgean CA, Coche EE. Right ventricle function assessment by MDCT. *AJR Am J Roentgenol.* January 2011;196(1):77-86.

Tsai IC, Tsai WL, Wang KY, et al. Comprehensive MDCT evaluation of patients with pulmonary hypertension: diagnosing underlying causes with the updated Dana Point 2008 classification. *AJR Am J Roentgenol.* September 2011;197(3):W471-W481.

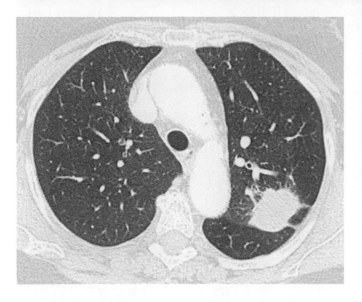 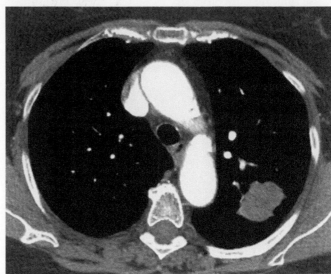

1. What are the findings?

2. What is the differential diagnosis?

3. What features would favor squamous cell carcinoma?

4. What is the radiographic sign that describes a central airway obstructive lesion causing upper lobe collapse?

5. Which primary lung neoplasm is most commonly associated with hypercalcemia?

Squamous cell lung carcinoma

Case ranking/difficulty: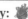

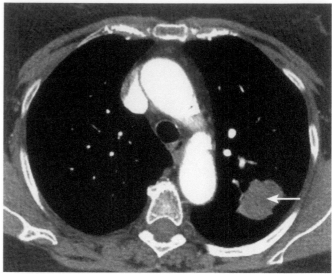

CT in lung window shows a left upper lobe parafissural mass (*arrow*).

CT in mediastinal window shows that the left upper lobe lesion is solid (*arrow*).

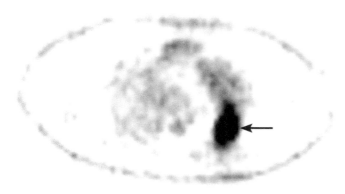

PET demonstrates a hypermetabolic left upper lobe mass (*arrow*).

Answers

1. There is a solitary left upper lobe parafissural mass.

2. All types of nonsmall cell lung neoplasia, including adenocarcinoma, squamous cell carcinoma, large cell carcinoma, carcinoid, and pulmonary lymphoma, can present as a solitary peripheral nodular lesion. Additional differential diagnostic considerations for a solitary pulmonary nodule/mass include solitary pulmonary metastasis, pulmonary hamartoma, granuloma, lung abscess, rheumatoid nodule, plasma cell granuloma, round pneumonia, arteriovenous malformation, bronchogenic cyst, pulmonary atresia/obstruction with mucoid impaction, pulmonary infarct, intrapulmonary lymph node, pulmonary hematoma, and pulmonary amyloidosis.

3. Squamous cell carcinoma typically causes bronchial obstruction and is the most common cell type to cavitate.

4. A central neoplasm may obstruct the upper lobar bronchus and cause upper lobar collapse. Since the medial aspect of the fissure typically has a convex shape due to the bulge created by the neoplasm, this has been termed the "Golden S" sign.

5. Hypercalcemia is most commonly associated with squamous cell carcinoma.

Pearls

- The two broad classes of lung cancer are small cell lung carcinoma and nonsmall cell lung carcinoma (NSCLC).
- NSCLC comprises three main subtypes: adenocarcinoma, squamous cell carcinoma (SCC), and large cell carcinoma.
- SCC commonly presents as a central bronchial lesion causing distal obstruction.
- SCC is the most common lung cancer cell type to cavitate.
- SCC is strongly associated with cigarette smoking.

Suggested Reading

Rosado-de-Christenson ML, Templeton PA, Moran CA. Bronchogenic carcinoma: radiologic-pathologic correlation. *Radiographics*. March 1994;14(2):429-446; quiz 447-8.

Dyspnea

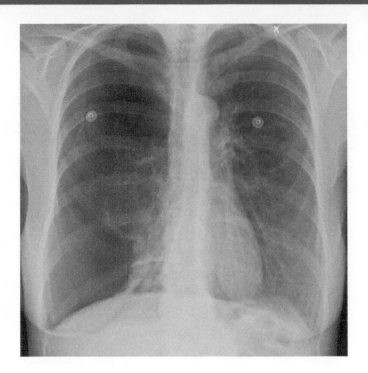

1. What are the findings?

2. What are the most common signs of
    pneumothorax on an erect chest radiograph?

3. What possible diseases should be suspected in
    cases of spontaneous pneumothorax?

4. What findings are suggestive of tension
    pneumothorax?

5. What can be done to ease detection of
    pneumothorax on chest x-ray?

Case ranking/difficulty: 🐾

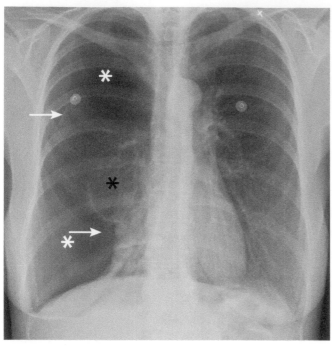

Frontal chest radiograph shows large areas of hyperlucency with absent vascular markings in the right hemithorax (*white asterisks*), atelectasis of the right lung (*black asterisk*), and visceral pleural line (*arrows*). There is mild mediastinal shift to the left.

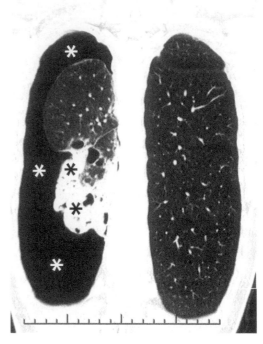

Coronal reformation of CT chest shows a large right pneumothorax (*white asterisks*) and right lung atelectasis (*black asterisks*).

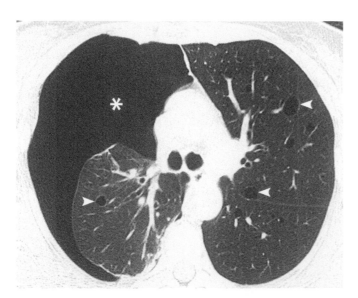

Axial CT chest redemonstrates the right pneumothorax (*asterisk*), but also shows multiple bilateral well-defined pulmonary cysts (*arrowheads*). The patient is known for lymphangioleiomyomatosis.

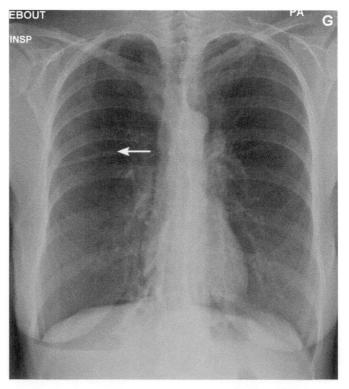

Frontal chest radiograph post chest tube (*arrow*) placement demonstrates marked regression of the pneumothorax and reexpansion of the right lung.

Answers

1. There is a large right pneumothorax (PTX), causing right lung atelectasis and mild mediastinal shift to the left. There is no sizeable pleural effusion and no evidence of cystic lung disease.

2. On erect chest radiograph, a PTX usually presents as a visceral pleural line and lack of lung markings peripheral to that line.

3. Spontaneous PTX can be seen with following pleuroparenchymal diseases: bullae/blebs, emphysema, asthma, cystic lung diseases (*Pneumocystis jiroveci* pneumonia, lymphangiomyomatosis, Langerhans cell histiocytosis), with certain infections (necrotic pneumonia, fungal diseases, tuberculosis), neoplasia (cavitating neoplasm, metastatic osteogenic sarcoma), and catamenial pneumothorax (pleural endometriosis).

4. The radiographic features of tension PTX include ipsilateral hyperinflation of the hemithorax, downward displacement of the diaphragm, and contralateral shift of the mediastinum. Atelectasis and subcutaneous emphysema can occur without tension PTX.

5. Detection of PTX is greatly limited in the semierect or supine positions. The patients should be imaged in erect or decubitus positions. The conspicuity of a PTX is increased on expiratory films, in which normal lung decreases in volume and increases in density relative to the fixed pleural air. Artifacts from tubing, sheets, or other extrinsic opacities can mimic a PTX, and should be removed if possible.

Pearls

- Primary spontaneous PTX occurs more frequently in young, tall, thin males.
- Secondary spontaneous PTX is due to underlying, usually cystic, lung disease.
- An expiratory view enhances the visualization of PTX.
- Tension PTX is a medical emergency and when suspected should be treated empirically without delay for imaging.

Suggested Reading

Slone RM, Gutierrez FR, Fisher AJ. *Thoracic Imaging. A Practical Approach.* McGraw-Hill; 1999:168. USBN: 0-07-058223-8.

Coughing

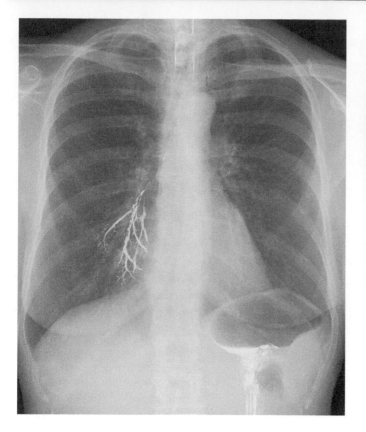 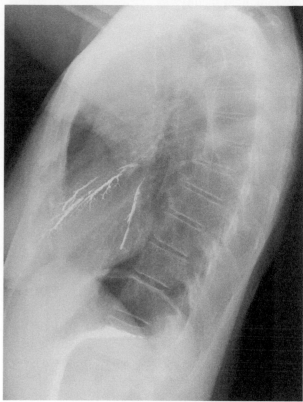

1. What are the findings?

2. What is the diagnosis?

3. What is the differential diagnosis of spontaneously hyperdense linear and branching densities in the lungs?

4. What are the most commonly involved lung zones with aspiration in erect position?

5. What factors predispose to aspiration?

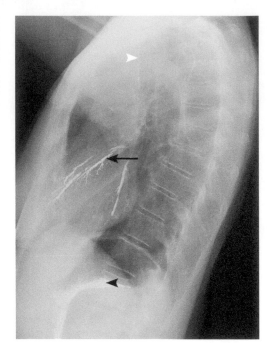

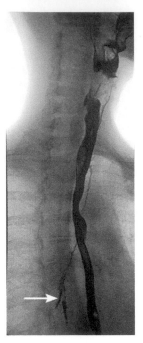

There are branching linear hyperdensities in the right lung base (*arrow*), hyperdense material outlining tracheal walls (*white arrowhead*), and contrast material in stomach (*black arrowhead*).

There are branching linear hyperdensities in the right middle lobe (*arrow*), hyperdense material outlining tracheal walls (*white arrowhead*), and contrast material in stomach (*black arrowhead*).

Imaging from a barium swallow study demonstrating barium aspiration (*arrow*).

Answers

1. The findings include branching linear hyperdensities in the right middle lobe, hyperdense material outlining tracheal walls, and contrast material in stomach.

2. The findings are pathognomonic of barium contrast aspiration.

3. The differential diagnosis of spontaneously hyperdense linear and branching densities in the lungs should include aspirated barium, bronchioliths, dendriform pulmonary ossifications, polymethyl methacrylate (vertebroplasty cement) pulmonary emboli, and embolized intravenously injected mercury.

4. The basal segments of the lower lobes are commonly involved when the patient is in the erect position. The middle lobe might be involved, if the patient leans forward.

5. Predisposing factors for aspiration include the extremes of age, swallowing disorders, neuromuscular dysfunction, broncho-oesophageal fistula, alcoholism, and head and neck cancer.

Pearls

- Barium aspiration is a known complication of upper gastrointestinal barium swallow/meal.
- The basal segments of the lower lobes are commonly involved when aspiration occurs with the person in the erect position. The middle lobe might be involved, if the person leans forward, and the posterior segments of the upper lobes or superior segments of the lower lobes are involved in the recumbent position.
- Usually no lung damage ensues following barium aspiration. On the other hand, aspiration of undiluted Gastrografin, because of its hyperosmolarity, can result in acute pulmonary edema, chemical pneumonitis, respiratory failure and death.

Suggested Readings

Tamm I, Kortsik C. Severe barium sulfate aspiration into the lung: clinical presentation, prognosis and therapy. *Respiration.* 1999;66(1):81-84.

Voloudaki A, Ergazakis N, Gourtsoyiannis N. Late changes in barium sulfate aspiration: HRCT features. *Eur Radiol.* September 2003;13(9):2226-2229.

Wani B, Yeola M. Aspiration of barium sulphate in swallow study. *Internet Journal of Pulmonary Medicine.* 2008;10(2). https://ispub.com/IJPM/10/2/9355

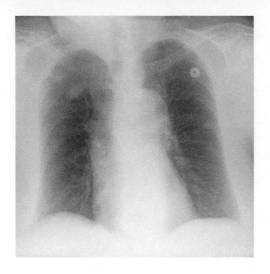 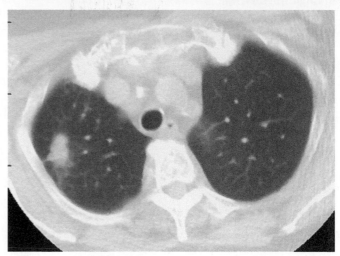

1. What are the findings?

2. What is the next step?

3. If a chest radiograph from 2 years ago was normal, what should be the next step?

4. Based on imaging, what is the most likely diagnosis?

5. What factors would favor malignancy?

Case ranking/difficulty:

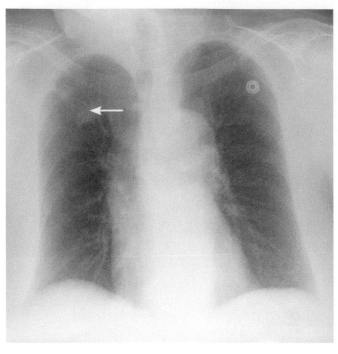

The anteroposterior radiograph shows a right upper lobe nodular opacity (*arrow*).

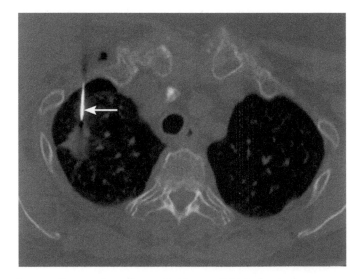

Image of a transthoracic needle biopsy of the lesion is shown, demonstrating the biopsy needle (*arrow*).

Answers

1. There is an irregular, solid, peripheral right upper lobe nodule.

2. Correlation with previous chest imaging should be the next step.

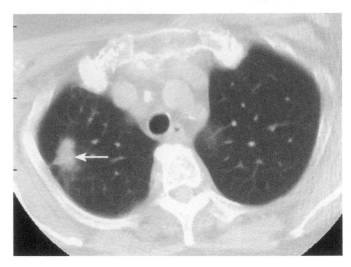

CT chest confirms a right upper lobe irregular nodule (*arrow*).

3. A newly developed lung nodule requires further investigation. PET-CT, transthoracic or transbronchial biopsy and short-term radiological follow-up are all valid options.

4. A peripheral nodule with irregular borders is most suspicious of a nonsmall cell lung cancer.

5. Cigarette smoking, exposure to asbestos and carcinogens such as uranium are among lung cancer risk factors.

Pearls

- The four major cell types of lung cancer are adenocarcinoma, squamous cell carcinoma, undifferentiated large cell carcinoma, and small cell carcinoma.
- Adenocarcinoma is the most common histological type of nonsmall cell lung cancer.
- Adenocarcinoma is the most common cell type seen in women and nonsmokers.
- Pulmonary adenocarcinoma typically presents as a peripheral nodule or mass.

Suggested Reading

Rosado-de-Christenson ML, Templeton PA, Moran CA. Bronchogenic carcinoma: radiologic-pathologic correlation. *Radiographics*. March 1994;14(2):429-446; quiz 447-8.

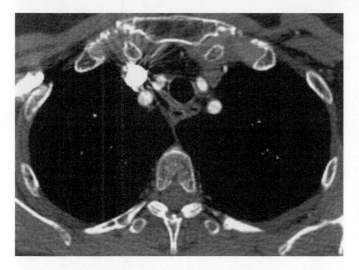 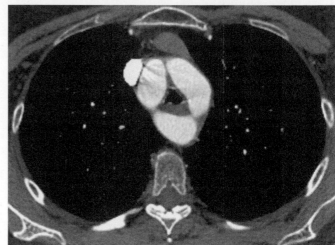

1. What is abnormal on the first CT image?

2. What is the abnormality on the second CT image?

3. What is the most common clinical presentation of this abnormality?

4. What is the branching pattern of the double aortic arch?

5. What is the most common vascular ring resulting in symptoms?

Case ranking/difficulty:

Category: Mediastinum

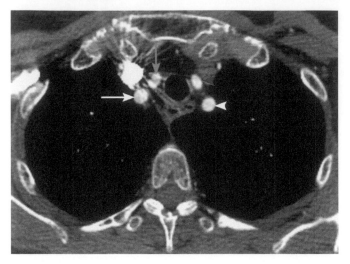

Axial CT image at the level of upper mediastinum demonstrates the "four vessel" sign: right subclavian (*white arrow*), right common carotid (*green arrow*), left common carotid (*red arrowhead*), and left subclavian (*white arrowhead*) arteries are seen on the same slice.

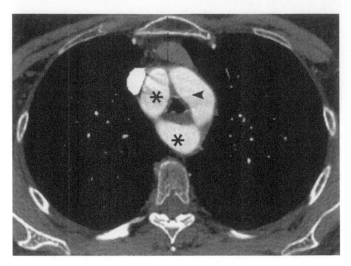

A CT image at a lower level shows that there are left (*arrowhead*) and right (*asterisks*) aortic arches.

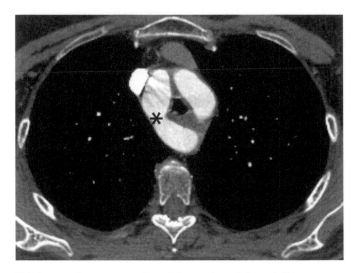

This image shows a complete right aortic arch (*asterisk*).

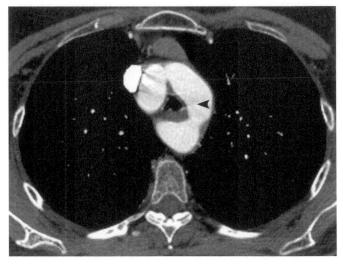

There is a complete left aortic arch (*arrowhead*), communicating both anteriorly and posteriorly with the right aortic arch.

Answers

1. The abnormality is the unusual configuration of the aortic arch vessels: there are four separate arteries arising from the aortic arch—"four vessel" sign.

2. The second image clearly shows two aortic arches, that is, a double aortic arch.

3. Possible symptoms related to a double aortic arch include stridor, dysphagia, and recurrent respiratory infections.

4. With a double aortic arch, the subclavian and carotid arteries arise from their respective arches, resulting in the "four vessel" sign on cross-sectional imaging.

5. Although right aortic arch with aberrant left subclavian artery and left ductus is the most common vascular ring, the most common symptomatic vascular ring is double aortic arch.

Pearls

- The most common vascular ring is right aortic arch with aberrant left subclavian artery, whereas the double aortic arch is the most common symptomatic vascular ring.
- Classical finding on cross-sectional imaging of the double aortic arch in the upper mediastinum is the "four vessel" sign.
- Symptomatic patients with double aortic arch present in early life with stridor and dysphagia.

Suggested Readings

Türkvatan A, Büyükbayraktar FG, Olçer T, Cumhur T. Congenital anomalies of the aortic arch: evaluation with the use of multidetector computed tomography. *Korean J Radiol*. July 2009;10(2):176-184.

Weinberg P. Aortic arch anomalies. *J Cardiovasc Magn Reson*. 2006;8(4):633-643.

Incidental chest radiograph finding in patient with previous history of long-standing peripherally inserted central catheters

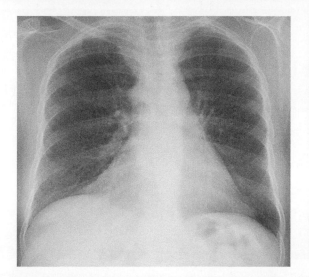
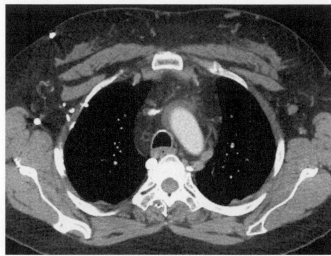
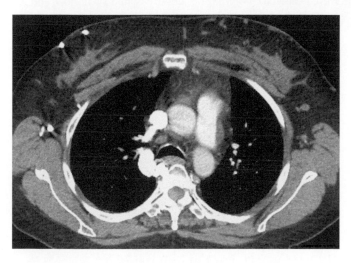
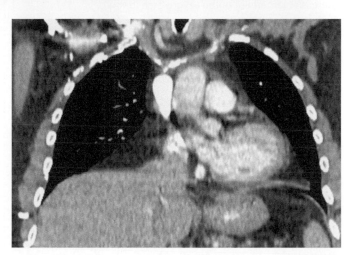

1. What is the major chest radiograph abnormality?

2. What vessel is abnormal?

3. What is the normal size of the azygos arch on a frontal chest radiograph?

4. What is the differential diagnosis of an enlarged azygos vein?

5. What is the diagnosis based on the CT findings?

Case ranking/difficulty: 🐾

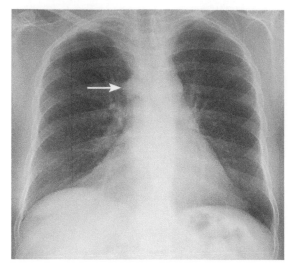

There is enlargement of the azygos arch (*arrow*).

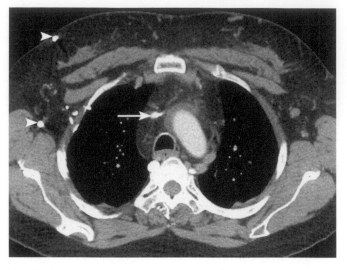

The CT shows a chronically occluded, calcified SVC (*arrow*) and multiple chest wall collateral vessels (*arrowheads*).

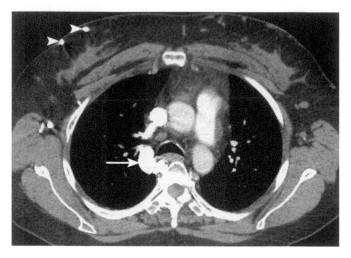

There is enlargement of the azygos vein (*arrow*). There are multiple chest wall collateral vessels (*arrowheads*).

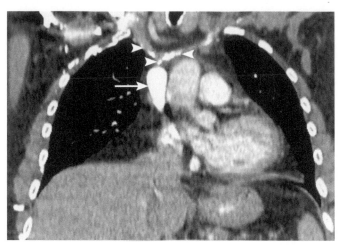

Coronal reformation shows enlarged azygos vein (*arrow*) and chronically occluded and calcified right and left brachiocephalic veins and proximal SVC (*arrowheads*).

Answers

1. The major radiographic abnormality is a focal bulge of the right mediastinal contour at the level of the right tracheobronchial angle.

2. The mediastinal contour abnormality is due to an enlarged azygos arch.

3. The transverse diameter of the azygos arch is normally <10 mm in the upright position and <15 mm in the supine position.

4. The differential diagnosis of an enlarged azygos vein includes: technical causes (supine position), obstructive causes (venous obstruction of SVC, IVC or other systemic veins), congestive causes (right heart strain/failure, tricuspid valve disease, pericardial tamponade, constrictive pericarditis or restrictive cardiomyopathy), increased cardiac output (pregnancy, fever or thyrotoxicosis), congenital causes (azygos continuation of an interrupted IVC or anomalous pulmonary venous return to azygos vein), and portal hypertension.

5. The CT images demonstrate chronic occlusion and calcifications of both brachiocephalic veins and proximal SVC, presumably secondary to long-standing use of indwelling central lines.

Pearls

- On frontal chest radiograph, the azygos venous arch appears as a knob at the right tracheobronchial angle.
- Azygos arch should be <10 mm on CXR in the upright position and <15 mm in supine position.
- The differential diagnosis of an enlarged azygos vein includes: technical causes (supine position), obstructive causes (venous obstruction of SVC, IVC or other systemic veins), congestive causes (right heart strain/failure, tricuspid valve disease, pericardial tamponade, constrictive pericarditis or restrictive cardiomyopathy), increased cardiac output (pregnancy, fever or thyrotoxicosis), congenital causes (azygos continuation of an interrupted IVC or anomalous pulmonary venous return to azygos vein), and portal hypertension.

Suggested Readings

Demos TC, Posniak HV, Pierce KL, Olson MC, Muscato M. Venous anomalies of the thorax. *AJR Am J Roentgenol.* May 2004;182(5):1139-1150.

Kapur S, Paik E, Rezaei A, Vu DN. Where there is blood, there is a way: unusual collateral vessels in superior and inferior vena cava obstruction. *Radiographics.* January 2010;30(1):67-78.

Follow-up in patient with treated lung cancer

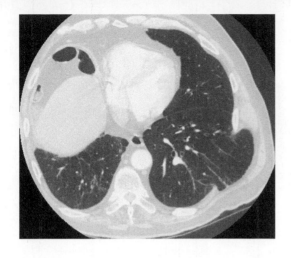 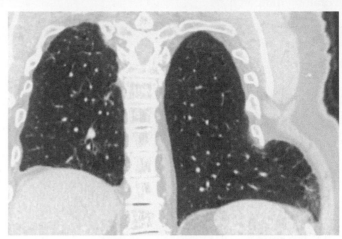

1. What is the finding?

2. What are the recognized types of this entity?

3. What type of this abnormality is the most common?

4. What are possible etiologies of this abnormality?

5. What are possible complications related to this entity?

Case ranking/difficulty: 🌑

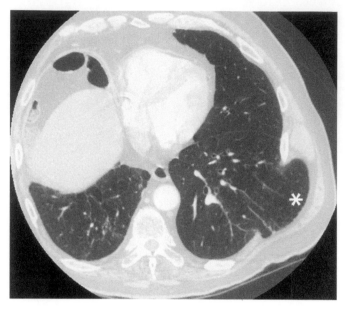

Axial CT image at the level of lung bases shows a focal protrusion of the posterolateral left lower lobe parenchyma between posterolateral ribs, outside the confines of the rib cage (*asterisk*).

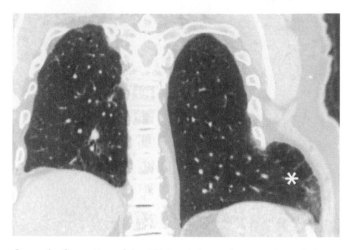

Coronal reformation of the CT chest shows the extrathoracic lung protrusion (*asterisk*) at the left lung base.

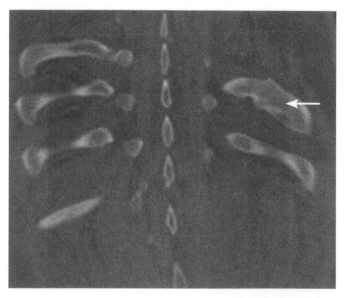

Coronal reformation CT in bone window shows an old fracture of a left posterior rib (*arrow*).

Answers

1. There is a left lateral intercostal lung hernia.

2. The lung hernias are classified as cervical, intercostal, and diaphragmatic.

3. Intercostal type of lung hernia is the most common.

4. Lung hernia can be congenital. Acquired lung hernias can be secondary to chest wall trauma, thoracic surgery, secondary to tuberculous empyema or empyema necessitans, or result from abnormally high intrathoracic pressures in certain occupations such as weightlifting or playing a wind instrument.

5. Lung hernia may undergo incarceration and strangulation, with resultant hemoptysis and pain at the site of the herniation.

Pearls

- Lung hernias are classified as cervical, intercostal, and diaphragmatic.
- Intercostal hernias are the most common type of lung hernias and are usually iatrogenic, posttraumatic or secondary to inflammation.
- Spontaneous lung hernias are associated with increased intrathoracic pressures related to certain occupations, such as weightlifting or playing a wind instrument.

Suggested Reading

Bhalla M, Leitman BS, Forcade C, Stern E, Naidich DP, McCauley DI. Lung hernia: radiographic features. *AJR Am J Roentgenol*. January 1990;154(1):51-53.

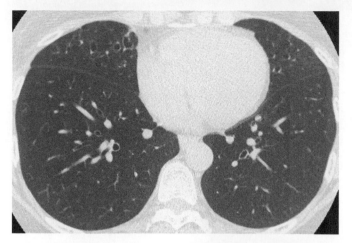 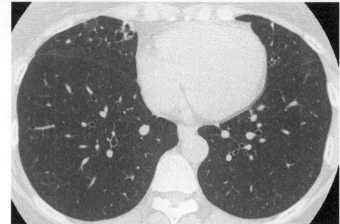

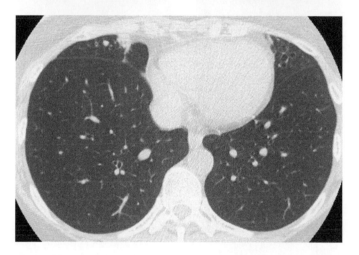

1. What are the findings?

2. What are the recognized morphologic types of bronchiectasis?

3. What are the recognized etiologies of bronchiectasis?

4. What eponym is used for indolent pulmonary infection resulting in bronchiectasis and nodules in middle-aged and elderly women?

5. Who is the author of the Lady Windermere character?

Case ranking/difficulty:

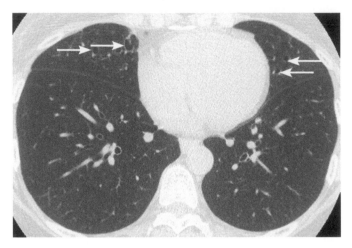

There is bronchiectasis in the right middle lobe and lingula (*arrows*).

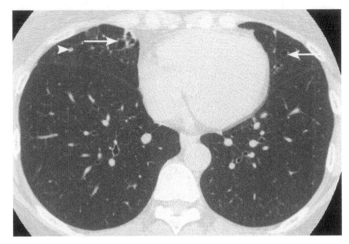

In addition to bronchiectasis (*arrows*), there is a right middle lobe nodule (*arrowhead*).

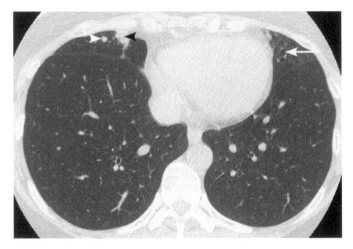

There is lingular bronchiectasis (*arrow*), a right middle lobe nodule (*white arrowhead*), and subsegmental atelectasis (*black arrowhead*).

Answers

1. The CT findings include right middle lobe (RML) and lingula bronchiectasis, several RML centrilobular nodules, and RML subsegmental atelectasis.

2. The morphological types of bronchiectasis are: cylindrical—dilated bronchi have a uniform caliber and parallel walls, varicose—beaded appearance, dilated bronchi with sites of relative narrowing, and cystic—cyst-like bronchi that extend to the pleural surface.

3. Bronchiectasis can be secondary to an infection (bacterial pneumonia, tuberculosis, *Mycobacterium avium* complex), allergic bronchopulmonary aspergillosis, cystic fibrosis, Kartagener syndrome, Williams-Campbell syndrome, Mounier-Kuhn

syndrome, bronchial obstruction, and fibrosis (ie, traction bronchiectasis).

4. The *Mycobacterium avium complex* (MAC) infection resulting in bronchiectasis, subsegmental atelectasis, and bronchiolocentric nodules, preferentially involving the RML and lingula, in middle-aged and elderly women is referred to as Lady Windermere syndrome.

5. "Lady Windermere's Fan, A Play About a Good Woman" is a four-act comedy by Oscar Wilde, 19th-century Irish author, which satirizes the morals of Victorian society.

   It was hypothesized that since Victorian females did not cough, they would collect the sputum and therefore be predisposed to getting pneumonia (or MAC).

Pearls

- *Mycobacterium avium* and *Mycobacterium intracellulare* are collectively referred to as *Mycobacterium avium* complex (MAC). They are nontuberculous mycobacteria, ubiquitously present in water.
- Infection with MAC occurs probably via aerosolized contaminated water.
- Symptoms of MAC infection are usually mild.
- There are two recognized subtypes of the disease in immunocompetent hosts: upper lobe cavitary disease, seen in males with chronic obstructive pulmonary disease, and nodular bronchiectatic disease seen in older females. The latter usually involves the right middle lobe and lingua, and is referred to as Lady Windermere syndrome.

- Disseminated MAC disease may occur in immunocompromised patients, and present as diffuse pulmonary opacities and lymphadenopathy.
- MAC may also cause hypersensitivity pneumonitis, referred to as "hot tub lung."

Suggested Readings

Field SK, Fisher D, Cowie RL. Mycobacterium avium complex pulmonary disease in patients without HIV infection. *Chest*. August 2004;126(2):566-581.

Levin DL. Radiology of pulmonary Mycobacterium avium-intracellulare complex. *Clin Chest Med*. September 2002;23(3):603-612.

Song JW, Koh WJ, Lee KS, et al. High-resolution CT findings of Mycobacterium avium-intracellulare complex pulmonary disease: correlation with pulmonary function test results. *AJR Am J Roentgenol*. October 2008;191(4):1070.

Post pacemaker insertion

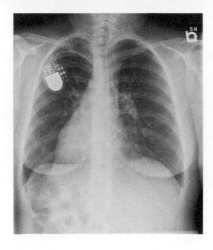 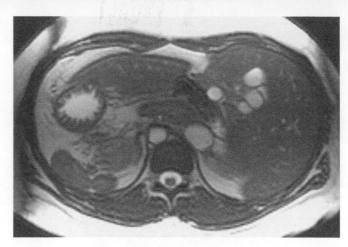

1. What structures are not in their normal anatomical position?

2. What are the recognized types of anatomical situs?

3. What thoracic structures will determine the situs?

4. What defines the anatomical right lung?

5. What syndrome is associated with bilateral trilobed lungs and bilateral eparterial bronchial position?

Case ranking/difficulty:

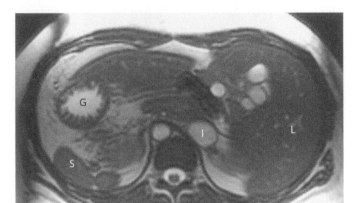

The MRI image of the upper abdomen shows that the spleen (S) and the gastric body (G) are located on the right, while the liver (L) and the IVC (I) are located on the left.

The cardiac apex (C), the aortic arch (*arrowhead*), and the gastric bubble (*asterisk*) are located on the right. The tip of atrial lead of the right transvenous dual-lead pacemaker is in the left-sided anatomical right atrial appendage (*arrow*).

Answers

1. The chest radiograph shows right-sided cardiac apex, aortic arch and gastric bubble, and left-sided right atrial appendage (confirmed by position of the tip of the pacemaker atrial lead). The MRI shows right-sided spleen and stomach, and left-sided liver and IVC.

2. The terms used to describe the anatomical situs are solitus, inversus, and ambiguous.

3. The cardiac atria are used to determine the situs.

4. The following define the anatomical right lung: three lobes, early origin of the upper lobe bronchus from the main stem bronchus, and eparterial bronchial position (the pulmonary artery lies in front of the main bronchus).

5. Bilateral trilobed lung and bilateral eparterial bronchial position is associated with asplenia syndrome, also known as Ivemark syndrome.

Pearls

- Situs inversus totalis results in mirror image of normal anatomical arrangement: right atrium, liver and trilobed lung on the left, and left atrium, spleen, stomach, and bilobed lung on the right.
- When situs inversus is detected, Kartagener and polysplenia/asplenia syndromes should be considered.
- Recognition of situs inversus is important for preventing surgical mishaps and for awareness of reversed anatomy and resulting atypical pathological presentations (eg, appendicitis with left lower quadrant abdominal pain, cholecystitis with left upper quadrant abdominal pain).

Suggested Readings

Lapierre C, Déry J, Guérin R, Viremouneix L, Dubois J, Garel L. Segmental approach to imaging of congenital heart disease. *Radiographics*. March 2010;30(2):397-411.

Maldjian PD, Saric M. Approach to dextrocardia in adults: review. *AJR Am J Roentgenol*. June 2007;188(6 suppl): S39-S49; quiz S35-8.

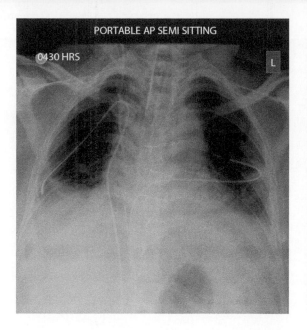
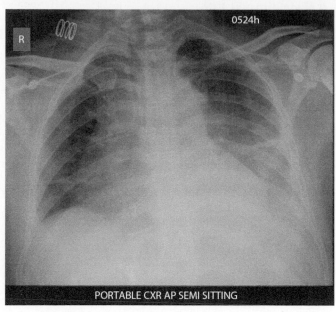

1. What is the major radiographic abnormality Left figure on the first postoperative day and right figure on the tenth postoperative day?

2. What is the main diagnosis?

3. List all the possible radiographic findings seen with the presented entity?

4. What should you consider, if the presented entity occurs after the second postoperative week?

5. What is the typical time span between recognizing the presented entity on imaging and identifying it clinically?

Case ranking/difficulty:

Category: Chest wall/Extrapleural

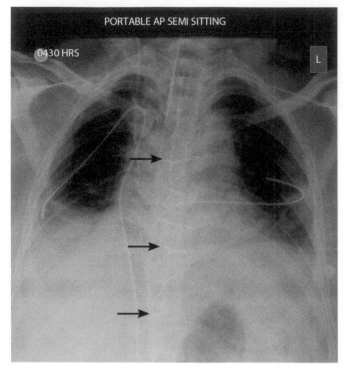

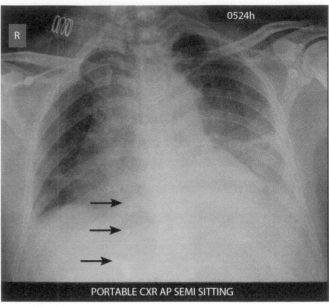

The radiograph on the tenth postoperative day shows interval displacement and malalignment of the lower sternal wires (*arrows*).

The radiograph on the first postoperative day demonstrates intact and well-aligned median sternotomy wires (*arrows*). Additionally, there are support equipment and a right pleural effusion.

Answers

1. The radiographs show progressive interval displacement and malalignment of the lower sternal wires (*arrows*).

2. The main diagnosis is that of sternal dehiscence.

3. Progressive postoperative displacement, rotation, and fracture of the sternal wires on serial chest radiography are all reliable signs of sternal dehiscence. A sternal defect lucent strip of a width that exceeds 3 mm is another sign, rarely seen on radiography.

4. If sternal dehiscence occurs after the second postoperative week, sternal osteomyelitis and/or mediastinitis should be considered.

5. Sternal dehiscence is typically identified on radiography about 3 days before it is recognized clinically.

Pearls

- Assessment of the integrity and alignment of the sternal wires is crucial in the postoperative period.
- Progressive sternal wire displacement, rotation, or fracture on chest radiographs is indicative of dehiscence.
- Sternal dehiscence may be associated with sternal or mediastinal infections.
- Radiologically, sternal dehiscence can be detected 3 days before it is recognized clinically.

Suggested Readings

Molina JE, Lew RS, Hyland KJ. Postoperative sternal dehiscence in obese patients: incidence and prevention. *Ann Thorac Surg*. September 2004;78(3):912-917; discussion 912-917.

Restrepo CS, Martinez S, Lemos DF, et al. Imaging appearances of the sternum and sternoclavicular joints. *Radiographics*. May-June 2009;29(3):839-859.

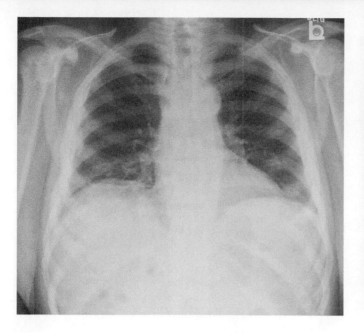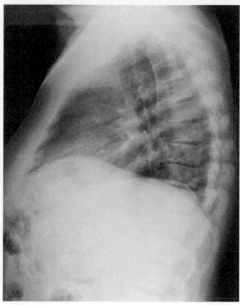

1. What are the radiographic abnormalities?

2. What should be included in the differential diagnosis of a bone scintigraphy superscan?

3. What three primary cancers account for 80% of cases of bone metastases?

4. What is the differential diagnosis of diffusely sclerotic bones?

5. What primary malignancies give rise to sclerotic bone metastases?

Case ranking/difficulty:

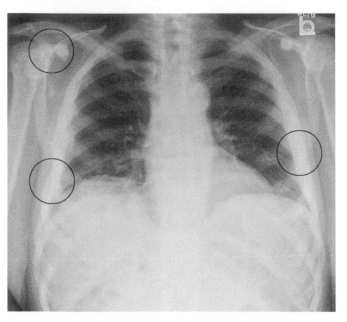

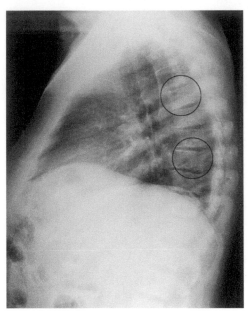

There are diffuse sclerotic bone lesions involving all the ribs, the entire spine, coracoid processes, and proximal humeri (*circles outline some of the lesions*).

Lateral chest radiograph shows diffusely sclerotic vertebrae and ribs (*circles outline some of the lesions*).

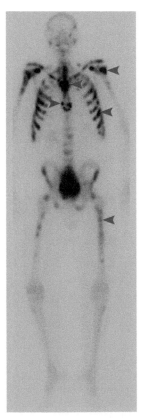

Bone scan in anterior projection confirms innumerable foci of increased activity throughout the axial skeleton and bilateral upper and lower proximal appendicular skeleton (*arrowheads*).

Answers

1. There are diffuse sclerotic lesions involving bilateral ribs, humeri, dorsal vertebrae, and coracoid processes.

2. A superscan refers to intense symmetric activity in the bones with diminished renal and soft tissue activity on a Tc99m diphosphonate bone scan. The differential diagnosis of superscan includes diffuse metastatic disease (particularly from prostate, breast, and transitional cell carcinoma), multiple myeloma, lymphoma, renal osteodystrophy, hyperparathyroidism, osteomalacia, myelofibrosis, mastocytosis, and Paget disease.

3. Lung, breast, and renal cell carcinomas account for 80% of cases of metastatic disease to the bone.

4. The differential diagnosis of diffusely sclerotic bones includes osteoblastic metastases, renal osteodystrophy, lymphoma, leukemia, myelofibrosis, mastocytosis, Paget disease, hyperthyroidism, hypoparathyroidism, osteopetrosis, pyknodysostosis, fluorosis, and hypervitaminosis D.

5. The cancers giving rise to sclerotic bone metastases include prostate carcinoma (most common), breast carcinoma (may be mixed), transitional cell carcinoma, carcinoid, medulloblastoma, neuroblastoma, mucinous adenocarcinoma of the gastrointestinal tract, and lymphoma.

Pearls

- Prostate cancer is the most common cause of diffuse sclerotic bone metastases.
- Patients with a prostate-specific antigen (PSA) >20 ng/mL have a high likelihood of bone metastases.
- The differential diagnosis of diffusely sclerotic bones includes osteoblastic metastases, renal osteodystrophy, lymphoma, leukemia, myelofibrosis, mastocytosis, Paget disease, hyperthyroidism, hypoparathyroidism, osteopetrosis, pyknodysostosis, fluorosis, and hypervitaminosis D.

Suggested Reading

Kundra V, Silverman PM, Matin SF, Choi H. Imaging in oncology from the University of Texas M.D. Anderson Cancer Center: diagnosis, staging, and surveillance of prostate cancer. *AJR Am J Roentgenol*. October 2007;189(4):830-844.

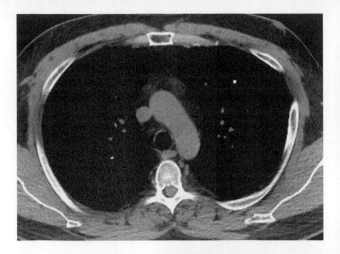
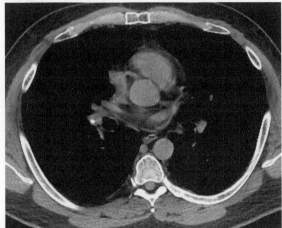
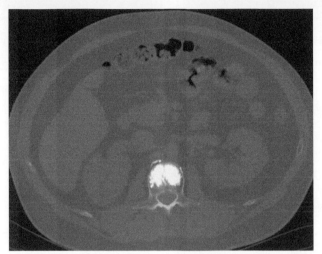

1. What are the findings?

2. What is the differential diagnosis of spontaneously hyperdense linear and branching densities in the lungs?

3. Which material will appear the densest on CT: calcium, barium, polymethyl methacrylate, talc, mercury?

4. What are indications for percutaneous vertebroplasty?

5. What are complications of percutaneous vertebroplasty?

Case ranking/difficulty:

Category: Lungs

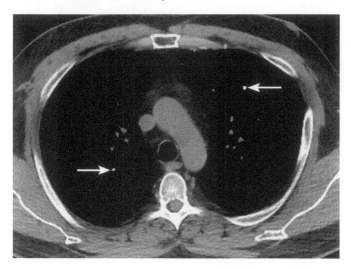

There are bilateral punctate hyperdensities (*arrows*).

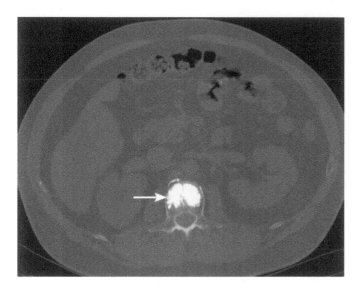

CT in bone window shows lumbar vertebroplasty (*arrow*).

Answers

1. There are bilateral pulmonary hyperdensities, one of which clearly localizes to the right interlobar pulmonary artery. The patient is also status post lumbar vertebroplasty.

2. The differential diagnosis of spontaneously hyperdense linear and branching pulmonary densities includes aspirated barium, bronchioliths, polymethyl methacrylate pulmonary emboli, and embolized IV injected mercury.

3. Barium and mercury will be denser than calcium, polymethyl methacrylate, and talc.

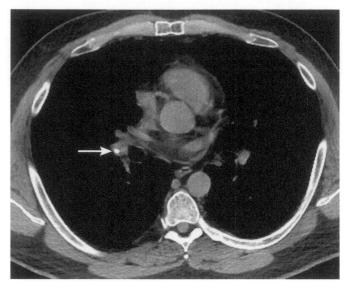

One hyperdensity clearly localizes to the right interlobar pulmonary artery (*arrow*).

4. Possible indications for vertebroplasty are painful osteoporotic fractures, vertebral destruction caused by hemangiomas, pathological fractures caused by tumors, and burst fractures. Unstable fractures are not an indication for vertebroplasty.

5. Complications of vertebroplasty include refractures of the stabilized vertebrae, fractures of neighboring vertebrae, persisting pain, compression of nerve roots due to cement leakage, and pulmonary cement embolisms.

Pearls

- Pulmonary cement embolism (PCE) is a known complication of percutaneous vertebroplasty.
- The true incidence of PCE is unknown; the reported incidence ranges between 4.6% and 26%.
- Most cases of PCE are asymptomatic.
- No clear treatment strategies exist for PCE.
- Linear and branching pulmonary hyperdensities are the typical radiographic findings of PCE.

Suggested Reading

Krueger A, Bliemel C, Zettl R, Ruchholtz S. Management of pulmonary cement embolism after percutaneous vertebroplasty and kyphoplasty: a systematic review of the literature. *Eur Spine J*. September 2009;18(9):1257-1265.

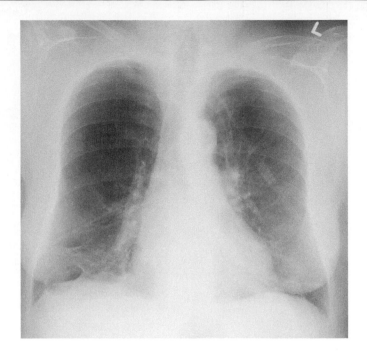

1. What is the main finding?

2. What should be the next step?

3. If the nodule is new, what should be the next step?

4. What should be included in the differential diagnosis of a solitary well-defined pulmonary nodule on radiography?

5. What can simulate a pulmonary nodule on chest radiography?

Case ranking/difficulty:

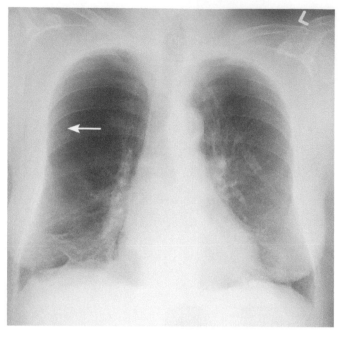

Frontal chest radiograph demonstrates a well-defined right upper lung zone nodule (*arrow*), as well as findings of emphysema, right lung base scarring, and mild cardiomegaly.

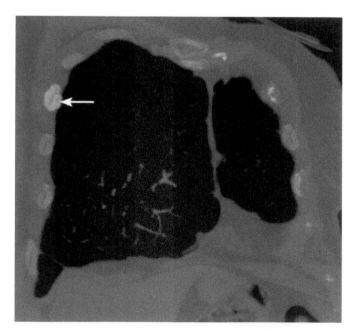

Coronal reformation in bone window again shows callous formation around a right anterior rib fracture (*arrow*).

Answers

1. The chest radiograph demonstrates a well-defined, dense right upper lung zone nodule. There are also findings of emphysema and nonspecific bibasilar opacities.

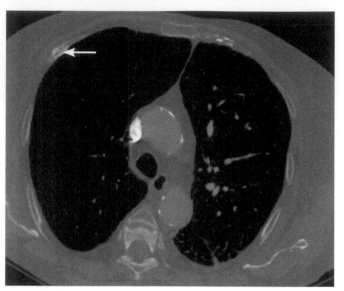

CT in bone window shows that the nodule seen on the radiograph corresponds to callous formation around a right anterior rib fracture (*arrow*).

2. Comparison to previous chest radiographs should be the next step in evaluation of the nodule.

3. If the nodule is new, CT chest without contrast would be the most appropriate next step.

4. Granuloma, hamartoma, solitary metastasis, lung carcinoma, carcinoid, and arteriovenous malformation are all part of the differential diagnosis of a solitary pulmonary nodule.

5. Nipple, electrocardiographic electrode, skin lesion, healing rib fracture, and bone island can all simulate a pulmonary nodule on chest radiography.

Pearls

- Given the two-dimensional nature of chest radiographs, findings outside the lung parenchyma may simulate pulmonary lesions. In certain cases, correlation with a lateral radiograph can determine the extraparenchymal nature of the abnormality.
- Correlation with prior imaging is a sine qua non of a good radiological practice, as demonstration of long-term stability of a suspected lesion might obviate the need for further investigations.
- Nipples, electrocardiographic electrodes, skin lesions (eg, moles, calcified sebaceous cysts, scars), healing rib fractures, and bone islands commonly simulate pulmonary nodules on chest radiography.

- When a rib fracture cannot be reliably differentiated from a pulmonary nodule on a chest radiograph, dedicated oblique radiographs of the ribs can be obtained.
- If nipple shadow needs to be excluded as the reason of the apparent nodule, chest radiographs with nipple markers should be obtained.

Suggested Reading

Guttentag AR, Salwen JK. Keep your eyes on the ribs: the spectrum of normal variants and diseases that involve the ribs. *Radiographics*. September-October 1999;19(5):1125-1142.

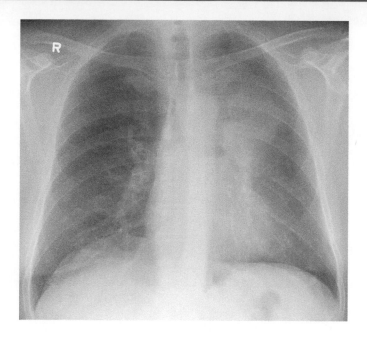

1. What are the radiographic findings?

2. What is the diagnosis?

3. What is the "veil sign?"

4. What is the "Luftsichel sign?"

5. In an adult with persistent lobar collapse on chest radiographs, what would be your recommendations?

Case ranking/difficulty: 🐾

Category: Lungs

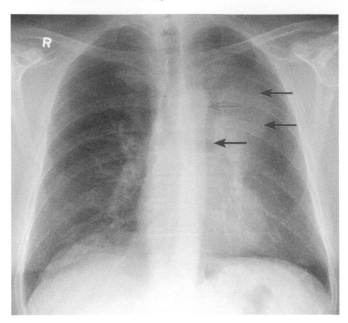

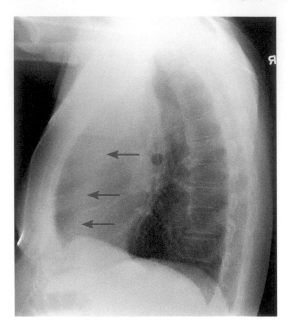

A homogenous opacity projects over the left paramediastinal border and is well defined laterally by a displaced major fissure (*red arrows*). In addition, the left hemithorax shows diffuse vague opacification (*the veil sign*). There is associated leftward cardiomediastinal shift and upward displacement of the left hilum, features supporting left upper lobe collapse. Note that the aortic arch is exceedingly well defined, representing a "Luftsichel sign" (*green arrow*). Also note the abrupt termination of the left main bronchial air column (*blue arrow*), which raises the possibility of an endobronchial obstructive lesion.

The collapsed left upper lobe appears on this lateral radiograph as a homogenous retrosternal band-like opacity, which is well defined by the anteriorly displaced left major fissure (*arrows*).

Answers

1. The radiographs show a homogenous opacity that projects over the left paramediastinal border and is well defined laterally by a displaced major fissure. The left hemithorax shows diffuse vague opacification overall. Despite of that, the aortic arch is very well defined. There is associated leftward cardiomediastinal shift and upward displacement of the left hilum. Additionally, there is abrupt termination of the left main bronchus air column.

2. The diagnosis is that of left upper lobe (LUL) collapse.

3. The "veil sign" describes the left hemithoracic hazy opacification and associated partial ill definition of the left cardiomediastinal border that occur with LUL collapse. This is a result of anterior and medial displacement of the collapsed LUL toward the mediastinum.

4. The "Luftsichel sign" describes paradoxical well definition of the aortic arch in the face of LUL collapse, due to insinuation of a hyperinflated left lower lobar superior segment between the collapsed lobe and aortic arch. "Luftsichel" means "air crescent" in German.

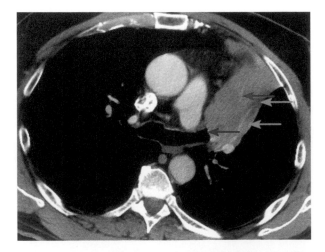

There is total collapse of the left upper lobe (*red arrow*), with leftward cardiomediastinal shift and anterior displacement of the left major fissure (*green arrows*). Note the abrupt termination of the left upper lobe bronchus (*blue arrow*), where an obstructive endobronchial squamous cell carcinoma was confirmed during surgery.

5. An adult with persistent lobar collapse on chest radiography should be further evaluated with CT, since intrinsic or extrinsic neoplastic bronchial occlusion is the major concern. If no obvious culprit lesion is seen, bronchoscopy would be the next step, since neoplasms can be obscured or missed on CT in the presence of adjacent lobar collapse.

Pearls

- Active search for possible lobar collapse should be part of the routine interpretation of chest radiographs.
- LUL collapse is in the differential diagnostic list of increased left hemithoracic density (ie, the "veil sign").
- Although LUL collapse is expected to obscure the aortic arch, it commonly leads to the opposite effect (ie, the "Luftsichel sign").

Suggested Readings

Ajlan AM, Belley G, Kosiuk J. "V V O I": a swift hand motion in detecting atelectasis on frontal chest radiographs. *Can Assoc Radiol J*. May 2011;62(2):146-150.

Parker MS, Chasen MH, Paul N. Radiologic signs in thoracic imaging: case-based review and self-assessment module. *AJR Am J Roentgenol*. March 2009;192(3 suppl):S34-S48.

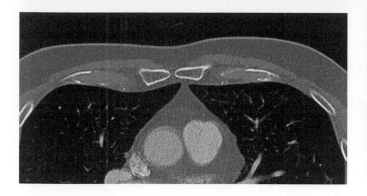 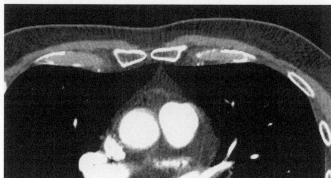

1. Describe the CT finding.

2. What is the diagnosis?

3. What abnormalities can be seen in association with a sternal cleft?

4. What is ectopia cordis?

5. What is pentalogy of Cantrell?

Case ranking/difficulty: 🌰

Category: Chest wall/Extrapleural

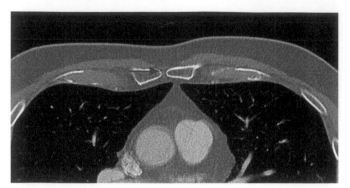

This is a magnified transverse image of the sternal body in bone window. There is a small midline defect in the sternal body (*arrow*), showing a sclerotic border and an appearance which resembles a bow tie.

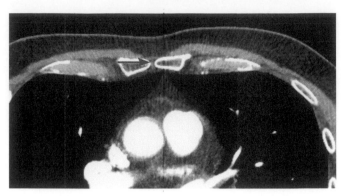

This is a magnified transverse image of the sternal body in soft tissue window. The midline defect has a fat-filled gap (*arrow*). No aggressive soft tissue components are seen.

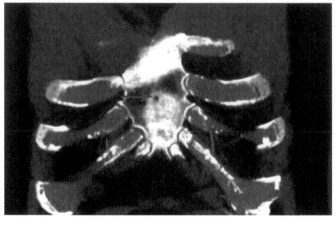

This magnified coronal image of the sternal body redemonstrates the sternal foramen (*arrow*).

Pearls

- A sternal foreman is a common finding in a busy CT chest practice.
- Sternal foramen has a classic appearance and should not be confused for sinister abnormalities.
- A sternal cleft is an uncommon finding that can be associated with other congenital abnormalities (such as ectopia cordis or pentalogy of Cantrell).

Answers

1. There is a small midline defect in the sternal body, showing a sclerotic border and an appearance which resembles a bow tie. The midline defect has a fat-filled gap and no aggressive soft tissue components.

2. Diagnosis: sternal foramen.

3. Sternal bands, ectopia cordis, and pentalogy of Cantrell may be seen in association with a sternal cleft.

4. Ectopia cordis is a very rare congenital abnormality where there is partial or complete extrathoracic location of the heart.

5. Pentalogy of Cantrell is an exceedingly rare congenital abnormality where there are defects of the abdominal wall, lower sternum, pericardium, and anterior diaphragm. This abnormality is associated with congenital heart diseases.

Suggested Readings

Morales JM, Patel SG, Duff JA, Villareal RL, Simpson JW. Ectopia cordis and other midline defects. *Ann Thorac Surg*. July 2000;70(1):111-114.

Restrepo CS, Martinez S, Lemos DF, Washington L, McAdams HP, Vargas D, Lemos JA, Carrillo JA, Diethelm L. Imaging appearances of the sternum and sternoclavicular joints. *Radiographics*. May-June 2009;29(3):839-859.

Singh N, Bera ML, Sachdev MS, Aggarwal N, Joshi R, Kohli V. Pentalogy of Cantrell with left ventricular diverticulum: a case report and review of literature. *Congenit Heart Dis*. September-October 2010;5(5):454-457.

Acute retrosternal pain

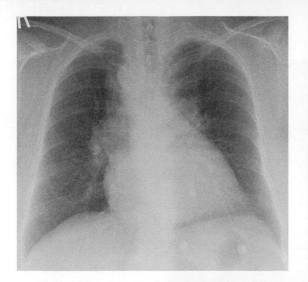
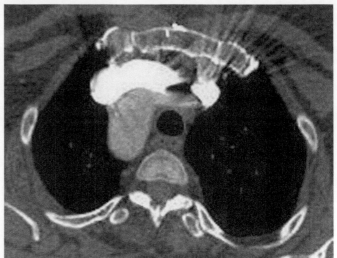
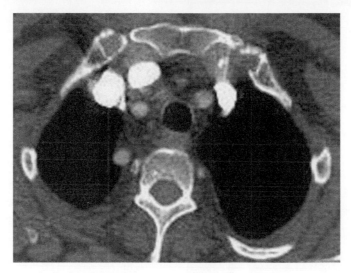

1. What are the findings?

2. What is the possible association between the right aortic arch and the presence of sternal wires in this patient?

3. What eponym describes the hypothetical double aortic arch system in developing embryo?

4. What aortic arch variant is most frequently associated with congenital heart disease?

5. What thoracic vascular abnormalities represent true vascular rings?

Case ranking/difficulty:

Category: Basic interpretation

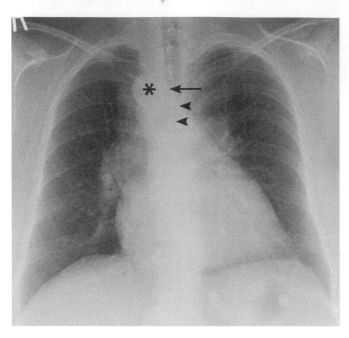

The chest radiograph shows a right aortic arch (*asterisk*), indenting the trachea on the right side (*arrow*). There are small sternal wires (*arrowheads*), in keeping with heart surgery at pediatric age.

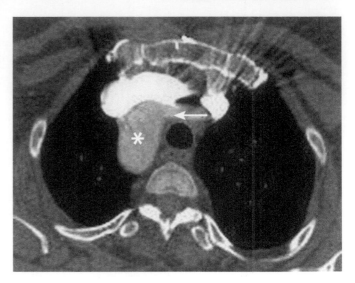

The CT confirms that the aortic arch is on the right side of the trachea (*asterisk*). The first vessel off the arch is the left brachiocephalic artery (*arrow*).

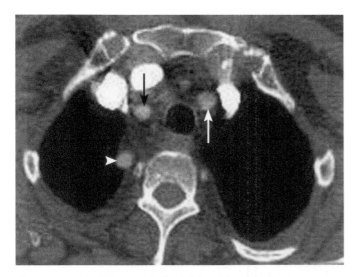

The first vessel off the arch is the left brachiocephalic artery (*white arrow*), the second branch is the right common carotid artery (*black arrow*), and the last vessel is the right subclavian artery (*arrowhead*).

Answers

1. There is a right aortic arch with mirror image branching pattern. There are small median sternotomy wires.

2. Right-sided arch is often associated with congenital heart disease (CHD) requiring surgery. The most common CHD associated with right arch is tetralogy of Fallot.

3. According to Edward's hypothetical double aortic arch system, there is an aortic arch on each side of the developing embryo; the right carotid and subclavian arteries arise from the right arch and the left carotid and subclavian arteries from the left arch. Interruption of this arch system at different locations helps to explain the various aortic arch anomalies.

4. Right aortic arch with mirror image branching pattern is the variant most frequently associated with CHD.

5. The true vascular rings include double aortic arch, pulmonary sling, and right arch with aberrant left subclavian (ie, ligamentum arteriosum between the arch at the level of the left subclavian artery and the left pulmonary artery completes the ring).

Pearls

- The two major branching patterns of the right aortic arch are right arch with aberrant left subclavian and right arch with mirror image.
- In the case of right aortic arch with aberrant left subclavian, the first vessel off the arch is the left common carotid artery. In the case of right arch with mirror image branching pattern, the first vessel off the arch is the left brachiocephalic artery.
- Right aortic arch with mirror image branching is associated with congenital heart disease, especially with tetralogy of Fallot.
- Left aortic arch with aberrant right subclavian is not a vascular ring.
- Right aortic arch with aberrant left subclavian artery, double aortic arch, and pulmonary sling are the most common types of true vascular rings.

Suggested Readings

Türkvatan A, Büyükbayraktar FG, Olçer T, Cumhur T. Congenital anomalies of the aortic arch: evaluation with the use of multidetector computed tomography. *Korean J Radiol.* Jul 2009;10(2):176-184.

Weinberg P. Aortic Arch Anomalies. *J Cardiovasc Magn Reson.* 2006;8(4):633-643.

Cough and dyspnea for several weeks

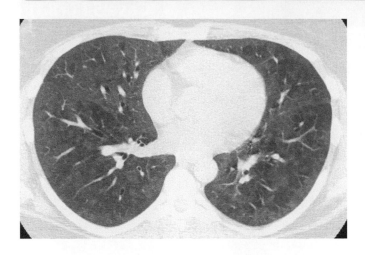 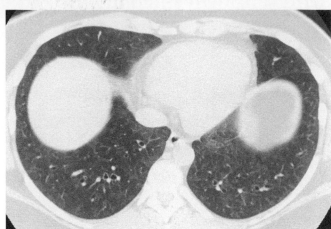

1. Describe the CT abnormalities.

2. What is this pattern called?

3. What are the major pathological categories that can lead to such an appearance?

4. What is the value of an expiratory CT scan in such a case?

5. What is the "headcheese sign?"

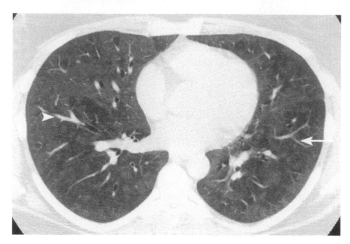

Bilateral geographic areas of hypo- and hyperattenuated lung parenchyma are seen. Note the smaller vascular caliber in the hypodense regions (*arrow*) and the larger vascular caliber in the hyperdense areas (*arrowhead*).

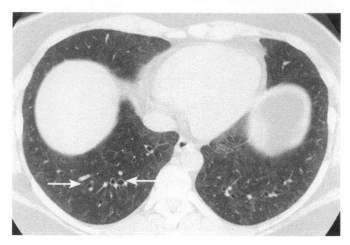

Minimal bilateral basal bronchiectasis is seen as denoted by the "signet ring sign" (*arrows*), suggesting a small airways process.

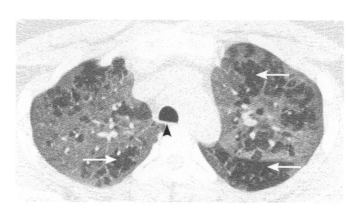

The posterior wall of the trachea is flat (*arrowhead*), denoting an expiratory image. The hypoattenuated lung regions do not change in density or volume compared to CT images performed in inspiration (*arrows*), while the hyperattenuated areas undergo volume loss–related changes. This is in keeping with air trapping, which denotes small airways abnormality.

Answers

1. The CT images show bilateral geographic areas of hypo- and hyperattenuated lung parenchyma and bilateral basal bronchiectasis. The vascular caliber is smaller in hypodense regions compared to vessels seen in hyperdense areas.

2. The pattern is that of mosaic attenuation.

3. The major pathological categories to consider when mosaic attenuation is seen are small airways disease, vascular disease, and primary parenchymal disease.

4. The value of an expiratory CT scan is in its ability to demonstrate air trapping.

5. When ground-glass opacities are superimposed on mosaic attenuation, the appearance has been termed the "headcheese sign." This appearance denotes a mixture of infiltrative and obstructive disease.

Pearls

- When mosaic attenuation (MA) pattern is seen, the next step is to determine if the vessels are smaller in the dark lung areas. If not, the MA is probably due to primary parenchymal disease. If the vessels are smaller, then the likely cause of MA is small airways or vascular disease. In the latter case, an expiratory CT scan should be obtained and if it shows air trapping, small airways disease (which is by far the most common of the three categories) is the cause of MA. If no air trapping is seen, MA is likely due to vascular disease.

- Bronchial wall thickening, bronchial dilatation, centrilobular nodules, and tree-in-bud pattern are additional clues to small airways disease as the cause of mosaic attenuation.

- Pulmonary vascular filling defects, beading, pruning, tapering, and dilatation are clues to vascular causes of mosaic attenuation.

Suggested Readings

Hansell DM. Small airways diseases: detection and insights with computed tomography. *Eur Respir J*. June 2001;17(6):1294-1313.

Stern EJ, Swensen SJ, Hartman TE, Frank MS. CT mosaic pattern of lung attenuation: distinguishing different causes. *AJR Am J Roentgenol*. October 1995;165(4): 813-816.

Worthy SA, Müller NL, Hartman TE, Swensen SJ, Padley SP, Hansell DM. Mosaic attenuation pattern on thin-section CT scans of the lung: differentiation among infiltrative lung, airway, and vascular diseases as a cause. *Radiology*. November 1997;205(2):465-470.

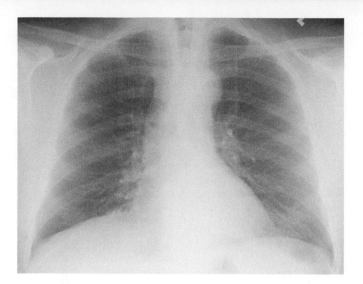

1. What is the most important imaging finding?

2. What is the differential diagnosis?

3. What are the most common primary tracheal tumors?

4. What are the risk factors for developing squamous cell carcinoma of the trachea?

5. When a primary tracheal neoplasm is seen in an adult, what is the chance of it being malignant?

Case ranking/difficulty:

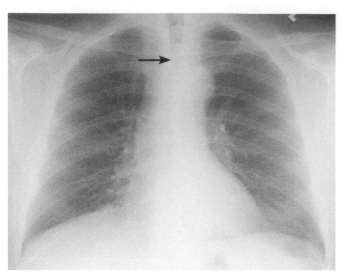

There is minimal narrowing of the tracheal air column due to a subtle right-sided irregularity just above the aortic arch level (*arrow*).

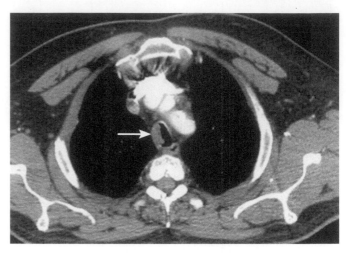

A soft tissue mural-based right-sided tracheal mass is seen (*arrow*). The mass disrupts the normal tracheal wall contour and has a minimally irregular surface. Only mild tracheal luminal narrowing is noted.

3. Primary tracheal neoplasms are generally rare, but the most common are SCC and ACC.

4. Smoking and alcoholism are known risk factors for developing tracheal SCC.

5. Ninety percent of primary tracheal neoplasms seen in adults are malignant.

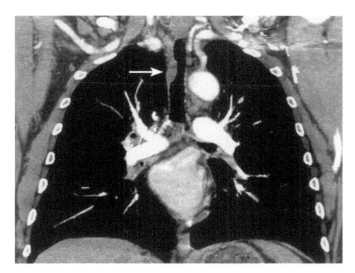

The coronal image better depicts the craniocaudal extension of the tracheal lesion and also shows an extraluminal exophytic component (*arrow*).

Pearls

- Always check the tracheal air column on frontal and lateral radiographs.
- Since SCCs are typically seen in smokers, always check for a possible associated lung cancer on the same chest CT!
- Mucus can mimic a tracheobronchial tumor, but should be differentiated on the basis of low attenuation, bubbly appearance, and dependent location. If adherent and nondependent, mucus will disappear or change in shape when CT is repeated after coughing.

Answers

1. The most important imaging finding is that of subtle right-sided tracheal irregularity just above the aortic arch level.

2. The major considerations for focal thickening of the trachea are squamous cell carcinoma (SCC) and adenoid cystic carcinoma (ACC). Metastasis is possible as well. Carcinoid, especially of the atypical type, is rare in the trachea. Mucoepidermoid carcinoma (MED) usually affects the lobar or segmental bronchi.

Suggested Readings

Marom EM, Goodman PC, McAdams HP. Diffuse abnormalities of the trachea and main bronchi. *AJR Am J Roentgenol*. March 2001;176(3):713-717.

Marom EM, Goodman PC, McAdams HP. Focal abnormalities of the trachea and main bronchi. *AJR Am J Roentgenol*. March 2001;176(3):707-711.

Park CM, Goo JM, Lee HJ, Kim MA, Lee CH, Kang MJ. Tumors in the tracheobronchial tree: CT and FDG PET features. *Radiographics*. January-February 2009;29(1): 55-71.

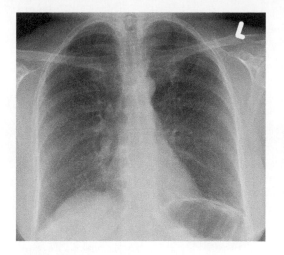
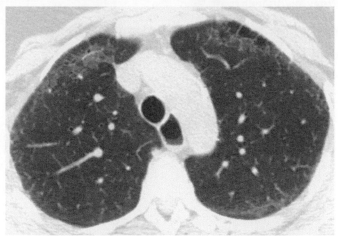
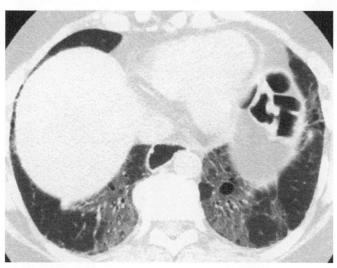
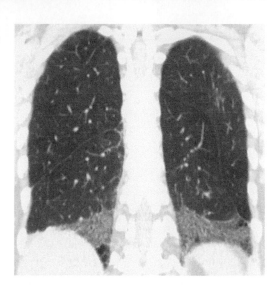

1. What are the radiographic findings?

2. What are the CT findings?

3. What is the differential diagnosis?

4. What are the recognized pathological types of this entity?

5. What are the major causes of this disease?

Case ranking/difficulty:

Category: Lungs

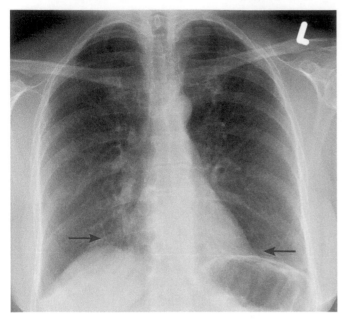

Subtle bibasilar lung reticulations are noted (*arrows*).

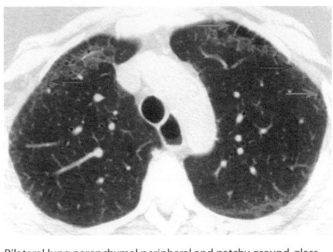

Bilateral lung parenchymal peripheral and patchy ground-glass opacities are present (*red arrows*), with minimal honeycombing (*green arrows*).

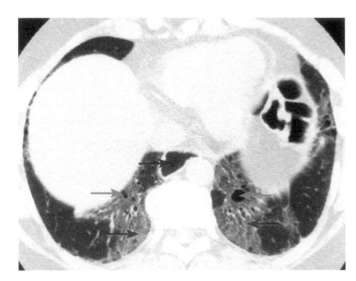

Bilateral lung parenchymal ground-glass opacities are present (*red arrows*), with associated mild traction bronchiectasis, architectural distortion, and lower lobar volume loss. A few lower lung nonpredominant scattered thin-walled cysts are seen (*green arrows*), which is a well-described but atypical feature of nonspecific interstitial pneumonia (NSIP). Note the dilated esophagus (*blue arrow*).

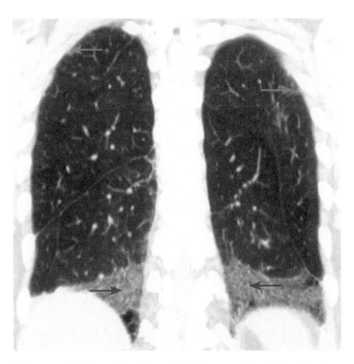

This coronal reformation shows that the upper lung is involved by minimal patchy changes (*green arrows*), while the lower lungs show severe involvement (*red arrows*).

Answers

1. There are subtle bibasilar reticulations on the radiograph.

2. The CT shows bilateral lung parenchymal patchy ground-glass opacities in the upper lung zones, with minimal honeycombing. More lung parenchymal ground-glass opacities are present at the lung bases, with mild traction bronchiectasis, architectural distortion, and lower lobar volume loss. A few lower lung scattered thin-walled cysts are seen. There is a dilated esophagus with an intraluminal air-fluid level.

3. The differential diagnosis is mainly that of nonspecific interstitial pneumonia (NSIP) versus usual interstitial pneumonia (UIP). Desquamative interstitial pneumonia (DIP) may be considered in a smoker with emphysema. Lymphoid interstitial pneumonia (LIP) could be considered in Sjögren or HIV patients.

4. *Fibrotic* and *cellular* NSIP are the recognized pathological types of this entity. A third type called *mixed* NSIP may be considered when both cellular and fibrotic patterns are present.

5. The most common cause of NSIP is collagen vascular disease. NSIP could be idiopathic, a manifestation of hypersensitivity pneumonitis or caused by a drug reaction.

Pearls

- NSIP pattern on CT should initiate the search for collagen vascular disease, hypersensitivity pneumonitis, or a drug reaction. NSIP can be designated as *idiopathic*, if such entities are excluded.
- Differentiating fibrotic NSIP from UIP might be difficult, but honeycombing, peribronchovascular involvement, subpleural sparing, craniocaudal gradient of abnormalities, and temporal progression are helpful distinguishing points.
- If consolidation predominates in what appears to be an NSIP pattern, the following should be considered: superimposed aspiration pneumonitis (note that a dilated esophagus in the context of progressive systemic sclerosis is a risk factor), superimposed pneumonia, and acute exacerbation of NSIP.

Suggested Readings

Kligerman SJ, Groshong S, Brown KK, Lynch DA. Nonspecific interstitial pneumonia: radiologic, clinical, and pathologic considerations. *Radiographics*. January-February 2009;29(1):73-87.

Mueller-Mang C, Grosse C, Schmid K, Stiebellehner L, Bankier AA. What every radiologist should know about idiopathic interstitial pneumonias. *Radiographics*. May-June 2007;27(3):595-615.

Silva CI, Müller NL. Idiopathic interstitial pneumonias. *J Thoracic Imaging*. November 2009;24(4):260-273.

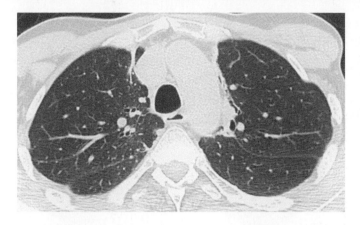
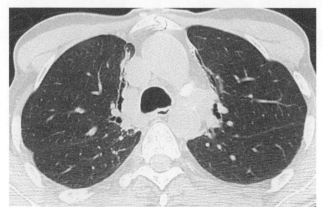
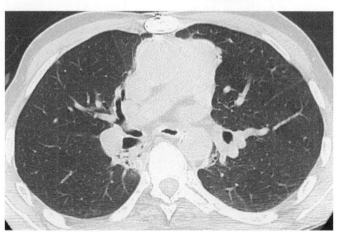
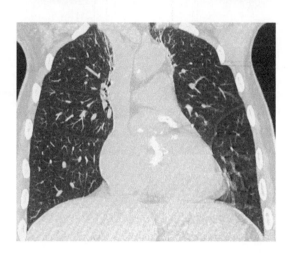

1. What are the CT findings?

2. What is the most likely diagnosis?

3. How are radiation-induced lung changes classified?

4. What is the reference point in time for dating radiation-induced lung changes?

5. How is PET useful in assessing for tumor recurrence in the context of prior radiation therapy?

Case ranking/difficulty:

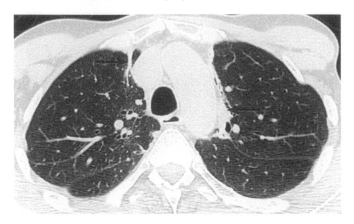

There is bilateral paramediastinal lung parenchymal architectural distortion and traction bronchiectasis (*arrows*).

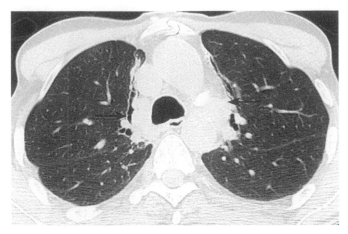

Similar bilateral paramediastinal changes and focal volume loss are seen at a lower CT slice, consistent with focal fibrosis (*arrows*).

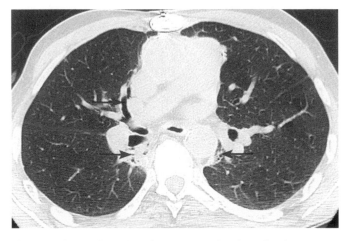

The lower lungs show sharply marginated and confined paramediastinal fibrotic lung changes (*arrows*).

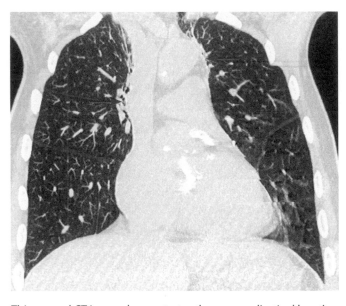

This coronal CT image demonstrates the paramediastinal location of the lung fibrosis (*arrows*), sparing the remainder of lungs.

Answers

1. Bilateral sharply marginated paramediastinal lung fibrosis is present on CT.

2. The most likely diagnosis is that of radiation-induced lung fibrosis.

3. Radiation-induced lung changes are generally divided into stages of acute *pneumonitis* and late *fibrosis*.

4. Radiation-induced lung changes should be dated from the time of completion of radiotherapy. Radiation pneumonitis occurs in the 1 to 6 months after completion of therapy, while fibrosis occurs in the following 6 to 12 months. However, radiation fibrosis may still progress 24 months after therapy completion. Radiation-induced lung changes typically stabilize after 24 months from completion of therapy.

5. Since PET has a high negative predictive value for postradiation tumoral recurrence, a normal or near-normal PET study virtually excludes a neoplastic process.

Pearls

- Radiation-induced lung changes manifest as *pneumonitis* in the early stage and *fibrosis* later on.
- Radiation-induced lung changes are confined to the radiation port, which may have complex configurations with newer ways of delivering targeted radiation.

- Pulmonary features that do not conform to the expected timeline of radiation-induced changes or that have unexpected morphology should raise the concern for neoplastic or infectious etiologies.

Suggested Readings

Choi YW, Munden RF, Erasmus JJ, et al. Effects of radiation therapy on the lung: radiologic appearances and differential diagnosis. *Radiographics*. July-August 2004;24(4):985-997; discussion 998.

Larici AR, del Ciello A, Maggi F, et al. Lung abnormalities at multimodality imaging after radiation therapy for non-small cell lung cancer. *Radiographics*. May-June 2011;31(3):771-789.

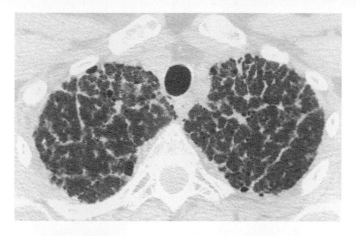
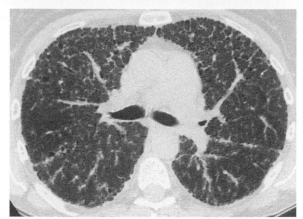
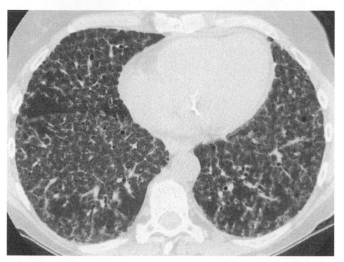
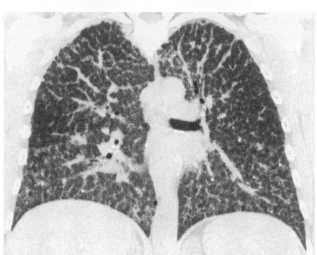

1. What are the CT findings?

2. What is the differential diagnosis based on the imaging findings?

3. What is the most common lung parenchymal imaging manifestation of sarcoidosis?

4. Describe the imaging-based staging system for pulmonary sarcoidosis.

5. Is the staging system of sarcoidosis based on radiography, CT, or MRI?

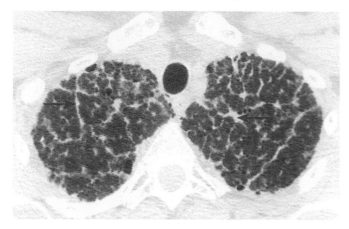

The upper lung demonstrates bilateral diffuse nodular septal thickening (*arrows*).

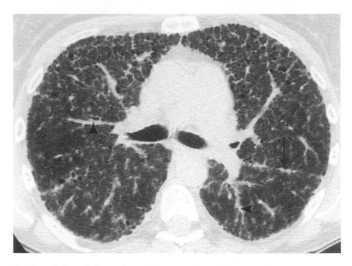

Similar diffuse bilateral midlung peribronchovascular (*arrowheads*) and fissural (*arrow*) involvement is seen.

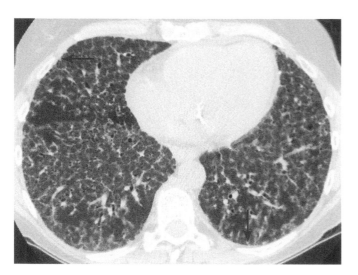

Diffuse involvement is also noted in the lower lungs, including nodularity of the subpleural regions (*arrows*). The overall appearance is consistent with a perilymphatic distribution.

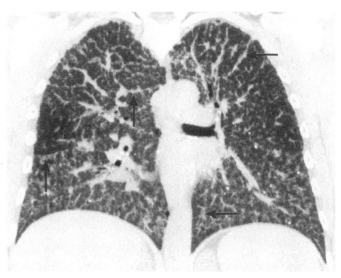

Diffuse bilateral perilymphatic nodularity is demonstrated on this coronal image (*arrows*), which also shows that the lung volumes are relatively preserved.

Answers

1. There is bilateral diffuse lung parenchymal nodular septal thickening, with peribronchovascular, fissural, and subpleural micronodularity, consistent with a perilymphatic distribution.

2. The differential diagnosis of perilymphatic nodularity is sarcoidosis, lymphangitic carcinomatosis, pneumoconiosis (ie, silicosis), and lymphoma.

3. Although the most common intrathoracic manifestation of sarcoidosis is lymphadenopathy, the most common lung parenchymal manifestation is that of perilymphatic nodularity.

4. The pulmonary sarcoidosis staging system consists of five stages: no abnormalities (stage 0), isolated lymphadenopathy (stage 1), lymphadenopathy with parenchymal lung changes (stage 2), parenchymal lung changes without lymphadenopathy (stage 3), and end-stage lung fibrosis (stage 4).

5. The pulmonary sarcoidosis staging system is a radiographic one and does not apply to CT.

Pearls

- The most common intrathoracic manifestation of sarcoidosis is hilar and mediastinal lymphadenopathy.
- The most common lung parenchymal manifestation of sarcoidosis is perilymphatic nodularity.
- The staging system of pulmonary sarcoidosis is a radiographic one and should not be applied to CT.

Suggested Readings

Criado E, Sánchez M, Ramírez J, et al. Pulmonary sarcoidosis: typical and atypical manifestations at high-resolution CT with pathologic correlation. *Radiographics*. October 2010;30(6):1567-1586.

Kanne JP, Yandow DR, Haemel AK, Meyer CA. Beyond skin deep: thoracic manifestations of systemic disorders affecting the skin. *Radiographics*. October 2011;31(6):1651-1668.

Park HJ, Jung JI, Chung MH, et al. Typical and atypical manifestations of intrathoracic sarcoidosis. *Korean J Radiol*. November-December 2009;10(6):623-631.

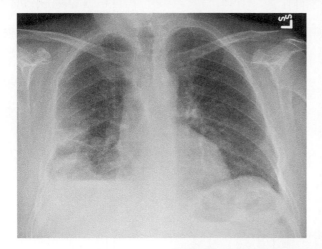
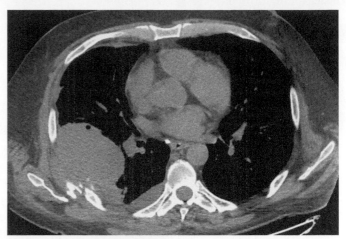
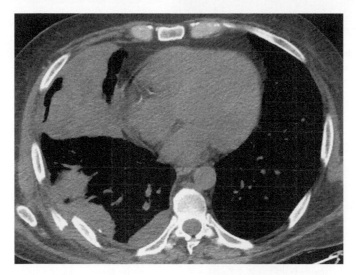

1. What are the radiographic findings?

2. What is the differential diagnosis based on the
   radiographic findings?

3. List a few malignant pleural pathologies?

4. What are the CT findings?

5. What is the final diagnosis?

Case ranking/difficulty:

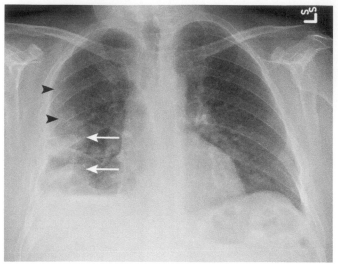

A relatively well-defined, lobulated, peripheral right basal opacity is seen (*arrows*) in proximity to a small pleural effusion. The opacity does not obscure the lung markings for the most part. Note the adjacent displaced rib fractures (*arrowheads*). A right central line is seen.

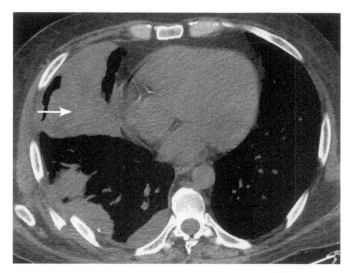

The collection is heterogeneous and has areas of relatively high attenuation (*arrow*), in keeping with a hemorrhagic component.

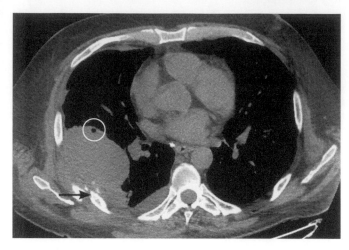

There are multiple displaced right-sided rib fractures (*arrow*). An associated multiloculated pleural collection is seen. A tiny bubble of pneumothorax is also seen (*circle*).

3. Mesothelioma, metastasis (from thymoma or extrathoracic malignancies), and lymphoma are the most common malignant pleural pathologies.

4. There are multiple displaced right-sided rib fractures and a multiloculated, heterogeneous, and high-density pleural collection. A tiny bubble of pneumothorax is also seen.

5. The final diagnosis is that of right hemothorax secondary to rib fractures.

Pearls

- Pleural or subpleural fluid collections can be mistaken for neoplasms on imaging.
- Whether history of trauma is provided or not, always check for osseous abnormalities.
- CT can easily differentiate fluid from soft tissue densities, which is important in further characterization of pleural-based abnormalities.

Answers

1. There is a relatively well-defined, peripheral right basal opacity in proximity to a pleural effusion. Note the adjacent displaced rib fractures.

2. Once the rib fractures are noted, a hemothorax would be the main diagnostic possibility. Otherwise, loculated pleural effusion, empyema, and malignant pleural processes should be considered. Primary lung carcinoma with a malignant effusion is also a concern.

Suggested Reading

Kuhlman JE, Singha NK. Complex disease of the pleural space: radiographic and CT evaluation. *Radiographics.* January-February 1997;17(1):63-79.

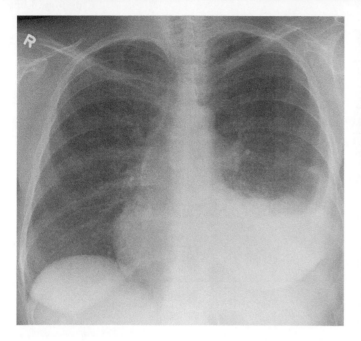
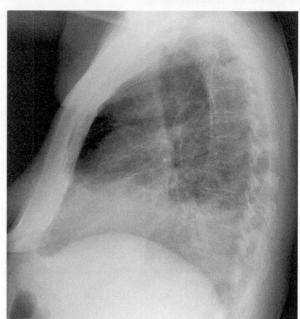
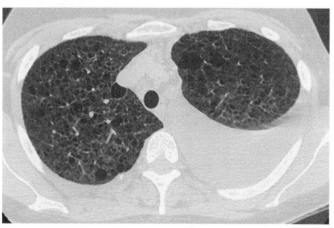
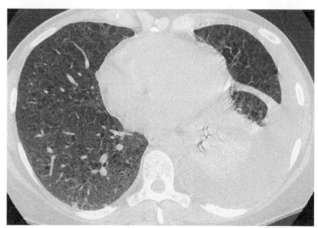

1. What are the radiographic findings?

2. What are the CT findings?

3. In this patient with cystic lung parenchymal changes, what would be your rationale in favoring one diagnosis over the others?

4. What is "Vogt triad?"

5. What cardiac finding would you expect to see on a chest CT of an adult with tuberous sclerosis?

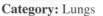
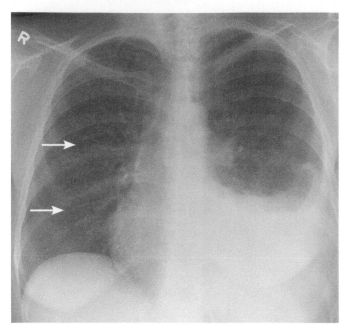

There is a moderate, left pleural effusion. An interstitial background of bilateral, diffuse, fine reticular opacities is seen (*arrows*). It is important to note that despite this striking interstitial pattern, the lung volumes are normal or even slightly increased.

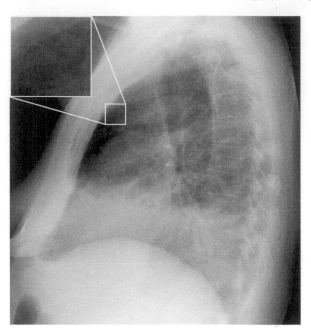

The lateral radiograph demonstrates the same findings seen on the frontal view. As a general rule of thumb, the better aerated retrosternal space is a good area to assess for possible interstitial lung changes (*magnified*).

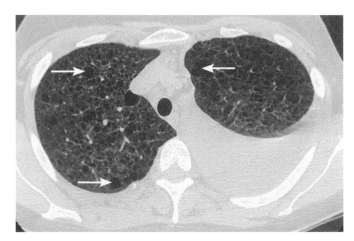

This upper lung zone image shows bilateral, diffuse, thin-walled small-to-medium cysts (*arrows*). A left pleural effusion is also seen, presumed to be chylous.

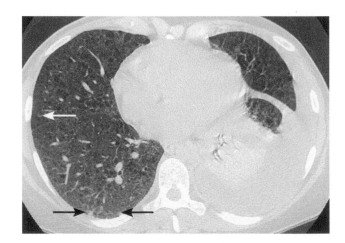

This more caudal image shows the same diffuse cystic findings and the left pleural effusion. Note the presence of a few scattered soft-tissue nodules, representing multifocal micronodular pneumocyte hyperplasia (MMPH) (*arrows*).

Answers

1. There is a moderate, left pleural effusion and diffuse bilateral fine reticular opacities, with normal or even slightly increased lung volumes.

2. There are bilateral, diffuse, thin-walled small-to-medium lung parenchymal cysts and a few scattered soft-tissue nodules. A left pleural effusion is also seen.

3. Since the cystic lung disease is seen together with a pleural effusion, and the patient is a female, sporadic lymphangioleiomyomatosis (LAM) or LAM with tuberous sclerosis (TS) should be the major considerations. Since the cysts are nearly uniform and no smoking history is given, pulmonary Langerhans cell histiocytosis becomes unlikely. Since the patient is not

immunocompromised and no ground-glass attenuation is present, *Pneumocystis jiroveci* pneumonia would not be favored. Given a large cystic burden and the lack of any history suggesting collagen vascular diseases (such as Sjögren syndrome) or immune deficiency disorders (such as human immune deficiency viral infection), lymphocytic interstitial pneumonia becomes less likely. Since the cysts are small and diffusely distributed, Birt-Hogg-Dubé syndrome becomes unlikely as well.

4. Less than 50% of TS patients present with "Vogt triad" of mental retardation, adenoma sebaceum, and seizures.

5. Intramyocardial fat foci are underrecognized in many TS cases. They represent myocardial hamartomas. Although cardiac rhabdomyomas are very common in the pediatric TS population, they spontaneously regress early in life and are not seen in adult TS patients.

Pearls

- The retrosternal area on lateral chest radiographs is an ideal region to assess for possible subtle interstitial lung changes.
- When renal tumors are seen together with cystic lung disease, consider the following: LAM, TS, and Birt-Hogg-Dubé syndrome.
- In TS patients, multifocal micronodular pneumocyte hyperplasia (MMPH) nodules should not be confused for metastatic disease.

Suggested Readings

Ajlan AM, Bilawich AM, Müller NL. Thoracic computed tomographic manifestations of tuberous sclerosis in adults. *Can Assoc Radiol J*. February 2012;63(1):61-68.

Umeoka S, Koyama T, Miki Y, Akai M, Tsutsui K, Togashi K. Pictorial review of tuberous sclerosis in various organs. *Radiographics*. November-December 2008;28(7):e32.

Weight loss in a human immunodeficiency virus (HIV)—positive patient

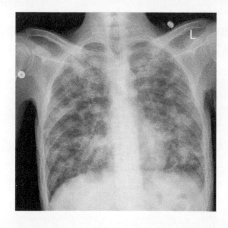
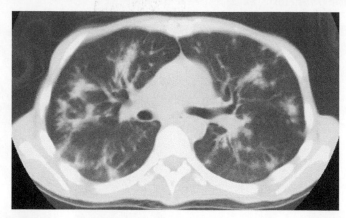
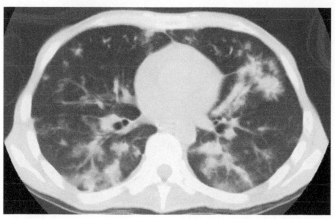
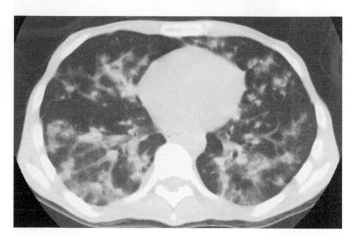

1. What are the radiographic findings?

2. What is the differential diagnosis based on the radiographic findings?

3. What are the CT findings?

4. What is the differential diagnosis based on the CT findings?

5. What are the acquired immune deficiency syndrome (AIDS)-defining neoplasms?

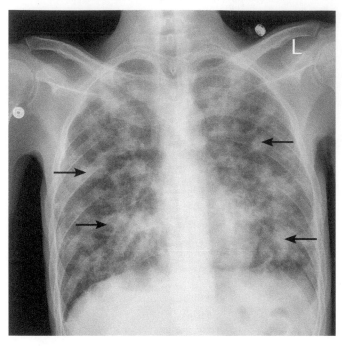

The radiograph shows bilateral diffuse, multifocal, irregular consolidations (*arrows*) with no obvious cavitations. No pleural effusions or lymphadenopathy are noted.

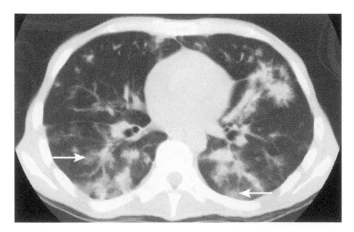

A few lesions are surrounded by ground-glass halos (*arrows*), suggesting perilesional hemorrhage.

Answers

1. The radiograph shows bilateral diffuse, multifocal, irregular consolidations with no obvious cavitations, pleural effusions, or lymphadenopathy.

2. The differential diagnosis based on the radiographic findings includes Kaposi sarcoma, lymphoma, metastases, and bacterial or fungal infections.

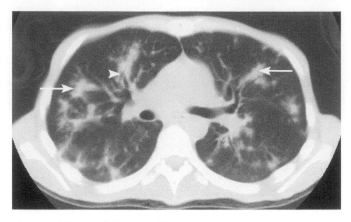

There are bilateral diffuse, multifocal, irregular consolidations (*arrows*) with some showing air bronchograms (*arrowhead*), but no cavitations. The abnormalities have peribronchovascular predominance, and the so-called "flame-shaped" appearance.

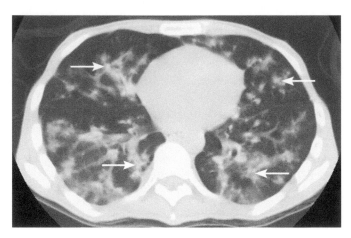

The same abnormality is seen in the lower lungs (*arrows*).

3. The CT shows bilateral diffuse, multifocal, irregular consolidations, with some showing air bronchograms, but no cavitations. The abnormalities have peribronchovascular predominance, and the so-called "flame-shaped" appearance. A few lesions are surrounded by ground-glass halos, suggesting perilesional hemorrhage.

4. The differential diagnosis based on the CT findings includes Kaposi sarcoma, lymphoma, and bacterial or fungal infections.

5. The AIDS-defining neoplasms are Kaposi sarcoma, lymphoma, and cervical carcinoma.

Pearls

- Kaposi sarcoma (KS) has been associated with human herpes virus 8 (HHV8).
- "Flame-shaped" appearance is an imaging buzz word for KS.
- Note that the presence of lymph node enlargement or pleural involvement in HIV patients argues against *Pneumocystis jiroveci* pneumonia and entertains the possibility of KS, lymphoma, and other HIV-related infections.
- When cavitary pulmonary nodules or consolidations are seen in an HIV patient, infections or other neoplasms are favored over KS.

Suggested Readings

Franquet T, Giménez A, Cáceres J, Sabaté JM, Nadal C. Imaging of pulmonary-cutaneous disorders: matching the radiologic and dermatologic findings. *Radiographics*. July 1996;16(4):855-869.

Restrepo CS, Martínez S, Lemos JA, et al. Imaging manifestations of Kaposi sarcoma. *Radiographics*. July-August 2006;26(4):1169-1185.

Shah RM, Kaji AV, Ostrum BJ, Friedman AC. Interpretation of chest radiographs in AIDS patients: usefulness of CD4 lymphocyte counts. Radiographics. January-February 1997;17(1):47-58; discussion 59-61. Erratum in: *Radiographics* May-June 1997;17(3):804.

Recurrent pneumonia

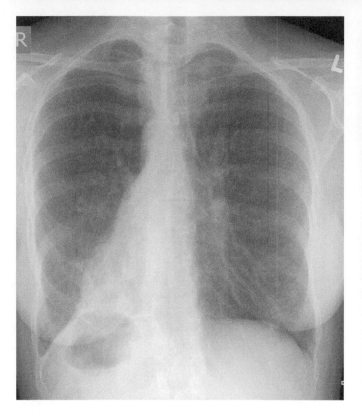 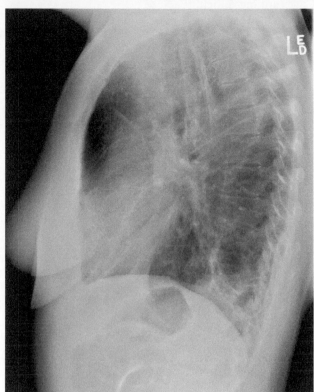

1. What are the radiographic findings?

2. What is the diagnosis based on the radiographic findings?

3. What percentage of patients with situs inversus have Kartagener syndrome?

4. What percentage of patients with Kartagener syndrome have primary ciliary dyskinesia?

5. What is the classic clinical triad of Kartagener syndrome?

Case ranking/difficulty: 🐾🐾

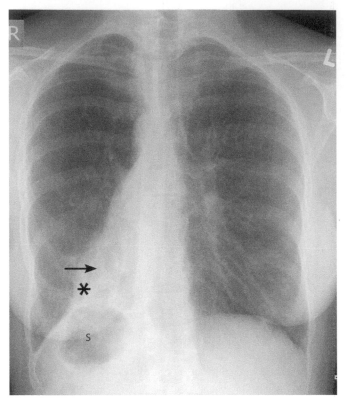

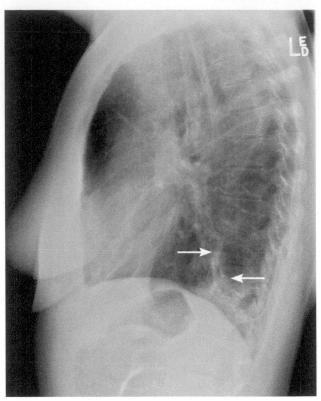

Situs inversus totalis is seen, as denoted by dextrocardia (*asterisk*) and a right-sided gastric gas bubble (S). The right lung base shows an irregular opacity and mild volume loss (*arrow*). Subtle rounded and linear lucencies are suspected in the left lower lung zone, raising the possibility of bronchiectasis.

The lower lungs demonstrate an irregular opacity as well as lucencies that raise the possibility of bronchiectasis (*arrows*).

Answers

1. The images show situs inversus totalis. The right lung base shows an irregular opacity and mild volume loss. Bronchiectasis is suspected in the left lower lung zone.

2. Situs inversus totalis and bronchiectasis raise the possibility of Kartagener syndrome.

3. Twenty percent of patients with situs inversus have Kartagener syndrome.

4. Fifty percent of primary ciliary dyskinesia patients have Kartagener syndrome.

5. The triad of chronic sinusitis, bronchiectasis, and situs inversus is characteristic of Kartagener syndrome.

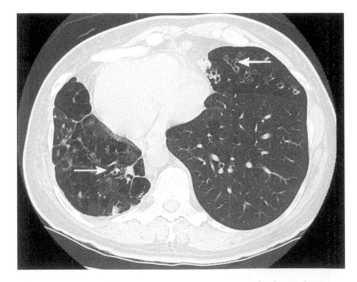

Bronchiectasis and mucus plugging are seen at the lower lungs (*arrows*).

> **Pearls**
>
> • Bronchiectasis can be classified according to congenital and acquired causes.
> • The triad of chronic sinusitis, bronchiectasis, and situs inversus is characteristic of Kartagener syndrome.

- When faced with what appears to be a case of situs inversus, the correct labeling and positioning of the radiograph should be checked.

Suggested Readings

Bent JP III. Kartagener syndrome. http://emedicine. medscape.com/article/299299-overview. Updated: February 28, 2014.

Kennedy MP, Noone PG, Leigh MW, et al. High-resolution CT of patients with primary ciliary dyskinesia. *AJR Am J Roentgenol*. May 2007;188(5):1232-1238.

Rossi SE, Franquet T, Volpacchio M, Giménez A, Aguilar G. Tree-in-bud pattern at thin-section CT of the lungs: radiologic-pathologic overview. *Radiographics*. May-June 2005;25(3):789-801.

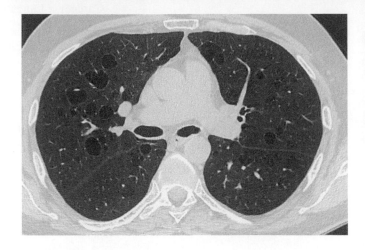 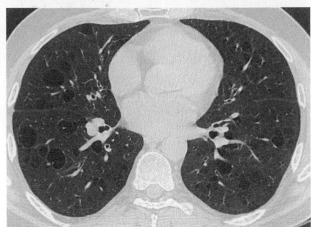

1. What are the imaging findings?

2. What is the differential diagnosis?

3. What is lymphocytic interstitial pneumonia (LIP) associated with?

4. What are the CT findings of LIP?

5. In the context of Sjögren syndrome with LIP, what imaging findings would be concerning for the development of lymphoma?

Case ranking/difficulty:

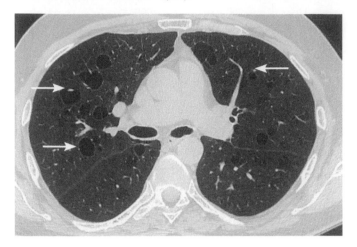

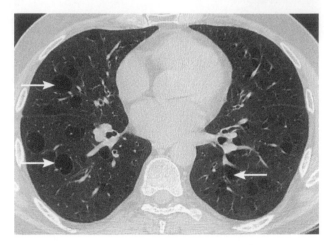

There are multiple bilateral scattered thin-walled cysts of variable sizes, with normal intervening lung parenchyma. Note that some cysts show a perivascular distribution (*arrows*).

This is a more caudal image showing the same findings (*arrows*), with no obvious zonal predominance.

Answers

1. The CT shows multiple bilateral scattered thin-walled cysts of variable sizes, with a perivascular distribution.

2. The major differential diagnosis of scattered lung cysts includes lymphangioleiomyomatosis (LAM), tuberous sclerosis (TS), pulmonary Langerhans cell histiocytosis (PLCH), *Pneumocystis jiroveci* pneumonia (PJP), lymphocytic interstitial pneumonia (LIP), and Birt-Hogg-Dubé syndrome (BHD).

3. LIP can be idiopathic or secondary to Sjögren syndrome, HIV, variable immune deficiency syndrome, and plasma cell Castleman disease.

4. LIP on CT can manifest as ground-glass opacities, cysts, septal thickening, peribronchovascular thickening, and centrilobular or peribronchovascular nodules.

5. In the context of Sjögren syndrome with LIP, the presence of pleural effusions, persistent consolidation, or nodules larger than 1 cm should raise the suspicion for developing lymphoma.

Pearls

- The major differential diagnosis of scattered lung cysts includes lymphangioleiomyomatosis (LAM), tuberous sclerosis (TS), pulmonary Langerhans cell histiocytosis (PLCH), *Pneumocystis jiroveci* pneumonia (PJP), lymphocytic interstitial pneumonia (LIP), and Birt-Hogg-Dubé syndrome (BHD).
- When LIP is suspected, HIV and Sjögren syndrome should be excluded.
- In the context of Sjögren syndrome with LIP, the presence of pleural effusions, persistent consolidation, and nodules larger than 1 cm should raise the suspicion for developing lymphoma.

Suggested Readings

Honda O, Johkoh T, Ichikado K, et al. Differential diagnosis of lymphocytic interstitial pneumonia and malignant lymphoma on high-resolution CT. *AJR Am J Roentgenol.* July 1999;173(1):71-74.

Lynch DA, Travis WD, Müller NL, et al. Idiopathic interstitial pneumonias: CT features. *Radiology.* July 2005;236(1):10-21.

Mueller-Mang C, Grosse C, Schmid K, Stiebellehner L, Bankier AA. What every radiologist should know about idiopathic interstitial pneumonias. *Radiographics.* May-June 2007;27(3):595-615.

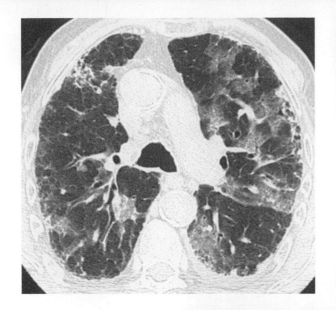
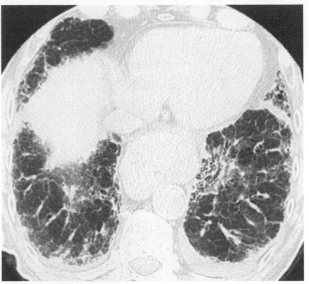

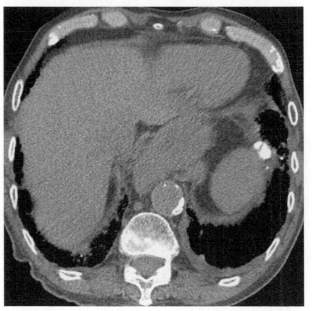

1. What are the CT findings?

2. What is the differential diagnosis?

3. What is the favored diagnosis?

4. How long does it typically take for lung
   fibrosis to develop after asbestos exposure?

5. What types of malignancies are associated with
   asbestos exposure?

Case ranking/difficulty:

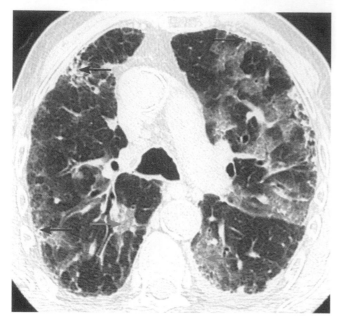

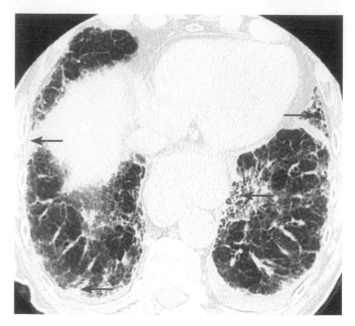

Bilateral subpleural reticulations are present (*red arrows*). In addition, subpleural and peribronchovascular ground-glass opacities are also seen (*green arrows*). These changes are associated with architectural distortion and traction bronchiectasis/ bronchiolectasis (*blue arrow*), in keeping with fibrosis.

This lower lung image demonstrates more subpleural fibrotic changes (*arrows*).

Answers

1. Bilateral subpleural reticulations are present, along with subpleural and peribronchovascular ground-glass opacities. The changes are associated with architectural distortion and traction bronchiectasis/bronchiolectasis. There is a left diaphragmatic-based calcified pleural plaque, indicative of prior asbestos exposure. Pleural thickening and pulmonary lung ossifications are also noted.

2. Given the peribronchovascular changes and predominance of ground-glass attenuation, nonspecific interstitial pneumonia (NSIP) is favored over usual intestinal pneumonia (UIP) in this case. Entities such as connective tissue disorders, asbestosis, drug reaction, idiopathic pulmonary fibrosis, and hypersensitivity pneumonitis should be excluded.

3. In the presence of asbestos-related pleural changes, the diagnosis of asbestosis becomes the major consideration. Of note, the fibrotic pattern in this case has features of NSIP rather than that of UIP.

4. Asbestosis (ie, fibrosis) typically develops 20 years or more from the time of exposure. On rare occasions, with heavier levels of exposure, fibrosis might start earlier.

5. Asbestos exposure is associated with mesothelioma. In addition, the risk of developing lung cancer is very high in asbestos-exposed smokers. Of note, the risk of developing lung cancer is increased in asbestos-exposed nonsmokers as well.

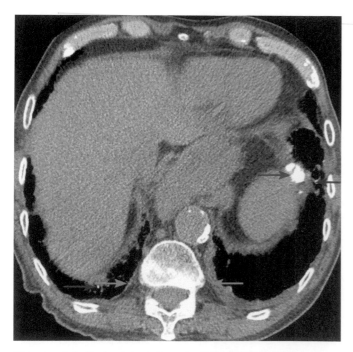

There is a left diaphragmatic-based calcified pleural plaque, in keeping with prior asbestos exposure (*red arrow*). There is also pleural thickening (*green arrows*) and a small left pleural effusion. Tiny fibrosis-related pulmonary lung ossifications are also noted (*blue arrows*).

Pearls

- Asbestosis is a term strictly applied to asbestos-induced fibrosis and not the mere presence of asbestos-related pleural changes.
- Although asbestosis typically presents with a UIP pattern, some cases might show NSIP or unusual fibrotic patterns.
- Meticulous attention should be paid to plural and lung abnormalities on CT scans of asbestosis patients, to ensure early detection of malignancies (eg, mesothelioma and lung cancer).

Suggested Readings

Roach HD, Davies GJ, Attanoos R, Crane M, Adams H, Phillips S. Asbestos: when the dust settles an imaging review of asbestos-related disease. *Radiographics*. October 2002;22 Spec No:S167-S184.

Roggli VL, Gibbs AR, Attanoos R, et al. Pathology of asbestosis—An update of the diagnostic criteria: report of the Asbestosis Committee of the College of American Pathologists and Pulmonary Pathology Society. *Arch Pathol Lab Med*. March 2010;134(3):462-480.

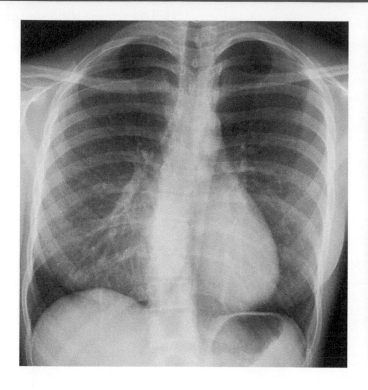 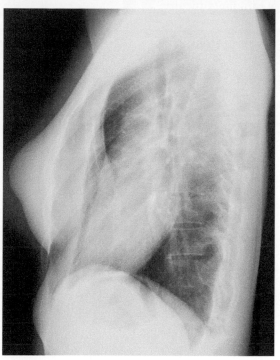

1. What are the radiographic findings?

2. What is the diagnosis?

3. List a few congenital or inherited entities that may be associated with this diagnosis.

4. What is the Haller index?

5. What is considered a clinically significant Haller index value?

Pectus excavatum

 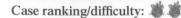

Category: Chest wall/Extrapleural

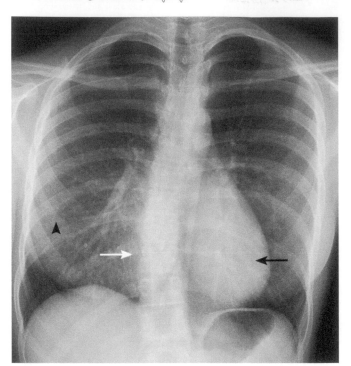

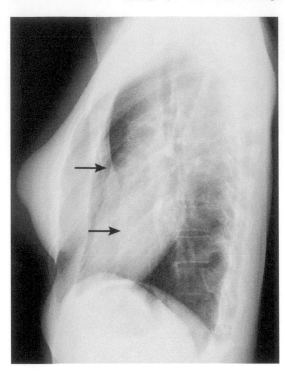

There is haziness and ill definition along the right cardiac border (*white arrow*), leftward displacement of the heart (*black arrow*), and a more vertical than usual orientation of the anterior ribs (*arrowhead*). Mild scoliosis is present.

The lateral radiograph shows marked posterior displacement of the lower sternum (*arrows*).

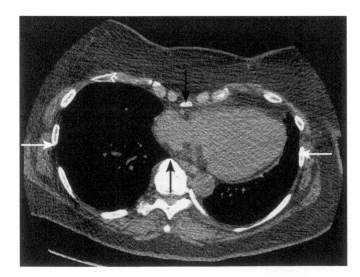

The sagittal chest diameter (*between black arrows*) is short, especially when compared to the coronal diameter (*between white arrows*). Note compression and displacement of the cardiac structures.

Answers

1. The frontal radiograph shows haziness and ill definition along the right cardiac border, leftward displacement of the heart, and a more vertical than usual orientation of the anterior ribs. Mild scoliosis is present. The lateral radiograph shows marked posterior displacement of the lower sternum.

2. The findings are consistent with the diagnosis of pectus excavatum.

3. Pectus excavatum may be associated with Marfan syndrome, Ehlers-Danlos syndrome, Poland syndrome, and congenital heart disease. Pectus excavatum may be a result of trauma, neuromuscular disorders, and chronic pulmonary diseases.

4. The Haller index is calculated on cross-sectional imaging by dividing the maximal transverse thoracic diameter by the anteroposterior thoracic diameter at the level of the most pronounced deformity.

5. A Haller index of 3.25 or more is considered clinically significant.

Pearls

- Pectus excavatum is the most common congenital sternal abnormality.
- Moderate and severe pectus excavatum can be associated with chest pain and cardiopulmonary compromise.
- The severity of pectus excavatum can be objectively determined based on Haller index, which is calculated from CT. A Haller index of 3.25 or more is an indication for surgery.
- The *Nuss procedure* is a minimally invasive approach, where a curved metallic bar is threaded under the sternum and then turned over to correct the pectus excavatum deformity.

Suggested Readings

Chu ZG, Yu JQ, Yang ZG, Peng LQ, Bai HL, Li XM. Correlation between sternal depression and cardiac rotation in pectus excavatum: Evaluation with helical CT. *AJR Am J Roentgenol.* July 2010;195(1):W76-W80.

Nuss D, Kelly RE, Croitoru DP, Katz ME. A 10-year review of a minimally invasive technique for the correction of pectus excavatum. *J Pediatr Surg.* April 1998;33(4):545-552.

Restrepo CS, Martinez S, Lemos DF, et al. Imaging appearances of the sternum and sternoclavicular joints. *Radiographics.* May-June 2009;29(3):839-859.

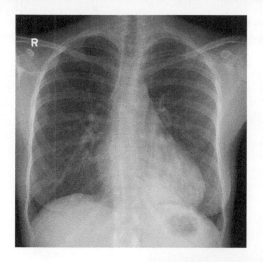
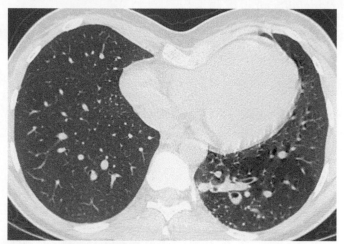

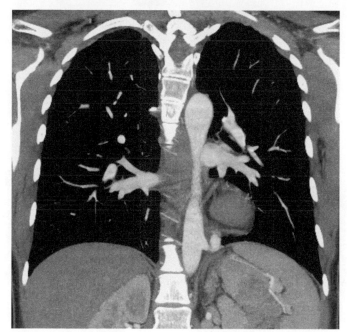

1. What are the radiographic findings?

2. What are the CT findings?

3. What is the diagnosis?

4. What are the types of pulmonary sequestration?

5. What type of sequestration is shown in the presented case?

Case ranking/difficulty:

Category: Lungs

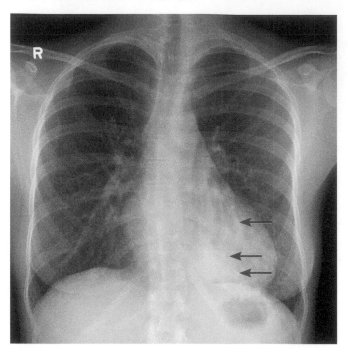

There is a left retrocardiac opacity (*arrows*).

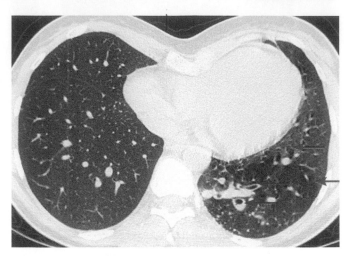

There is a left lower lung circumscribed lucency (*red arrows*), with dilated and impacted airways (*blue arrows*).

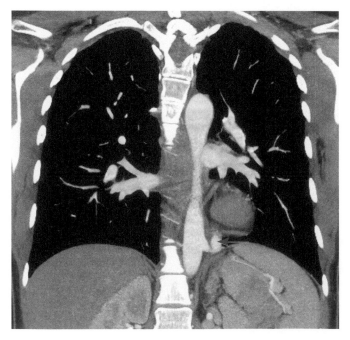

An accessory vessel arises from the descending thoracic aorta and feeds the left lower lobe lesion (*arrow*).

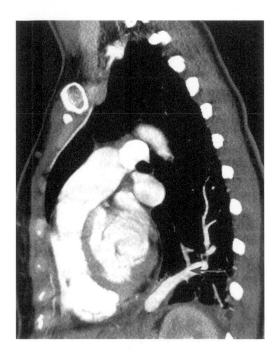

The course of the abnormal feeding artery is well seen on this sagittal view (*arrow*).

Answers

1. The radiograph shows a left retrocardiac opacity.

2. The CT shows left lower lobe circumscribed lucency, with dilated and impacted airways. An accessory vessel arises from the descending thoracic aorta and feeds the left lower lobe abnormality.

3. The diagnosis is that of pulmonary sequestration.

4. Pulmonary sequestrations are divided into intralobar and extralobar types.

5. Given the age, this is likely an intralobar type of pulmonary sequestration. Of note, pulmonary venous drainage into the left atrium is typical of intralobar pulmonary sequestrations (not shown here).

Pearls

- On a normal frontal chest radiograph, the retrocardiac region should be of equal density on each side of the midline.
- Intralobar sequestration should be a consideration when pneumonia recurs in the same location.
- Although systemic arterial supply to the lung is a hallmark of pulmonary sequestration, it can occasionally occur without associated pulmonary sequestration.
- Pulmonary sequestration can be associated with other malformations (eg, cystic adenomatoid malformation, bronchial atresia, or congenital lobar emphysema).

Suggested Readings

Do KH, Goo JM, Im JG, Kim KW, Chung JW, Park JH. Systemic arterial supply to the lungs in adults: spiral CT findings. *Radiographics*. March-April 2001;21(2):387-402.

Konen E, Raviv-Zilka L, Cohen RA, et al. Congenital pulmonary venolobar syndrome: spectrum of helical CT findings with emphasis on computerized reformatting. *Radiographics*. September-October 2003;23(5):1175-1184.

Riedlinger WF, Vargas SO, Jennings RW, et al. Bronchial atresia is common to extralobar sequestration, intralobar sequestration, congenital cystic adenomatoid malformation, and lobar emphysema. *Pediatr Dev Pathol*. Sepember-October 2006;9(5):361-373.

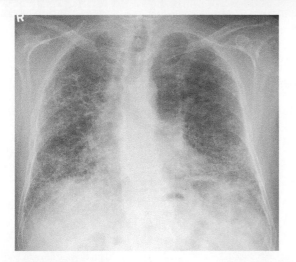
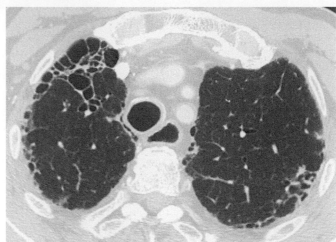
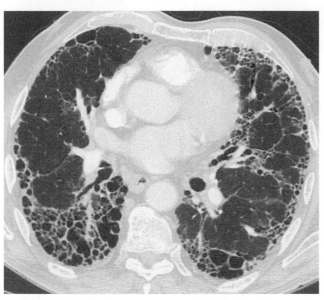
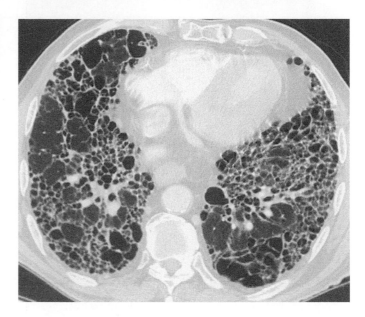

1. What are the radiographic findings?

2. What is the differential diagnosis based on the radiographic findings?

3. What are the CT findings?

4. What is the definition of acute exacerbation of idiopathic pulmonary fibrosis (IPF)?

5. List all the idiopathic interstitial pneumonias.

Case ranking/difficulty:

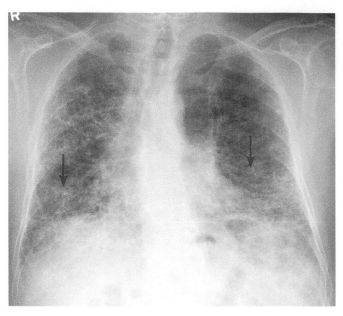

There are bilateral coarse reticulations, with bibasilar and peripheral predominance (*arrows*). There is associated volume loss (note the downward displacement of the hila).

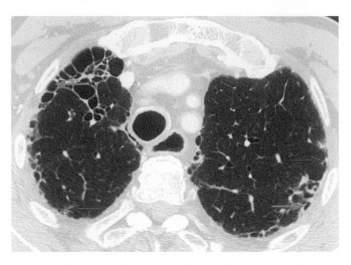

There are bilateral peripheral reticulations (*red arrows*) and honeycombing (*green arrows*).

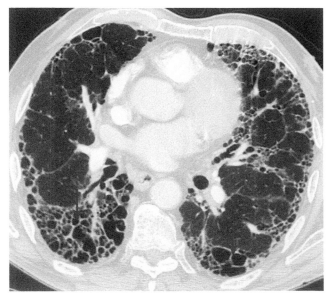

The same abnormalities have a bilateral and near-symmetrical distribution (*arrows*).

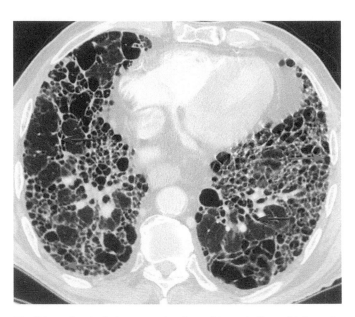

The bilateral reticulations, traction bronchiectasis/ bronchiolectasis (*red arrows*), architectural distortion, and honeycombing (*green arrows*) predominate at the lower lungs.

Answers

1. The radiograph shows bilateral coarse reticulations, with bibasilar and peripheral predominance. There is associated volume loss.

2. The appearance is most consistent with that of a usual interstitial pneumonia pattern, thus the following should be considered: idiopathic interstitial pneumonia, occupational lung diseases (asbestosis), connective tissue disorders (eg, rheumatoid arthritis or scleroderma), and drug toxicity (eg, bleomycin or methotrexate). Fibrotic nonspecific interstitial pneumonia and hypersensitivity pneumonitis may be included in the radiographic differential diagnosis as well.

3. The CT shows bilateral near-symmetrical reticulations, traction bronchiectasis/ bronchiolectasis, architectural distortion, honeycombing, and volume loss. The abnormalities are predominantly peripheral and bibasilar. There are a few small mediastinal and bilateral hilar lymph nodes.

4. The definition of acute exacerbation of IPF is deterioration in 30 days or less, in the absence of other explanatory causes, with new bilateral airspace opacities.

5. Idiopathic interstitial pneumonias include idiopathic pulmonary fibrosis (IPF), nonspecific interstitial pneumonia (NSIP), cryptogenic organizing pneumonia (COP), respiratory bronchiolitis-associated interstitial lung disease (RB-ILD), desquamative interstitial pneumonia (DIP), lymphocytic interstitial pneumonia (LIP), and acute interstitial pneumonia (AIP).

Pearls

- Honeycombing is associated with poor prognosis and should not be overcalled when faced with adjacent emphysema or cystic traction bronchiectasis/ bronchiolectasis in an IPF patient.
- Acute exacerbation of IPF should be considered when faced with new bilateral airspace opacities in a clinically deteriorating IPF patient.
- UIP is designated as typical IPF when it is idiopathic in a patient where all features of fibrosis (including honeycombing) are seen in a classic bilateral peripheral and basilar distribution.
- When the clinical and imaging picture is typical of IPF, surgical biopsy can be avoided.

Suggested Readings

Kligerman SJ, Groshong S, Brown KK, Lynch DA. Nonspecific interstitial pneumonia: radiologic, clinical, and pathologic considerations. *Radiographics*. January-February 2009;29(1):73-87.

Silva CI, Müller NL. Idiopathic interstitial pneumonias. *J Thorac Imaging*. November 2009;24(4):260-273.

Travis WD, Costabel U, Hansell DM, et al. An official American Thoracic Society/European Respiratory Society statement: Update of the international multidisciplinary classification of the idiopathic interstitial pneumonias. *Am J Respir Crit Care Med*. September 2013;188(6):733-748.

Long-standing smoker and intravenous drug abuser, presenting with shortness of breath

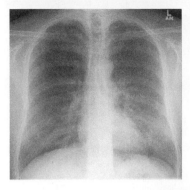
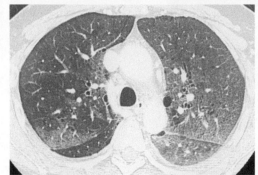
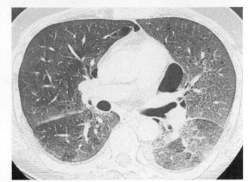
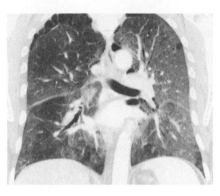
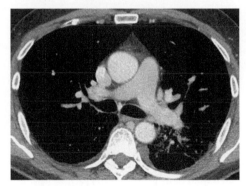

1. What are the radiographic findings?

2. What are the CT findings?

3. What is (1,3)-β-D-glucan?

4. What is the most common pulmonary infection in HIV patients?

5. What is the most common opportunistic infection in HIV patients?

Case ranking/difficulty: 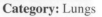   **Category:** Lungs

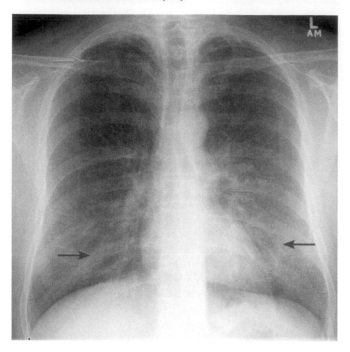

Vague areas of airspace opacification are noted bilaterally, being more pronounced on the left (*red arrows*). Subtle round and lucent areas are also seen (*green arrows*), raising the possibility of lung parenchymal cysts or paraseptal emphysema.

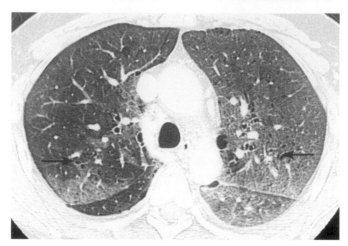

Bilateral, diffuse, and heterogenous ground-glass lung parenchymal attenuation is noted. Centrilobular (*blue arrows*) and paraseptal (*green arrows*) emphysema is seen, consistent with the patient's long-standing history of smoking.

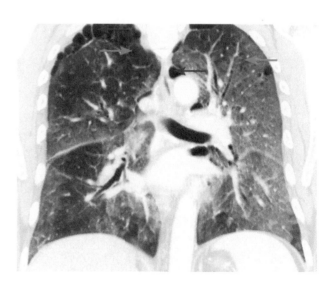

This coronal image shows the bilateral, diffuse, and heterogenous nature of the airspace abnormality. Note the centrilobular (*green arrows*) and paraseptal (*blue arrows*) emphysematous background.

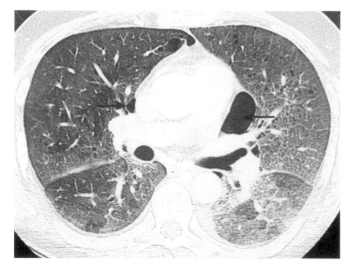

This image shows the same abnormalities; however, mild septal thickening is also noted in areas of ground-glass attenuation (*green arrows*). Paraseptal emphysema is redemonstrated (*blue arrows*).

Answers

1. The radiograph shows vague areas of airspace opacification. Subtle round and lucent areas are also seen, raising the possibility of lung parenchymal cysts or paraseptal emphysema.

2. The CT shows bilateral, diffuse, and heterogenous ground-glass lung parenchymal attenuation, with superimposed mild septal thickening. Centrilobular and paraseptal emphysema is seen. There is no lymphadenopathy.

3. (1,3)-β-D-glucan (BDG) is a fungal protein that is found in the wall of *Pneumocystis jiroveci* organism. This substance can be detected in the serum of many patients with *Pneumocystis jiroveci* pneumonia (PJP).

4. Bacterial pneumonia is the most common pulmonary infection in HIV patients.

5. PJP is the most common opportunistic infection in HIV patients.

Pearls

- Serum lactate dehydrogenase and (1,3)-β-D-glucan levels are useful diagnostic markers in PJP patients.
- PJP can present with mosaic attenuation or crazy paving patterns.
- Consider apical blebs or cystic lung diseases (including PJP) in a young patient presenting with a "spontaneous" pneumothorax.

Suggested Readings

Shah RM, Kaji AV, Ostrum BJ, Friedman AC. Interpretation of chest radiographs in AIDS patients: usefulness of CD4 lymphocyte counts. *Radiographics*. January-February 1997;17(1):47-58; discussion 59-61. Erratum in: *Radiographics*. May-June 1997;17(3):804.

Sider L, Gabriel H, Curry DR, Pham MS. Pattern recognition of the pulmonary manifestations of AIDS on CT scans. *Radiographics*. July 1993;13(4):771-784; discussion 785-786.

Tasaka S, Tokuda H, Sakai F, et al. Comparison of clinical and radiological features of pneumocystis pneumonia between malignancy cases and acquired immunodeficiency syndrome cases: a multicenter study. *Intern Med*. 2010;49(4):273-281.

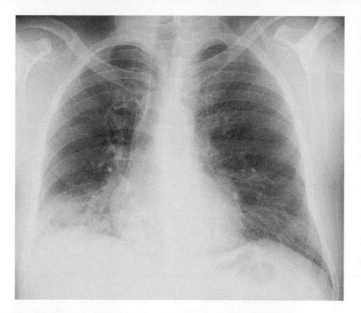

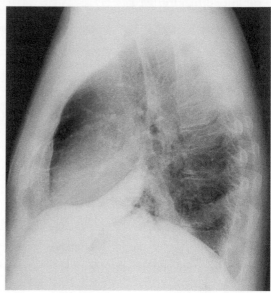

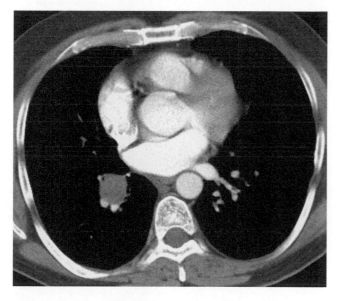

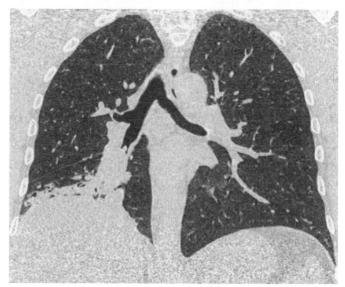

1. What are the radiographic findings?

2. What are the CT findings?

3. What is the most common bronchopulmonary neuroendocrine tumor?

4. Why would hilar lymph nodes be enlarged in the context of pulmonary carcinoids?

5. What does DIPNECH stand for?

Case ranking/difficulty: **Category:** Airways

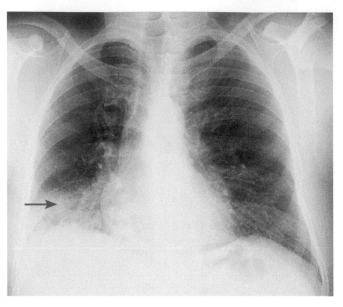

Right basal consolidation and volume loss are noted (*arrow*). No obvious hilar lesion is identified.

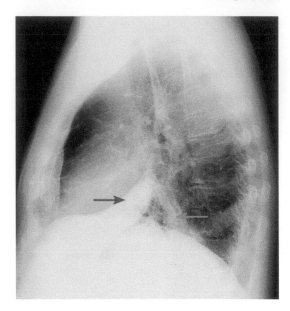

Total right middle lobe collapse (*red arrow*) and partial right lower lobar consolidation (*green arrow*) are seen.

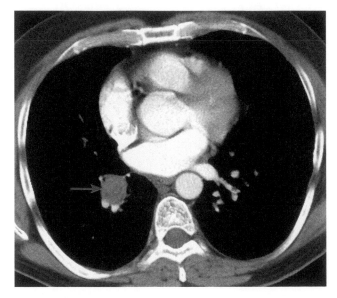

There is well-defined right lower lobe lesion of soft tissue attenuation (*arrow*).

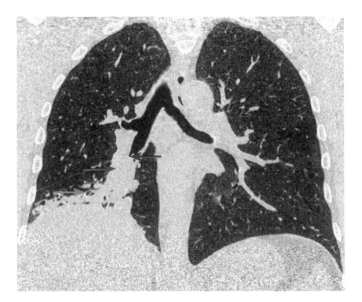

There is a lesion in the right lower lobe (*red arrow*), and an endoluminal tumoral component is suspected (*blue arrow*). There are secondary postobstructive changes of the right lower lobe (*green arrow*). The right middle lobe atelectasis identified on the preceding lateral chest radiograph was possibly due to mucus plugging.

Answers

1. Total right middle lobe collapse and partial right lower lobar consolidation are seen.

2. There is a soft tissue lesion in the right lower lobe, with secondary postobstructive changes. An endoluminal tumoral component is suspected.

3. Typical carcinoid is the most common bronchopulmonary neuroendocrine tumor.

4. Hilar or mediastinal lymph node enlargement in the context of pulmonary carcinoid raises the concern for metastatic involvement, but can also be reactive due to recurrent pneumonia.

5. DIPNECH stands for diffuse idiopathic pulmonary neuroendocrine cell hyperplasia. DIPNECH is a rare condition in which endobronchial mucosal neuroendocrine cells undergo hyperplasic proliferation, without invasion of the basement membrane.

Pearls

- Consider postobstructive lung changes in the context of persistent airspace opacities or recurrent focal pneumonia.
- Hilar or mediastinal lymph node enlargement in the context of pulmonary carcinoid raises the concern for metastatic involvement, but can also be reactive due to recurrent pneumonia.
- There are a few clinical and imaging features distinguishing typical from atypical carcinoids, but their definitive differentiation based on imaging alone is not usually possible, since both types have overlapping imaging findings.

Suggested Readings

Jeung MY, Gasser B, Gangi A, et al. Bronchial carcinoid tumors of the thorax: spectrum of radiologic findings. *Radiographics*. March-April 2002;22(2):351-365.

Park CM, Goo JM, Lee HJ, Kim MA, Lee CH, Kang MJ. Tumors in the tracheobronchial tree: CT and FDG PET features. *Radiographics*. January-February 2009;29(1): 55-71.

Scarsbrook AF, Ganeshan A, Statham J, et al. Anatomic and functional imaging of metastatic carcinoid tumors. *Radiographics*. March-April 2007;27(2):455-477.

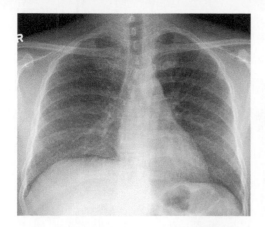
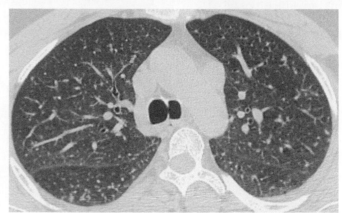

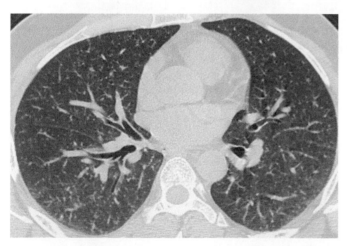
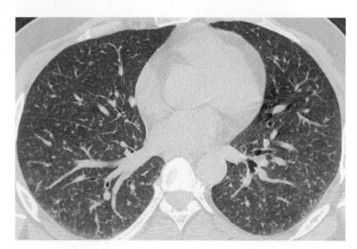

1. What is the radiographic finding?

2. What is the differential diagnosis based on the radiographic finding?

3. What are the CT findings?

4. What is the differential diagnosis based on the CT findings?

5. Given the pattern seen on CT, how did this disease spread to the lungs?

Case ranking/difficulty: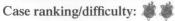

Category: Lungs

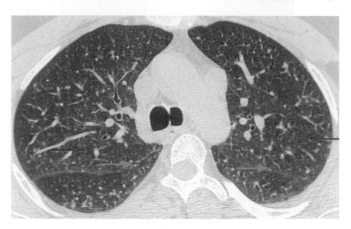

Bilateral, diffuse micronodules are seen. Some nodules are related to the vessels in the center of the secondary lobule, in keeping with a "centrilobular" location (*red arrows*). Other nodules are abutting fissures, in keeping with a "perilymphatic" location (*green arrows*). This mixture of locations is consistent with a "random" distribution. Since the nodules are 3 mm or less in size, the appearance is classified as a "miliary" pattern.

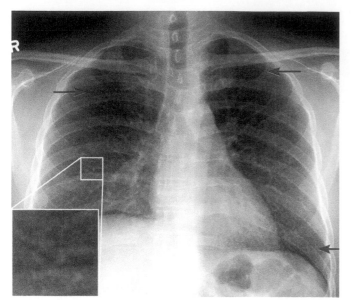

Scattered and faint tiny nodular opacities are seen in both lungs (*arrows and magnification*), with no other abnormalities. This radiograph serves as an example of how subtle a miliary pattern can appear on a chest radiograph.

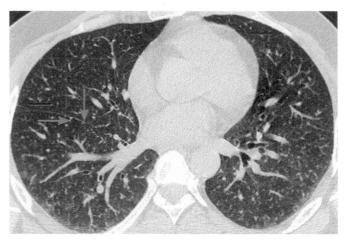

Perifissural (*green arrows*) and subpleural (*blue arrows*) nodules are well seen on this image.

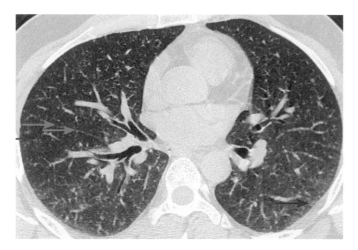

This image shows that some nodules are centrilobular (*red arrow*), while others are abutting pleura (*blue arrows*) and fissures (*green arrows*).

Answers

1. The radiographic finding is that of bilateral, diffuse and faint, tiny nodular opacities.

2. The differential diagnosis based on the radiographic finding includes infection (bacterial such as tuberculosis, fungal such as histoplasmosis, and viral such as varicella), neoplasms (metastases from thyroid cancer, renal cell carcinoma, melanoma, lung adenocarcinoma (previously known as bronchoalveolar carcinoma), choriocarcinoma, and sarcoma), sarcoidosis, pneumoconioses (silicosis and coal workers pneumoconiosis), hypersensitivity pneumonitis, and Langerhans cell histiocytosis.

3. Bilateral and diffuse micronodules are seen on CT in both centrilobular and perilymphatic locations, consistent with a random distribution. The picture is that of a miliary pattern.

4. The differential diagnosis based on the CT finding is limited to infectious and metastatic causes.

5. Given the miliary pattern seen on CT, the infection has spread to the lungs via hematogenous route.

Pearls

- Miliary TB can be extremely subtle and may be easily missed on chest radiographs.
- On chest radiographs, a miliary pattern cannot be differentiated from other distributions (ie, centrilobular or perilymphatic patterns), resulting in a relatively long differential diagnostic list.
- Once a miliary pattern is defined on CT, the differential diagnosis becomes limited to hematogenous spread of infection or metastases.

Suggested Readings

Burrill J, Williams CJ, Bain G, Conder G, Hine AL, Misra RR. Tuberculosis: a radiologic review. *Radiographics*. September-October 2007;27(5):1255-1273.

Jeong YJ, Lee KS. Pulmonary tuberculosis: up-to-date imaging and management. *AJR Am J Roentgenol*. September 2008;191(3):834-844.

Rossi SE, Franquet T, Volpacchio M, Giménez A, Aguilar G. Tree-in-bud pattern at thin-section CT of the lungs: radiologic-pathologic overview. *Radiographics*. May-June 2005;25(3):789-801.

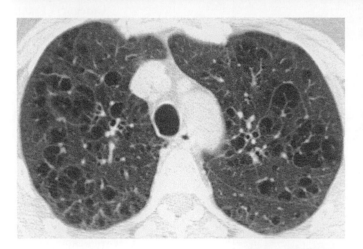
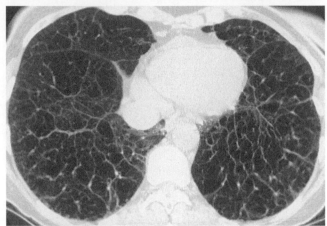
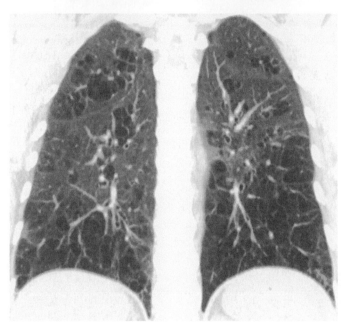

1. What are the CT findings?

2. What is the differential diagnosis?

3. What is the mode of inheritance of alpha-1-antitrypsin deficiency (AATD)?

4. List a few conditions that can be associated with AATD.

5. What are the typical characteristics of emphysema of AATD?

Case ranking/difficulty:

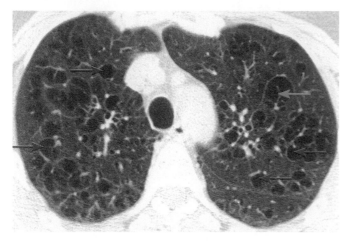

Marked upper lung centrilobular emphysema is seen (*red arrows*). Note that the lucency "surrounds" the centrilobular pulmonary artery (*green arrow*).

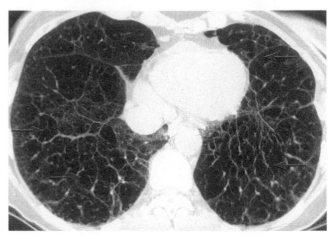

Marked lower lung panacinar emphysema is also present (*arrows*). Note that the lucencies involve the entire structure of the secondary pulmonary lobule.

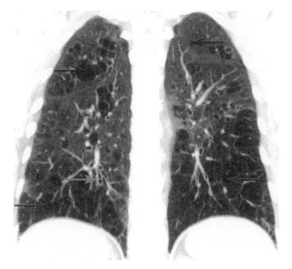

This coronal image clearly shows the distribution of the emphysematous lung changes. There is striking lower lung panacinar emphysema (*red arrows*). Note the less pronounced upper lung centrilobular emphysema (*blue arrows*). Also note the presence of mild central cylindrical bronchiectasis (*green arrow*).

4. A few conditions that can be associated with AATD are liver cirrhosis, hepatocellular carcinoma, pulmonary emphysema, bronchiectasis, c-ANCA small-vessel vasculitis, necrotizing panniculitis.

5. Emphysema of AATD is characteristically panacinar and lower lobar.

Pearls

- AATD can be suspected when imaging reveals basilar-predominant emphysema, emphysema at age of 45 years or younger, emphysema without recognized risk factors, or bronchiectasis unexplained by other causes.
- The differential diagnosis for bibasilar panacinar emphysema is AATD and IV Ritalin injection in drug abusers.
- Although AATD is notoriously associated with bibasilar panacinar emphysema, a component of centrilobular emphysema might be encountered as well.

Answers

1. The CT shows marked centrilobular upper lung and panacinar lower lung emphysema. There is mild central cylindrical bronchiectasis as well.

2. Although smoking-related emphysema is considered, the striking lower lung panacinar involvement is consistent with alpha-1-antitrypsin deficiency (AATD). If there is history of intravenous drug abuse, lung changes related to Ritalin injection should be considered.

3. The mode of inheritance of AATD is autosomal dominant.

Suggested Readings

Hartman TE, Tazelaar HD, Swensen SJ, Müller NL. Cigarette smoking: CT and pathologic findings of associated pulmonary diseases. *Radiographics*. March-April 1997;17(2):377-390.

Matsuoka S, Yamashiro T, Washko GR, Kurihara Y, Nakajima Y, Hatabu H. Quantitative CT assessment of chronic obstructive pulmonary disease. *Radiographics*. January 2010;30(1):55-66.

Meyer CA, White CS, Sherman KE. Diseases of the hepatopulmonary axis. *Radiographics*. May-June 2000;20(3):687-698.

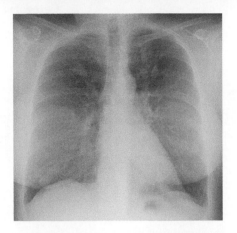
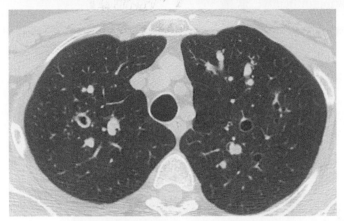
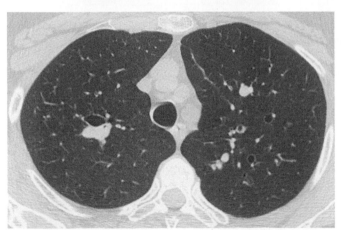
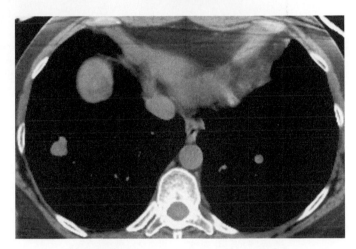

1. What are the radiographic findings?

2. What are the CT findings?

3. What is your main diagnostic consideration?

4. What is meant by dermal *Aspergillus* hypersensitivity?

5. What is bronchocentric granulomatosis (BG)?

Case ranking/difficulty:

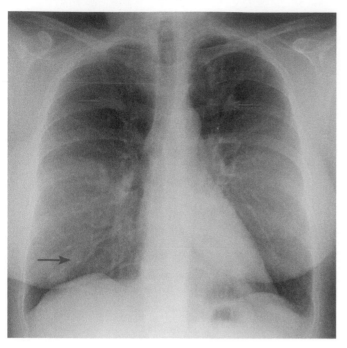

There are bilateral scattered, partially defined, tubular, and branching lung parenchymal opacities (*arrows*), with upper lung predominance.

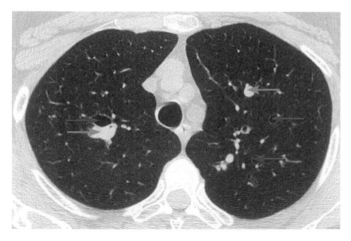

Bilateral bronchiectasis (*red arrows*) and mucus plugs (*green arrows*) are also seen on this more caudal image.

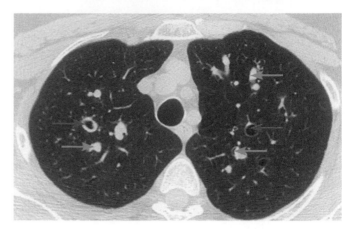

Bilateral segmental and subsegmental cylindrical bronchiectasis is present (*red arrows*), with areas of mucus impaction (*green arrows*) and without postobstructive lung parenchymal changes.

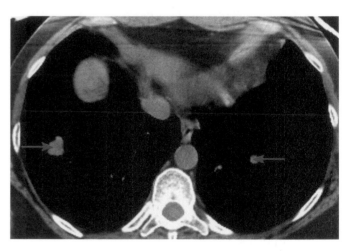

The impacted mucus is of relatively high density (*arrows*), when compared to adjacent soft tissue structures. This feature is characteristic of ABPA and has prognostic implications.

Answers

1. The radiograph shows bilateral scattered, partially defined, tubular, and branching lung parenchymal opacities, with upper lung predominance.

2. Bilateral segmental and subsegmental cylindrical bronchiectasis is present on CT, with areas of high-attenuation mucus plugging.

3. Allergic bronchopulmonary aspergillosis (ABPA) is the main diagnostic consideration.

4. *Aspergillus* hypersensitivity is an immediate skin hypersensitivity reaction to *Aspergillus* antigens. Only a small number of patients with this type of reaction will develop full-blown ABPA.

5. BG is a rare condition of necrotizing granulomatous reaction of airways with surrounding lung parenchyma inflammation. One-third of BG patients have clinical features of ABPA, while no clear etiology can be established in the remaining patients.

Pearls

- The differential diagnosis of waxing and waning (migratory or fleeting) parenchymal lung opacities includes organizing pneumonia, eosinophilic lung disease, ABPA, pulmonary hemorrhage, pulmonary vasculitis, and aspiration pneumonitis.
- When chest radiographic abnormalities are seen in an asthmatic patient, the following entities are considered: ABPA, chronic eosinophilic pneumonia, Churg-Strauss syndrome, and bronchocentric granulomatosis.
- High-attenuation mucus plugging is typical of ABPA and has important prognostic implications, since this finding is commonly associated with a more severe and relapsing disease course.

Suggested Readings

Agarwal R, Gupta D, Aggarwal AN, Saxena AK, Chakrabarti A, Jindal SK. Clinical significance of hyperattenuating mucoid impaction in allergic bronchopulmonary aspergillosis: an analysis of 155 patients. *Chest*. October 2007;132(4):1183-1190.

Franquet T, Müller NL, Giménez A, Guembe P, de La Torre J, Bagué S. Spectrum of pulmonary aspergillosis: histologic, clinical, and radiologic findings. *Radiographics*. July-August 2001;21(4):825-837.

Jeong YJ, Kim KI, Seo IJ, et al. Eosinophilic lung diseases: a clinical, radiologic, and pathologic overview. *Radiographics*. May-June 2007;27(3):617-637; discussion 637-639.

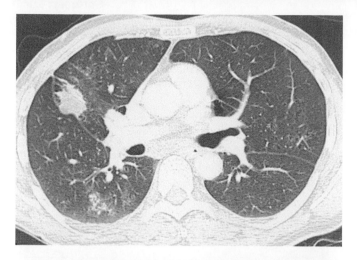
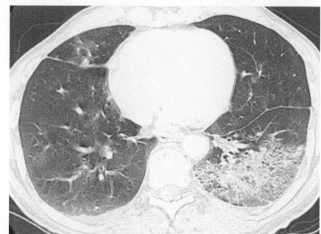
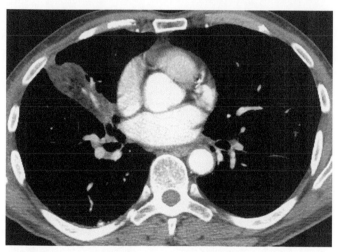
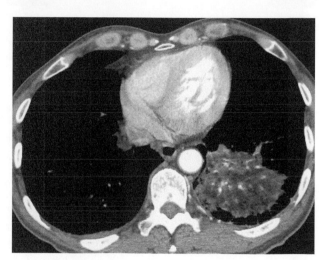

1. What are the CT findings?

2. What is the diagnosis?

3. How is this entity classified?

4. Which population is at risk of developing this condition?

5. How is a "crazy-paving pattern" different from "ground-glass attenuation" on CT?

Case ranking/difficulty:

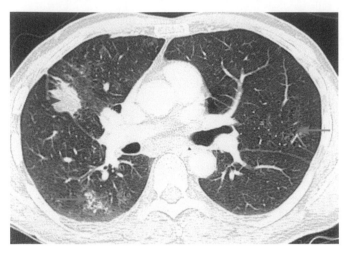

The right lung lesion is irregular and has minimal surrounding spiculations (*red arrow*), in an appearance that can be mistaken for lung cancer. Other airspace opacities are also noted bilaterally (*green arrows*).

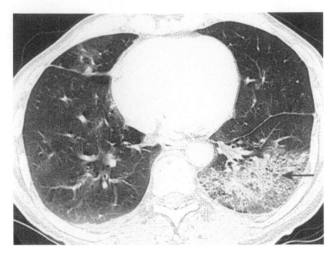

The largest lesion in the left lower lobe is of partial ground-glass attenuation and has minimal internal septal thickening (*arrow*), resulting in a crazy-paving appearance.

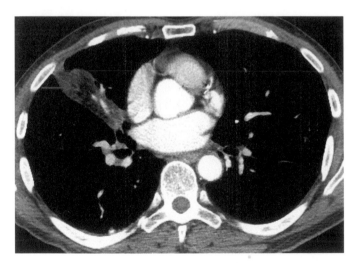

The middle lobe parenchymal lesion shows very low attenuation (*arrow*), consistent with fatty composition.

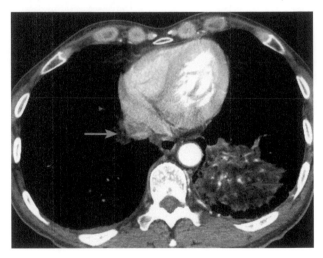

The left lower lobe parenchymal lesion shows very low attenuation (*red arrow*), consistent with fatty composition. Another similar lesion is seen in the right lung (*green arrow*).

Answers

1. The CT shows bilateral areas of lung parenchymal airspace opacification, with internal fat attenuation.

2. Given the internal fat density of the abnormality, the diagnosis is that of lipoid pneumonia.

3. Lipoid pneumonia can be divided into exogenous and endogenous types.

4. The population at risk of developing lipoid pneumonia includes patients with pharyngeal abnormalities, esophageal disorders, neurologic deficits, and chronic illnesses. Individuals using mineral oil as a topical moisturizer or as a laxative for constipation are a classic subgroup that may develop lipoid pneumonia.

5. Ground-glass attenuation represents increased lung attenuation without obscuration of the underlying lung markings, whereas crazy paving represents ground-glass attenuation with additional internal septal thickening.

Pearls

- Lipoid pneumonia can be divided into two types: exogenous (ie, aspiration or inhalation of oil- or fat-containing material) and endogenous (ie, changes distal to chronic airway obstruction).

- Many patients with lipoid pneumonia are asymptomatic or present with nonspecific symptoms.
- Chronic fibrotic lipoid pneumonia may be mistaken for lung cancer, a pitfall that can be avoided by recognizing intralesional fat attenuation.
- Assessing the attenuation of lung lesions on the soft tissue window should be part of routine CT reading.

Suggested Readings

Franquet T, Giménez A, Rosón N, Torrubia S, Sabaté JM, Pérez C. Aspiration diseases: findings, pitfalls, and differential diagnosis. *Radiographics*. May-June 2000;20(3):673-685.

Gaerte SC, Meyer CA, Winer-Muram HT, Tarver RD, Conces DJ. Fat-containing lesions of the chest. *Radiographics*. October 2002;22 Spec No:S61-S78.

Rossi SE, Erasmus JJ, Volpacchio M, Franquet T, Castiglioni T, McAdams HP. "Crazy-paving" pattern at thin-section CT of the lungs: radiologic-pathologic overview. *Radiographics*. November-December 2003;23(6): 1509-1519.

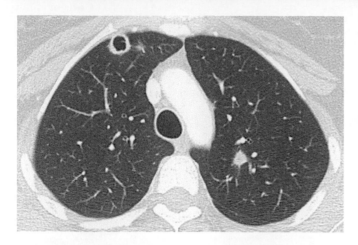
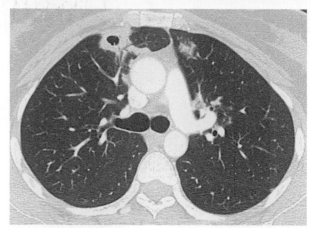
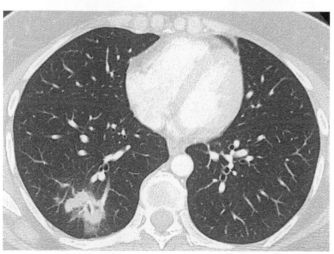
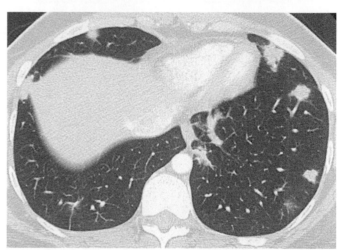

1. What are the CT findings?

2. What is the differential diagnosis based on the CT findings?

3. What is the differential diagnosis of multiple bilateral peripherally located opacities?

4. Which of these two signs can be seen with this pathological entity: the "halo sign" or the "reverse halo sign?"

5. Which antineutrophil cytoplasmic antibodies (ANCA) are more commonly positive with this pathological entity: cytoplasmic (c-ANCA) or perinuclear (p-ANCA)?

Case ranking/difficulty: 🌸🌸   **Category:** Lungs

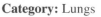

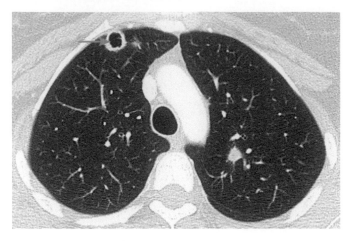

A peripheral thick-walled cavity is present in the right upper lobe (*arrow*).

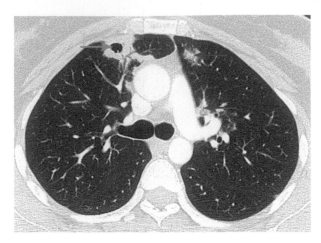

Irregular consolidations are seen (*red arrows*), with another cavitary lesion in the right upper lobe (*green arrow*).

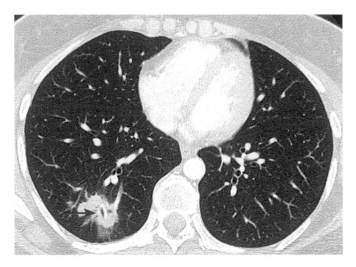

A large irregular right lower lobar nodular consolidation is also seen (*arrow*).

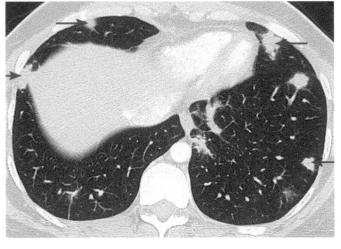

Multifocal peripheral, irregular, nodular consolidations are seen at the lung bases (*arrows*).

Answers

1. The CT shows bilateral multifocal, irregular, nodular consolidations in a peripheral distribution, with a few lesions demonstrating thick-walled cavities.

2. The CT findings are those of multiple bilateral cavitary lesions, for which the differential diagnosis includes metastases (eg, from squamous cell carcinoma, sarcoma, and transitional cell carcinoma), connective tissue disorders (eg, rheumatoid arthritis), vasculitis (eg, Wegener granulomatosis), infections (eg, *S aureus*, anaerobes, gram-negative organisms, tuberculosis, and fungi), septic emboli, and posttraumatic lung contusions/lacerations.

3. The differential diagnosis for multifocal peripheral (ie, subpleural) airspace opacities includes organizing

pneumonia, eosinophilic pneumonia, vasculitis (such as Wegener granulomatosis), septic emboli, and posttraumatic lung contusions. Pulmonary infarction in the context of pulmonary embolism is peripheral as well, but multifocality is unusual (ie, usually one or two). If the opacities are rounded and well defined, metastases and necrobiotic nodules of rheumatoid arthritis can be included.

4. Both the "halo sign" and the "reverse halo sign" can be seen with WG.

5. The c-ANCA serology is more sensitive and specific for WG. Positivity for p-ANCA can be seen in WG and several other vasculitides (including microscopic polyangiitis and Churg-Strauss syndrome).

Pearls

- In general, clinical presentations hinting to the diagnosis of vasculitis are diffuse pulmonary hemorrhage, acute glomerulonephritis, chronic refractory sinusitis or rhinorrhea, mononeuritis multiplex, and palpable purpura.
- There has been a recent ban on the term WG, due to the Nazi past of Dr Wegener, and the new accepted term is granulomatosis with polyangiitis.
- Increased parenchymal attenuation in WG can be a result of any of the following: parenchymal inflammation, pulmonary hemorrhage, organizing pneumonia, superadded infection, or mosaic attenuation secondary to airway or vascular diseases.
- WG can be a cause of persistent/chronic airspace disease.

Suggested Readings

Chung MP, Yi CA, Lee HY, Han J, Lee KS. Imaging of pulmonary vasculitis. *Radiology*. May 2010;255(2):322-341.

Marten K, Schnyder P, Schirg E, Prokop M, Rummeny EJ, Engelke C. Pattern-based differential diagnosis in pulmonary vasculitis using volumetric CT. *AJR Am J Roentgenol*. March 2005;184(3):720-733.

Mayberry JP, Primack SL, Müller NL. Thoracic manifestations of systemic autoimmune diseases: radiographic and high-resolution CT findings. *Radiographics*. November-December 2000;20(6):1623-1635.

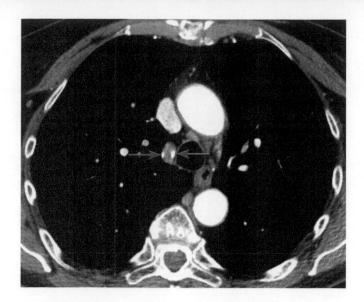

1. What are the arrows pointing at?

2. Why are the azygos valves hyperdense on this image?

3. How many cusps is the azygos valve composed of?

4. What are the factors that can increase the possibility of IV contrast refluxing into the azygos arch?

5. How do the azygos valve appear on unenhanced CT?

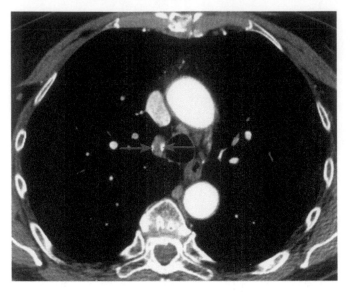

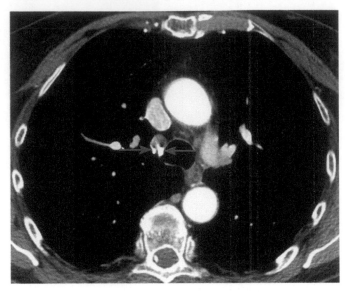

Two small rounded high-density areas are seen within the azygos arch (*arrows*).

A lower CT image shows that the two dense structures assume a cup-shaped appearance and demonstrate blood-contrast levels (*arrows*).

Answers

1. The arrows are pointing at the azygos valve.

2. The azygos valve is hyperdense on this image due to intravenous contrast refluxing into the azygos arch.

3. The azygos valve is bicuspid.

4. Higher contrast injection rates, shorter scanning delays, and right arm injections are factors that increase the chance of azygos arch veins visualization (secondary to increased chance of IV contrast refluxing into the azygos arch).

5. On an unenhanced CT, the azygos valve is not apparent, since it has the same soft tissue attenuation as the rest of the azygos arch.

Pearls

- Azygos arch valve may show dense contrast accumulation on contrast-enhanced CT.
- Opacified azygos valve may be mistaken for calcified lymph nodes or mediastinal masses.
- Knowledge of the typical location and appearances of the azygos arch valve, combined with proper window settings, would help avoid misinterpretation. Additionally, the noncalcified nature of the azygos valve can be confirmed on an unenhanced CT.

Suggested Readings

Ichikawa T, Endo J, Koizumi J, et al. Visualization of the azygos arch valves on multidetector-row computed tomography. *Heart Vessels*. March 2008;23(2):118-123.

Yeh BM, Coakley FV, Sanchez HC, Wilson MW, Reddy GP, Gotway MB. Azygos arch valves: prevalence and appearance at contrast-enhanced CT. *Radiology*. January 2004;230(1):111-115.

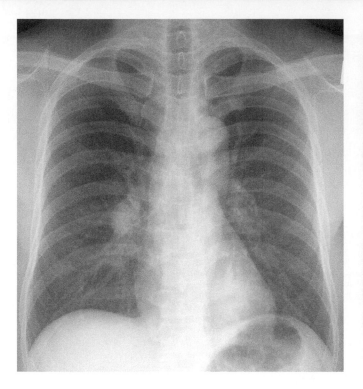
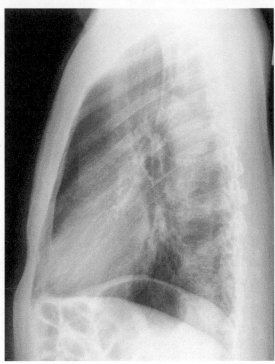

1. What is the imaging finding?

2. What is the differential diagnosis based on the main imaging finding?

3. What are the two broad categories of lung cancer?

4. What is the most common type of lung cancer?

5. Which type of cells gives origin to small cell lung cancer?

Case ranking/difficulty:

Category: Lungs

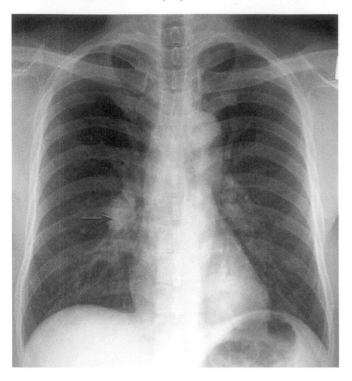

An abnormal well-defined and homogeneous right hilar density is present (*arrow*).

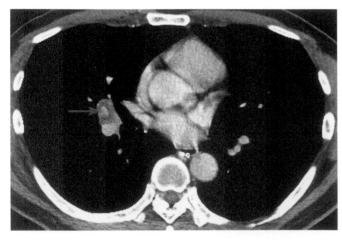

An irregular well-defined hypodense right hilar lesion is seen (*arrow*), with a central irregular hyperdense area that may represent contrast enhancement or calcifications. A feeding tube was placed (*arrowhead*), since the patient had severe locked jaw precluding normal feeding (a symptom that was later attributed to a paraneoplastic condition known as 'stiff man syndrome').

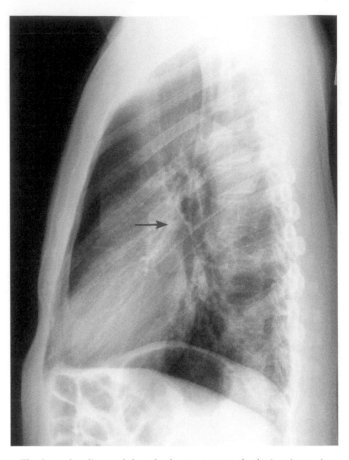

The lateral radiograph barely demonstrates the lesion (*arrow*).

Answers

1. An abnormal well-defined and homogeneous right hilar density is present.

2. The main causes of a unilateral hilar mass lesion include neoplastic (eg, lung cancer, carcinoid, metastasis, or lymphoma), infectious (eg, tuberculous, fungal, or bacterial organisms), inflammatory (ie, atypical sarcoid presentation).

3. Lung cancers are generally divided into nonsmall cell lung cancers (which include adenocarcinoma, squamous cell carcinoma, and large cell carcinoma) and small cell lung cancers.

4. Adenocarcinoma is the most common lung cancer type.

5. Small cell lung cancer arises from bronchial mucosal Kulchitsky neuroendocrine cells.

Pearls

- On chest radiography, the hila should be routinely assessed in terms of size, contour, position, and density.
- Evaluating for the symmetry of the hilar density is as important as assessing the other parameters.
- Lung cancers are divided into nonsmall cell and small cell types.
- Small cell lung cancer is the most aggressive lung cancer type and presents with local or distant metastases in the majority of patients.

Suggested Readings

Chong S, Lee KS, Chung MJ, Han J, Kwon OJ, Kim TS. Neuroendocrine tumors of the lung: clinical, pathologic, and imaging findings. *Radiographics*. January-February 2006;26(1):41-57; discussion 57-58.

Kazarian M, Laird-Offringa IA. Small-cell lung cancer-associated autoantibodies: potential applications to cancer diagnosis, early detection, and therapy. *Mol Cancer*. 2011;10(10):33.

UyBico SJ, Wu CC, Suh RD, Le NH, Brown K, Krishnam MS. Lung cancer staging essentials: the new TNM staging system and potential imaging pitfalls. *Radiographics*. September 2010;30(5):1163-1181.

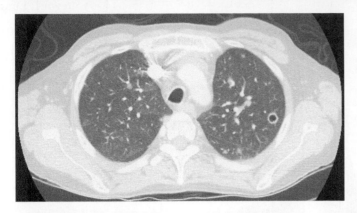
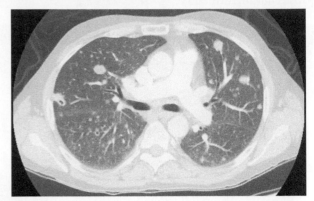
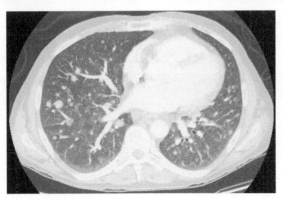
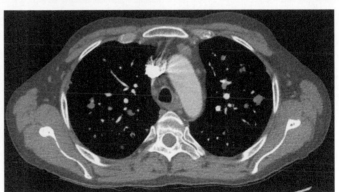

1. What are the CT findings?

2. What is the differential diagnosis in this HIV patient based on the CT findings?

3. What defines AIDS in an HIV-positive individual?

4. What type of lymphoma is more commonly seen in AIDS patients?

5. Is Hodgkin lymphoma an AIDS-defining illness?

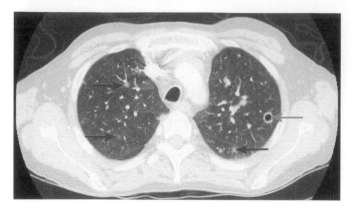

A thin-walled cavity is seen in the left upper lobe (*green arrow*) and small nodules are noted bilaterally (*red arrows*).

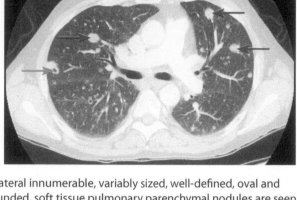

Bilateral innumerable, variably sized, well-defined, oval and rounded, soft tissue pulmonary parenchymal nodules are seen (*red arrows*), some of which show central cavitation (*green arrows*).

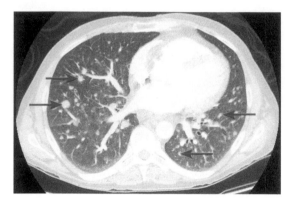

The bilateral nodules are also seen in this lower lung image (*arrows*).

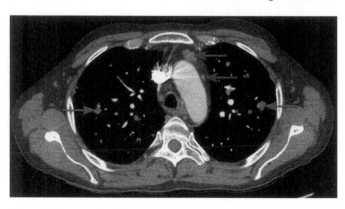

The nodules are of soft tissue attenuation (*red arrows*). Mediastinal lymph node enlargement is also noted (*blue arrows*).

Answers

1. Bilateral innumerable, variably sized, well-defined, oval and rounded, soft tissue pulmonary parenchymal nodules are seen, some of which show central cavitation. Mediastinal lymphadenopathy is also present.

2. The differential diagnosis is mainly that of lymphoma, Kaposi sarcoma, metastases, infection (eg, cytomegalovirus, mycobacterial, or fungal pneumonia), and septic emboli.

3. AIDS is diagnosed in HIV-seropositive individuals if the CD4 count is < 200 cells/mm³ or an AIDS-defining illness is acquired. AIDS-defining illnesses can be infectious (eg, *Pneumocystis jiroveci* pneumonia, cytomegalovirus, or Kaposi sarcoma) or noninfectious (eg, lymphoma).

4. Most of AIDS-related lymphomas are non-Hodgkin, high-grade B-cell type.

5. In contrast to non-Hodgkin lymphoma, the Hodgkin lymphoma type is not considered an AIDS-defining disease.

Pearls

- It is important to consider CD4 counts when interpreting imaging findings in HIV patients.
- AIDS-related lymphoma is commonly non-Hodgkin, of high-grade B-cell type, extranodal, and disseminated.
- In contrast to non-Hodgkin lymphoma, the Hodgkin lymphoma type is not considered an AIDS-defining disease.

Suggested Readings

Eisner MD, Kaplan LD, Herndier B, Stulbarg MS. The pulmonary manifestations of AIDS-related non-Hodgkin's lymphoma. *Chest*. September 1996;110(3):729-736.

Levine AM. Management of AIDS-related lymphoma. *Curr Opin Oncol*. September 2008;20(5):522-528.

Shah RM, Kaji AV, Ostrum BJ, Friedman AC. Interpretation of chest radiographs in AIDS patients: usefulness of CD4 lymphocyte counts. *Radiographics*. January-February 1997;17(1):47-58; discussion 59-61. Erratum in: *Radiographics* May-June 1997;17(3):804.

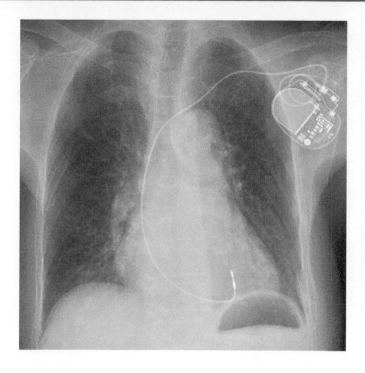
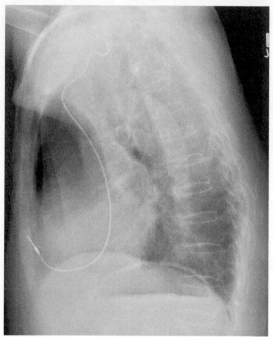

1. What is the most important radiographic finding in this patient?

2. List a few complications of pacemaker insertion.

3. What is twiddler's syndrome?

4. What is postcardiotomy syndrome?

5. What cardiac chamber is most commonly involved by pacemaker lead perforation?

Case ranking/difficulty:

Category: Basic interpretation

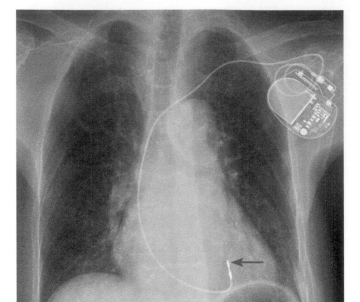

Although the integrity and course of the pacemaker lead are normal, the tip shows an unusual acute angle upward curvature (*arrow*). Cardiomegaly is also noted.

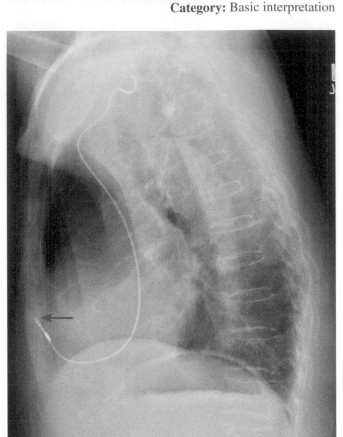

The lateral projection shows that the lead tip is clearly situated beyond the confines of the cardiac shadow and projects within the subcutaneous tissues of the anterior chest (*arrow*).

Answers

1. The tip of the pacemaker lead has an acute angle upward curvature and projects within the subcutaneous tissues of the anterior chest, denoting cardiac perforation by the lead.

2. Complications related to pacemaker insertion include lead malpositioning, lead dislodgment, lead fracture, pneumothorax, hemothorax, hemopericardium, pericardial tamponade, twiddler's syndrome, postcardiotomy syndrome, and infection.

3. Manipulation (usually rotation) by the patient of the pulse generator in its subcutaneous pocket might lead to proximal winding of the lead and tip dislodgment, known as twiddler's syndrome.

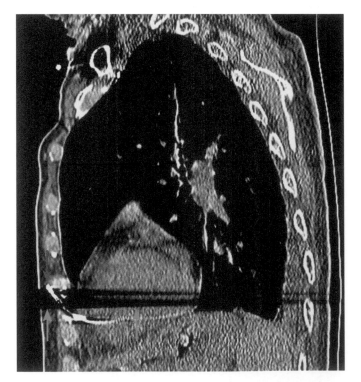

Sagittal reformat of a non-ECG-synchronized CT demonstrating pacemaker lead perforating the right ventricle, with the tip that resides in the anterior chest subcutaneous tissue (*red arrow*). Note the associated metallic-beam hardening artifacts (*green arrows*).

4. Postcardiotomy syndrome is a rare condition presumed to represent an autoimmune reaction secondary to pericardial injury. It is classically seen after surgery, but can be seen after myocardial infarction (in which case it is known as Dressler syndrome), coronary stenting, cardiac trauma, or pacemaker insertion. The condition presents as a painful febrile illness with a pericardial effusion.

5. The right atrial wall is the most common site of pacemaker lead perforation.

Pearls

- Permanent pacemakers and Implantable cardioverter defibrillators (ICDs) can be differentiated by the presence of a dense "shock coil" component on the lead. Both devices can be called cardiovascular implantable electronic devices (CIEDs) or cardiac conductive devices (CCDs) for the sake of simplicity.
- Evaluation of the position of a CIED is not complete unless both PA and lateral projections are available.
- A contralateral pneumothorax in the context of a newly inserted CIED raises the possibility of multiple bilateral insertion attempts or cardiac perforation with associated lung injury.

Suggested Readings

Lanzman RS, Winter J, Blondin D, et al. Where does it lead? Imaging features of cardiovascular implantable electronic devices on chest radiograph and CT. *Korean J Radiol.* September-October 2011;12(5):611-619.

Steiner RM, Tegtmeyer CJ, Morse D, et al. The radiology of cardiac pacemakers. *Radiographics.* May 1986;6(3): 373-399.

Takasugi JE, Godwin JD, Bardy GH. The implantable pace-maker-cardioverter-defibrillator: radiographic aspects. *Radiographics.* November 1994;14(6):1275-1290.

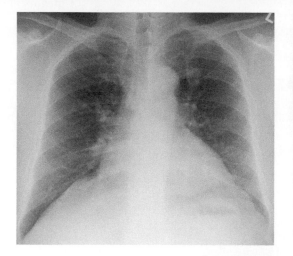

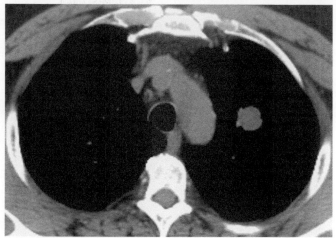

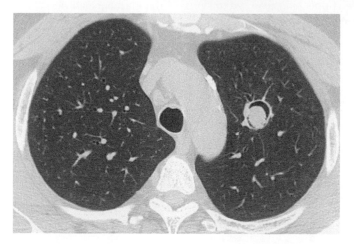

1. What are the radiographic findings?

2. What are the CT findings?

3. What is the differential diagnosis for an air-crescent sign?

4. What is "Monod sign?"

5. In which part of the lung does aspergilloma develop?

Case ranking/difficulty:

Category: Lungs

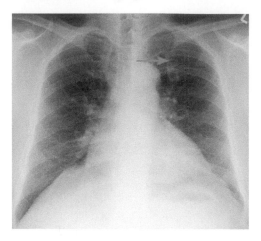

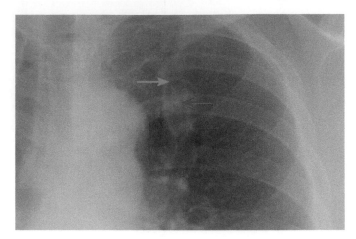

There is a nodular opacity in the left upper lung zone (*red arrow*), with a surrounding crescent of lucency (*green arrow*).

This is a magnified view of the abnormality (*red arrow*), which better shows the "air crescent sign" (*green arrow*).

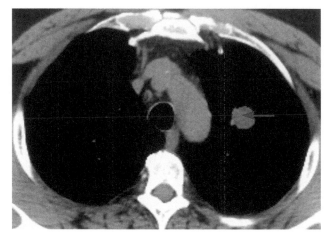

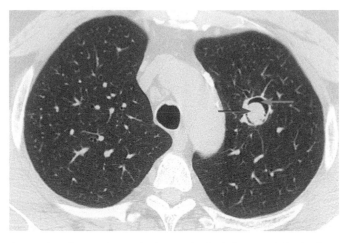

The left upper lobe abnormality is of homogenous soft tissue attenuation on CT (*arrow*).

A round and smooth opacity is seen in the left upper lobe (*red arrow*). The opacity is dependent within a thin-walled cavity, resulting in an "air crescent sign" (*green arrow*).

Answers

1. The radiograph shows a nodular opacity in the left upper lung zone, with a surrounding crescent of lucency.

2. The CT shows a round, smooth, homogenous, and soft tissue-attenuated opacity in the left upper lobe, residing in a dependent location within a thin-walled cavity, resulting in an "air crescent sign."

3. An air crescent can be seen in cases of aspergilloma, invasive aspergillosis, hydatid cyst, lung carcinoma, Rasmussen aneurysm in cavitary tuberculosis, lung abscess, and pulmonary hematoma.

4. "Monod sign" is a description of the lucency that surrounds a fungal ball that resides in a dependent portion of a preexisting lung space. Strictly speaking, "Monod sign" is not synonymous with "air crescent sign," since "air crescent sign" was actual description of necrotizing pneumonia (classically invasive aspergillosis) and not fungal balls.

5. Patients with abnormal preexisting lung parenchymal spaces (cavities, cysts, pneumatoceles, bronchiectasis, bronchogenic cysts, and pulmonary sequestrations) are at risk of developing fungal balls.

Pearls

- Any preexisting abnormal lung space has the potential to grow an aspergilloma.
- Be aware of interval pleural thickening or an increase in cavity/cyst wall thickness as an early sign of aspergilloma.
- Aspergillomas are often asymptomatic.
- In rare cases of life-threatening hemoptysis, aspergilloma may be treated with angioembolization or surgery.

Suggested Readings

Bruzzi JF, Rémy-Jardin M, Delhaye D, Teisseire A, Khalil C, Rémy J. Multi-detector row CT of hemoptysis. *Radiographics*. January-February 2006;26(1):3-22.

Franquet T, Müller NL, Giménez A, Guembe P, de La Torre J, Bagué S. Spectrum of pulmonary aspergillosis: histologic, clinical, and radiologic findings. *Radiographics*. July-August 2001;21(4):825-837.

Marshall GB, Farnquist BA, MacGregor JH, Burrowes PW. Signs in thoracic imaging. *J Thorac Imaging*. March 2006;21(1):76-90.

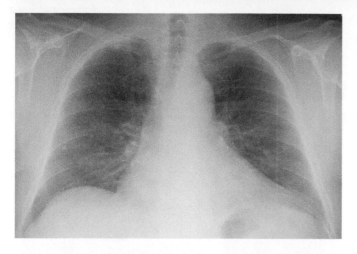
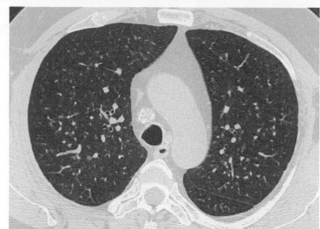
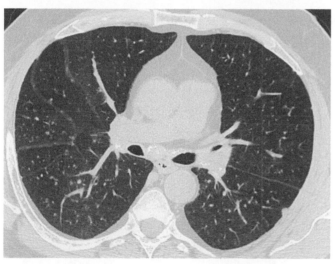
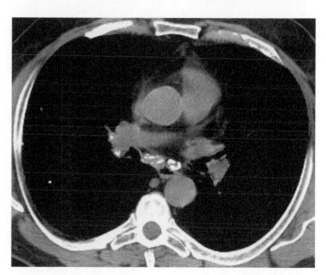

1. What are the radiographic findings?

2. What is the differential diagnosis based on the radiographic findings?

3. What are the CT findings?

4. How is silicosis classified based on imaging appearance?

5. What is Caplan syndrome?

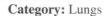

Case ranking/difficulty: 🐾 🐾

Category: Lungs

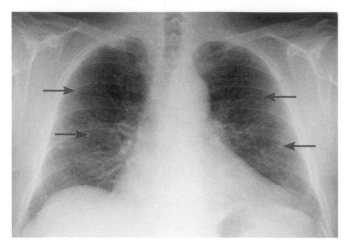

Numerous bilateral small nodular lung parenchymal opacities are present (*arrows*), some of which are of higher density in keeping with calcification. Note that the lung volumes are preserved, the hila appear normal in size, and no pleural effusions are seen.

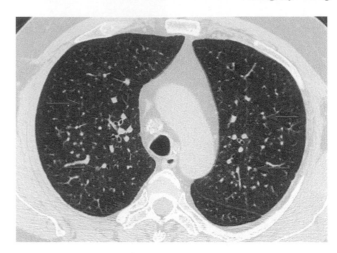

Numerous bilateral small lung parenchymal centrilobular nodules are present (*arrows*), with no volume loss or other fibrotic lung features.

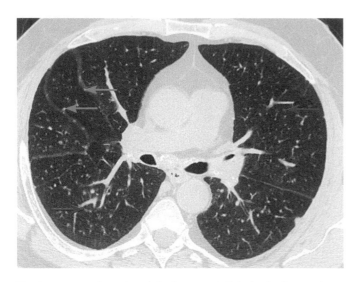

The lung parenchymal nodules have centrilobular (*red arrows*) and perifissural (ie, perilymphatic) (*green arrows*) distributions.

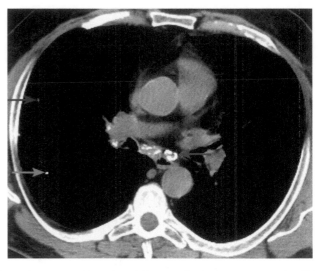

Some lung parenchymal nodules are of soft tissue attenuation (*blue arrow*), whereas others are densely calcified (*green arrow*). Calcified intrathoracic lymph nodes are also seen, with heterogeneous or peripheral (ie, eggshell) patterns of calcification (*red arrow*).

Answers

1. Numerous bilateral small lung nodules are present, some of which are calcified. No fibrotic lung features are present.

2. The differential diagnosis of multiple, small, bilateral, calcific lung nodules is mainly that of infectious granulomas (eg, from tuberculosis or histoplasmosis), sarcoid nodules, pneumoconiosis (eg, silicosis), and metastases (ie, mucin-producing or sarcomatous neoplastic primaries).

3. Numerous bilateral centrilobular and perilymphatic lung nodules are seen, some having soft tissue attenuation,

and some calcified. Heterogeneous and peripheral (ie, eggshell) lymph nodes calcifications are present as well.

4. Based on the nodular size of less or more than 1 cm, silicosis is classified as simple or complicated (ie, progressive massive fibrosis) forms.

5. Caplan syndrome is a syndrome of pneumoconiosis that coexists with rheumatoid arthritis. Thus, both rheumatic (ie, necrobiotic) nodules and silicotic nodules can be seen in patients with Caplan syndrome.

Pearls

- Many patients with occupational lung diseases are exposed to several pathogenic agents; thus, silicosis may coexist with other pneumoconioses (eg, asbestosis).
- Eggshell calcification in lymph nodes is highly suggestive of silicosis, but can occur with sarcoidosis, tuberculosis, histoplasmosis, and treated lymphoma.
- Silicosis patients are at a higher risk of developing tuberculosis and lung cancer.

Suggested Readings

Chong S, Lee KS, Chung MJ, Han J, Kwon OJ, Kim TS. Pneumoconiosis: comparison of imaging and pathologic findings. *Radiographics*. January-February 2006;26(1):59-77.

Marchiori E, Souza CA, Barbassa TG, Escuissato DL, Gasparetto EL, Souza AS. Silicoproteinosis: high-resolution CT findings in 13 patients. *AJR Am J Roentgenol*. December 2007;189(6):1402-1406.

Sirajuddin A, Kanne JP. Occupational lung disease. *J Thorac Imaging*. November 2009;24(4):310-320.

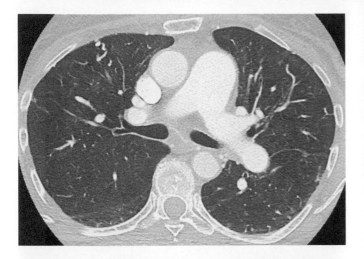
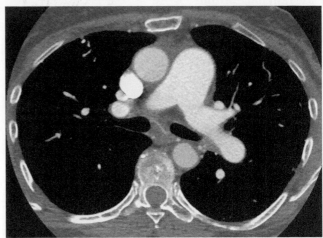
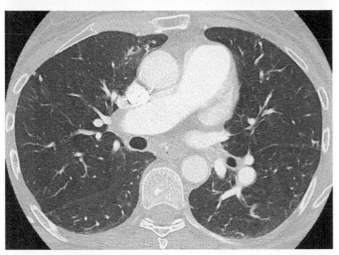
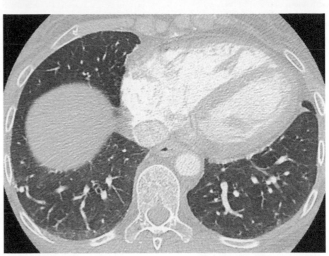

1. What are the CT findings?

2. What is the differential diagnosis?

3. What is the most likely diagnosis?

4. List a few possible sources of systemic arterial
   lung supply.

5. What is the most common source of systemic
   arterial supply to the lungs?

Case ranking/difficulty: **Category:** Lungs

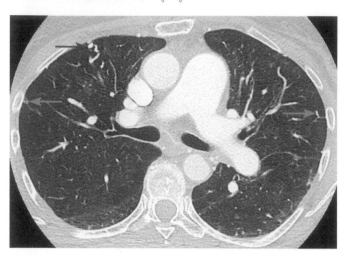

There is a large peripheral intraparenchymal serpentine structure in the right upper lobe (*red arrow*). Similar smaller peripheral abnormalities are also seen bilaterally (*green arrows*).

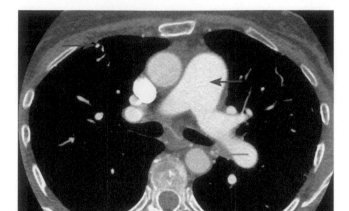

The right upper lobar serpentine abnormality is of aortic-equivalent attenuation (*red arrow*), consistent with an arterial collateral to the lung. There is enlargement of the pulmonary trunk (*blue arrow*) and dilatation of the bronchial arteries (*green arrow*).

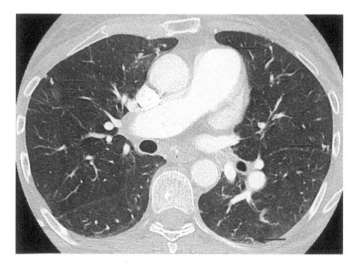

The systemic intraparenchymal arterial collaterals are peripheral (*arrows*).

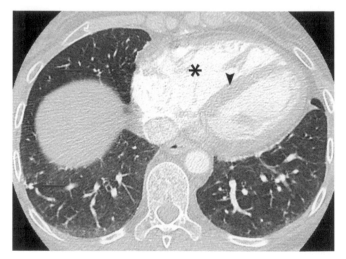

The abnormal intraparenchymal arterial collateral vessels are also seen in the lower lungs (*arrows*). The right ventricle is dilated and hypertrophied (*asterisk*), and the interventricular septum is straightened (*arrowhead*), features denoting right-sided cardiac strain.

Answers

1. Systemic arterial collateral lung supply is present, from both bronchial and nonbronchial arteries. There is dilatation of the pulmonary trunk and signs of right heart strain, all denoting pulmonary arterial hypertension (PAHTN).

2. The abnormal intraparenchymal pulmonary vasculature raises concern for the following entities: long-standing PAHTN, Osler-Weber-Rendu syndrome, and hepatopulmonary syndrome.

3. Given the overall appearance of the abnormal intraparenchymal pulmonary vessels and the associated secondary findings, the final diagnosis is that of systemic arterial collaterals secondary to long-standing PAHTN.

4. Systemic arterial blood supply to the lung can originate from the aorta or from the aortic branches, such, such as bronchial, intercostal, internal thoracic, and inferior phrenic arteries.

5. About 90% of the cases of systemic arterial supply to the lungs are from bronchial arteries.

Pearls

- The lung parenchymal findings in cases of PAHTN include mosaic attenuation, centrilobular ground-glass nodularity, and intraparenchymal systemic arterial collaterals/neovascularity.
- In long-standing PAHTN, the lung commonly shows dilated bronchial arteries, but systemic collaterals from nonbronchial arteries (eg, intercostal arteries) may be seen.
- The nonbronchial systemic pulmonary arterial collaterals in PAHTN should be differentiated from multiple arteriovenous malformations (AVMs) and hepatopulmonary syndrome.

Suggested Readings

Devaraj A, Hansell DM. Computed tomography signs of pulmonary hypertension: old and new observations. *Clin Radiol*. August 2009;64(8):751-760.

Do KH, Goo JM, Im JG, Kim KW, Chung JW, Park JH. Systemic arterial supply to the lungs in adults: spiral CT findings. *Radiographics*. March-April 2001;21(2):387-402.

Tsai IC, Tsai WL, Wang KY, et al. Comprehensive MDCT evaluation of patients with pulmonary hypertension: diagnosing underlying causes with the updated Dana Point 2008 classification. *AJR Am J Roentgenol*. September 2011;197(3):W471-W481.

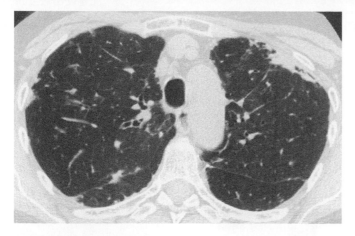
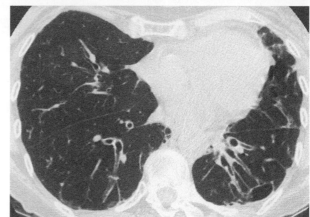
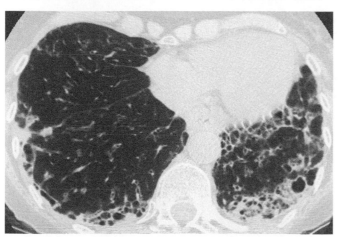
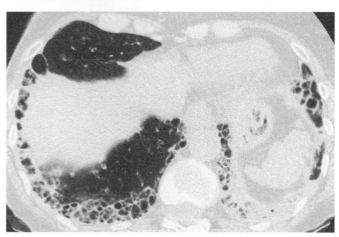

1. What are the CT findings?

2. What is the most likely diagnosis with regard to the presented fibrotic pattern?

3. What are the main causes of a usual interstitial pneumonia (UIP) pattern?

4. What are common patterns of lung involvement in rheumatoid arthritis (RA) patients?

5. What is the difference between follicular bronchiolitis (FB) and lymphocytic interstitial pneumonia (LIP)?

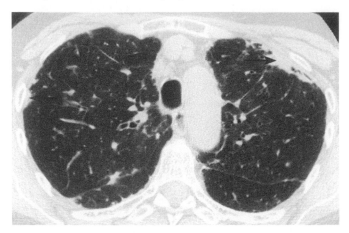

Bilateral multifocal subpleural consolidations are noted (*arrows*), suggesting organizing pneumonia.

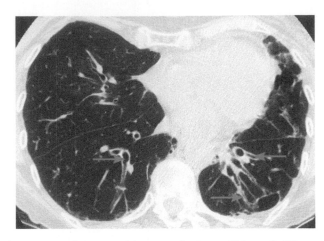

There are small airways changes in the form of bilateral diffuse cylindrical bronchiectasis and bronchial wall thickening (*arrows*).

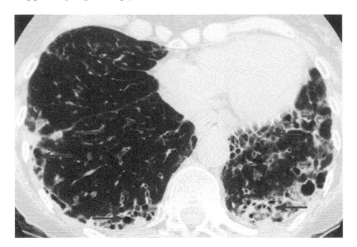

Bilateral basilar predominant areas of peripheral reticulations, architectural distortion, traction bronchiectasis, and volume loss (*arrows*) are seen.

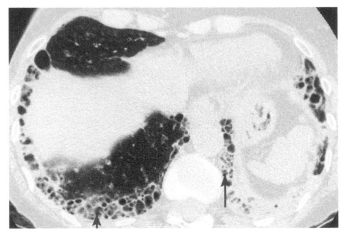

Subpleural stacks of variably sized cystic spaces are seen (*arrows*). These spaces share thin walls and do not communicate with the bronchiectatic airways, in keeping with honeycombing.

Answers

1. Bilateral basilar predominant areas of peripheral reticulations, architectural distortion, traction bronchiectasis, volume loss, and honeycombing are seen. There is bilateral diffuse cylindrical bronchiectasis and bronchial wall thickening. Bilateral multifocal subpleural consolidations are also noted.

2. Since reticulations, architectural distortion, traction bronchiectasis, volume loss, and honeycombing are all present, a usual interstitial pneumonia (UIP) pattern is the likely diagnosis.

3. The main causes of UIP are idiopathic pulmonary fibrosis, end-stage asbestosis, connective tissue disorders, and drug toxicity.

4. Usual interstitial pneumonia, airways changes (eg, bronchiectasis, bronchial wall thickening, mucus plugging, centrilobular nodules, tree-in-bud pattern, mosaic attenuation, and air trapping), and serositis are common thoracic manifestations of RA.

5. The radiology literature is somewhat confusing when it comes to explaining the difference between FB and LIP. In simple terms, both entities are lymphoproliferative disorders. However, the abnormality in FB is mainly centered on the bronchioles (ie, in the centrilobular region). Thus, FB presents with small airways disease features and centrilobular nodularity. In contrast, the lymphatic proliferation in LIP involves the alveolar interstitium in a more diffuse manner (ie, also involves the septa at the periphery of the secondary pulmonary lobule). Thus, LIP presents with septal nodules/thickening, ground-glass opacities, and cysts.

Pearls

- Similar to any other collagen vascular disorder, the thoracic manifestations of RA are a result of the disease itself, superadded infection, or drug toxicities.
- Usual interstitial pneumonia, airways changes, and serositis are common thoracic manifestations of RA.
- Focal airspace disease (ie, consolidation or ground-glass opacities) in RA can be a result of organizing pneumonia or infection.
- Necrobiotic (rheumatoid) nodules is an extremely rare RA lung manifestation that typically occurs late in the course of the disease.

Suggested Readings

Capobianco J, Grimberg A, Thompson BM, Antunes VB, Jasinowodolinski D, Meirelles GS. Thoracic manifestations of collagen vascular diseases. *Radiographics*. January-February 2012;32(1):33-50.

Kim EA, Lee KS, Johkoh T, et al. Interstitial lung diseases associated with collagen vascular diseases: radiologic and histopathologic findings. *Radiographics*. October 2002;22 Spec No:S151-S165.

Lynch DA. Lung disease related to collagen vascular disease. *J Thorac Imaging*. November 2009;24(4):299-309.

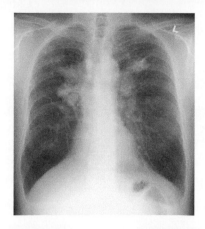
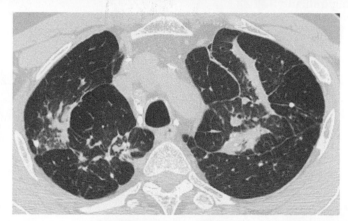
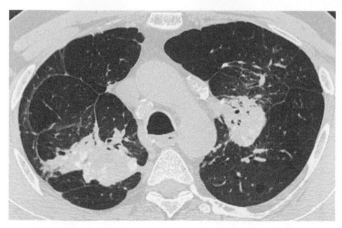
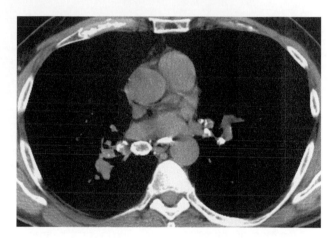

1. What are the radiographic findings?

2. What is the likely diagnosis based on the radiographic findings?

3. What are the CT findings?

4. What is the differential diagnosis based on the CT findings?

5. What does cavitation in progressive massive fibrosis (PMF) opacities usually indicate?

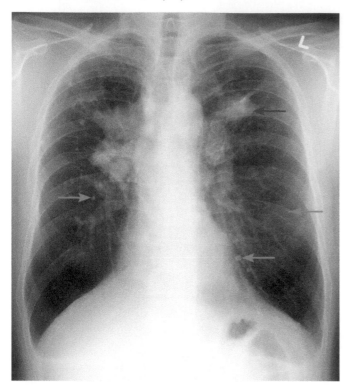

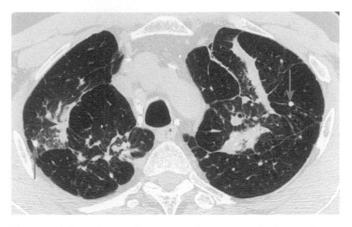

Bilateral paramediastinal, near-symmetric, relatively well-defined, irregular lung parenchymal opacities are seen (*red arrows*). The hila are elevated, in keeping with local volume loss. The lower lung zones are hyperlucent, likely due to compensatory hyperinflation. There are a few bilateral scattered small calcified lung nodules (*green arrows*).

There are bilateral upper lungs irregular opacities (*red arrows*) and associated fibrotic changes. Scattered small nodules are seen bilaterally as well (*green arrows*).

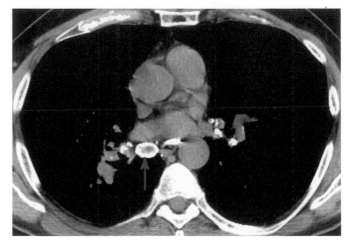

Bilateral calcified hilar and mediastinal lymph nodes are seen, with one enlarged lymph node demonstrating eggshell calcification (*arrow*).

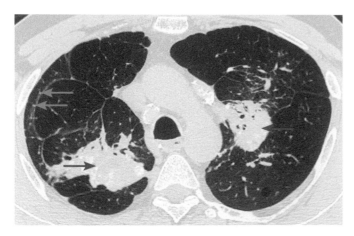

The size of the bilateral confluent lung opacities (*red arrows*) exceeds 1 cm, consistent with complicated silicosis. There are small perilymphatic nodules as well (*green arrows*).

Answers

1. Bilateral paramediastinal, irregular, relatively well-defined, lung parenchymal opacities are seen, with features of local lung volume loss. The lower lung zones show compensatory hyperinflation. There are a few bilateral scattered small calcified lung nodules as well.

2. Progressive massive fibrosis (PMF) is the most likely diagnosis.

3. There are large bilateral upper lung irregular opacities, with adjacent fibrotic changes and bilateral scattered small lung nodules. Bilateral calcified hilar and mediastinal lymph nodes are seen, with one lymph node demonstrating eggshell calcification.

4. The differential diagnosis of PMF is generally that of pneumoconiosis (eg, silicosis, coal worker's pneumoconiosis, hard-metal exposure, berylliosis, etc.) and injected or inhaled talcosis, but sarcoidosis is a known mimicker.

5. Cavitation in PMF denotes ischemic necrosis or superadded tuberculosis.

Pearls

- A 1 cm cutoff for size is the difference between simple versus complex silicosis on CT. When the opacities are >1 cm, the condition is referred to as "complicated silicosis" (also known as PMF).
- Cavitation in PMF can occur due to ischemic necrosis or superadded tuberculosis.
- MRI may be used to help differentiate PMF from lung cancer. Typically, PMF has low T2 signal intensity, whereas cancer has high T2 signal intensity.

Suggested Readings

Chong S, Lee KS, Chung MJ, Han J, Kwon OJ, Kim TS. Pneumoconiosis: comparison of imaging and pathologic findings. *Radiographics*. January-February 2006;26(1):59-77.

Marchiori E, Souza CA, Barbassa TG, Escuissato DL, Gasparetto EL, Souza AS. Silicoproteinosis: high-resolution CT findings in 13 patients. *AJR Am J Roentgenol*. December 2007;189(6):1402-1406.

Sirajuddin A, Kanne JP. Occupational lung disease. *J Thorac Imaging*. November 2009;24(4):310-320.

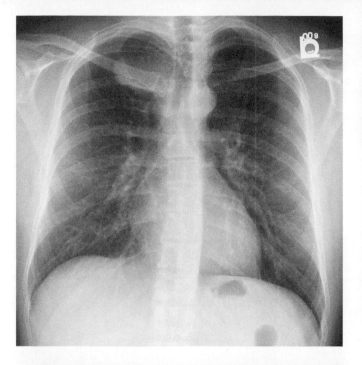

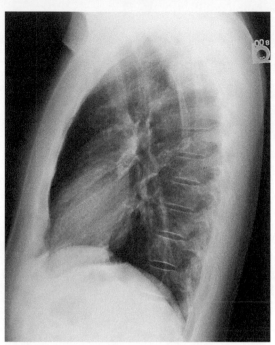

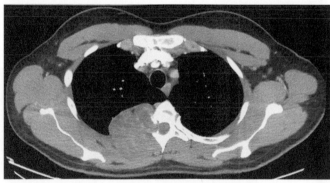

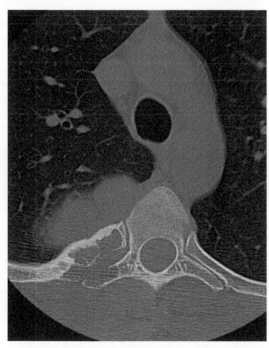

1. What are the radiographic findings?

2. What are the CT findings?

3. What is the differential diagnosis?

4. What is the most common posterior mediastinal tumor?

5. What is the most common intrathoracic neurogenic tumor?

Case ranking/difficulty: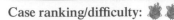

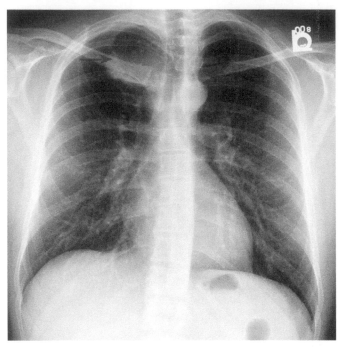

A homogenous and well-defined oval opacity projects over the medial right upper lung (*red arrow*), with no obvious cavitation or calcification. The superior cortex of the medial posterior right fifth rib is not well delineated (*green arrowhead*) and the adjacent intercostal space is splayed, denoting a posterior mediastinal location. It is difficult to assess the status of the adjacent thoracic vertebral body on this frontal radiograph.

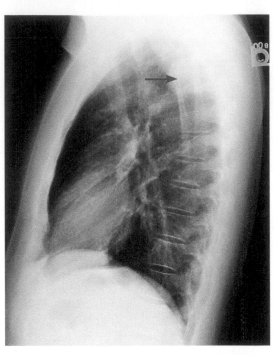

The lesion has a paravertebral location on this lateral chest radiograph (*arrow*).

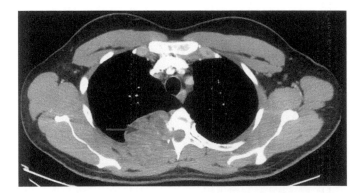

There is a large and heterogeneous right paravertebral mass of soft tissue density (*red arrow*), extending into the epidural spinal canal via a widened right neural foramen (*green arrowhead*) and exerting mild mass effect on the spinal cord.

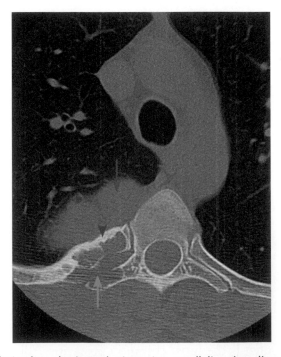

The lesion has a horizontal orientation, paralleling the adjacent rib (*red arrow*). The adjacent right vertebral transverse process and posterior rib are involved by expansile lytic osseous abnormalities (*green arrow*). Note that there are areas of osseous scalloping and hyperostosis (*blue arrowhead*), suggesting a long-standing abnormality.

Answers

1. There is a well-defined opacity in the medial right upper lung. The superior cortex of the medial part of the underlying rib is not well delineated.

2. There is a heterogeneous right paravertebral mass of soft tissue density, extending into the epidural spinal canal via a widened right neural foramen and exerting mild mass effect on the spinal cord. The adjacent vertebral transverse process and rib show expansile lytic changes. There is scalloping and hyperostosis of the involved rib as well.

3. The differential diagnosis of the presented abnormality includes neurogenic tumors, metastasis, multiple myeloma, sarcomas, and lymphoma.

4. Neurogenic tumors are considered the most common posterior mediastinal tumors.

5. Schwannomas are the most common intrathoracic neurogenic tumors.

Pearls

- A horizontal orientation paralleling an adjacent rib favors a peripheral nerve sheath tumor over other posterior mediastinal neurogenic tumors.
- Posterior mediastinal neurogenic tumors are commonly associated with long-standing bone changes, such as osseous scalloping and widened neural foramen.
- MRI is a useful tool in evaluating mediastinal neurogenic tumors and may show intraspinal extension as a "dumbbell shape" appearance.

Suggested Readings

De Waele M, Carp L, Lauwers P, Hendriks J, De Maeseneer M, Van Schil P, Blockx P. Paravertebral schwannoma with high uptake of fluorodeoxyglucose on positron emission tomography. *Acta Chir Belg*. September-October 2005;105(5):537-538.

Fierro N, D'ermo G, Di Cola G, Gallinaro LS, Galassi G, Galassi G. Posterior mediastinal schwannoma. *Asian Cardiovasc Thorac Ann*. March 2003;11(1):72-73.

Nakazono T, White CS, Yamasaki F, et al. MRI findings of mediastinal neurogenic tumors. *AJR Am J Roentgenol*. October 2011;197(4):W643-W652.

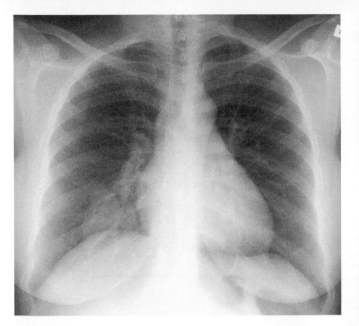
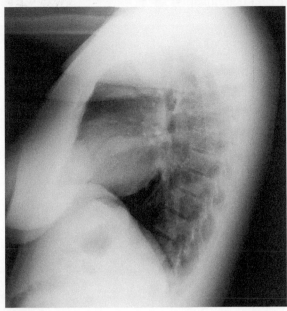
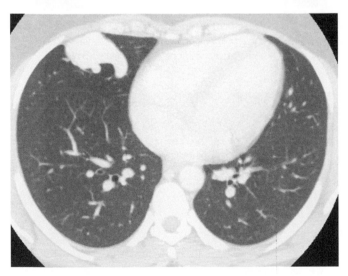
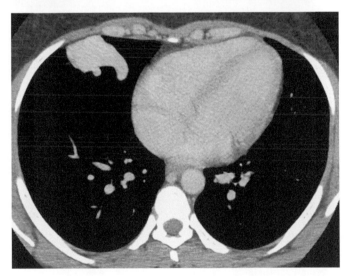

1. What are the radiographic findings?

2. What are the CT findings?

3. What is the final diagnosis?

4. What is the difference between a pulmonary arteriovenous malformation (AVM) and a pulmonary venous varix?

5. Which imaging finding was typically considered an indication for coil embolization of a pulmonary AVM?

Case ranking/difficulty:

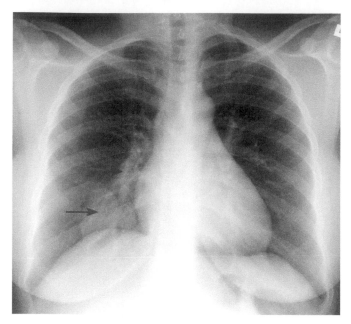

A well-defined opacity projects over the right lower lung zone (*arrow*). There is no obscuration of the adjacent hemidiaphragm, in keeping with a right middle lobe location. A large tubular opacity is seen in the right hilar region (*arrowhead*).

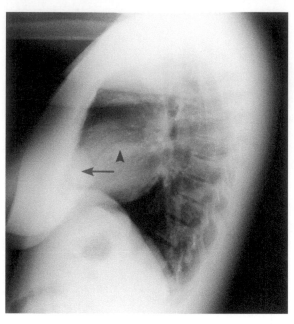

The lesion is seen in a middle lobe location on the lateral radiograph (*arrow*). A large tubular opacity is connecting the lesion to the hilum, suggesting a vascular abnormality (*arrowhead*).

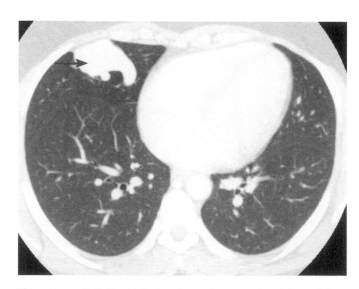

There is a well-defined lobulated mass lesion in the right middle lobe (*arrow*), with no surrounding airspace changes.

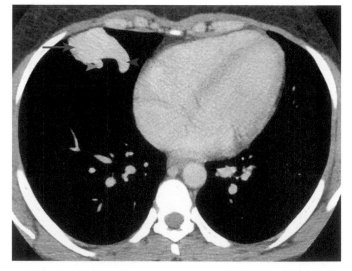

The lesion demonstrates uniform blood-pool-equivalent contrast enhancement (*arrow*). Two associated vascular structures are seen, representing a feeding pulmonary artery (*green arrowhead*) and a dilated draining pulmonary vein (*blue arrowhead*).

Answers

1. There is a well-defined right middle lobe lung opacity, connected to right hilar region by a large tubular density.

2. CT confirms the presence of a vascular enhancing lesion, with a feeding pulmonary artery and a draining vein.

3. The diagnosis is pulmonary arteriovenous malformation.

4. A pulmonary varix is a dilated vein with no nidus nor feeding artery.

5. The previously accepted indication for treating a pulmonary AVM was the diameter of its feeding vessel in excess of 3 mm. However, the current guidelines recommend treating pulmonary AVMs in adults of any feeding artery size, even if smaller than 3 mm in diameter.

Pearls

- A pulmonary varix is a dilated vein with no nidus nor feeding artery.
- The finding of pulmonary AVM on CT should prompt the search for clinical features of hereditary hemorrhagic telangiectasia.
- The previously accepted indication for treating a pulmonary AVM was the diameter of its feeding vessel in excess of 3 mm, but the new guidelines recommend treating pulmonary AVMs in adults of any feeding artery size.
- Pulmonary AVMs are treated by coil embolization.

Suggested Readings

Jaskolka J, Wu L, Chan RP, Faughnan ME. Imaging of hereditary hemorrhagic telangiectasia. *AJR Am J Roentgenol*. August 2004;183(2):307-314.

Martinez-Jimenez S, Heyneman LE, McAdams HP, et al. Nonsurgical extracardiac vascular shunts in the thorax: clinical and imaging characteristics. *Radiographics*. September 2010;30(5):e41.

Trerotola SO, Pyeritz RE. PAVM embolization: an update. *AJR Am J Roentgenol*. October 2010;195(4):837-845.

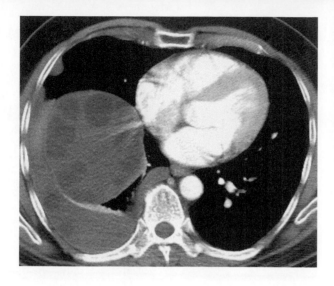
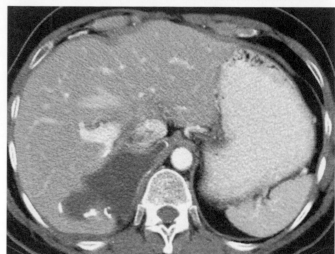

1. What are the imaging findings?

2. What are the two main types of hydatid disease that can affect humans?

3. What is the best modality to delineate intralesional membranes or daughter cysts of thoracic hydatid disease?

4. What is a *giant hydatid cyst*?

5. What is *capitonnage*?

Case ranking/difficulty: **Category:** Chest wall/Extrapleural

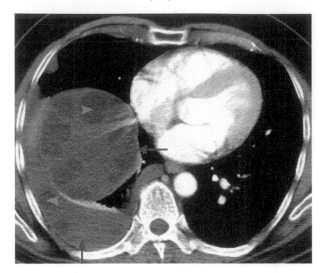

Two large and well-defined fluid-attenuated lesions are based on the right lower hemithoracic pleura (*arrows*). The abnormalities have several internal peripheral lower-attenuation cysts (*arrowheads*).

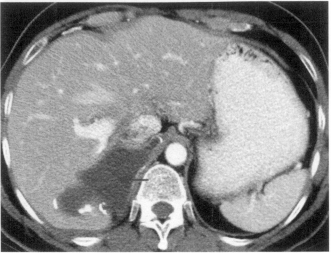

A cystic lesion involves the liver and demonstrates dense peripheral calcifications (*arrow*).

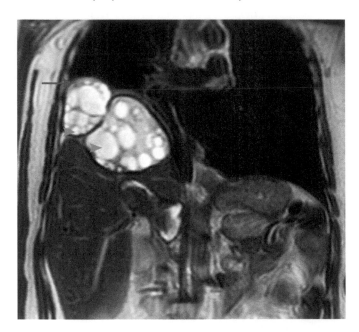

The abnormalities are depicted on this coronal T2-weighted image as intermediate-intensity lesions (*arrow*), with high-intensity internal cysts (*arrowheads*).

Answers

1. Two well-defined fluid-attenuated right pleural lesions are seen, with several internal peripheral lower-attenuation cysts. Additionally, a cystic lesion involves the liver and demonstrates dense peripheral calcifications.

2. The two main forms of hydatid disease that affect humans are caused by the parasites *Echinococcus granulosus* and *Echinococcus multilocularis*.

3. MRI is the best modality to delineate intralesional membranes or daughter cysts of thoracic hydatid disease.

4. Due to the soft and elastic consistency of the lung parenchyma, intraparenchymal hydatid cysts can grow to a large size in a short interval. Lesions 10 cm or larger are termed *giant hydatid cysts*.

5. Capitonnage is a procedure where a cystic cavity is obliterated by suturing opposing cyst walls together. This is considered an option in treating hydatid cysts.

Pearls

- Two types of parasites causing hydatid disease can affect humans and have different epidemiology: *Echinococcus granulosus* and *Echinococcus multilocularis*.
- Human infection by *Echinococcus* occurs by contact with a definite host (ie, carnivores) or by ingesting contaminated fluids or food.
- Similar to many other parasitic infestations, eosinophilia may be encountered with hydatid infection.

Suggested Readings

Martínez S, Restrepo CS, Carrillo JA, Betancourt SL, Franquet T, Varón C, Ojeda P, Giménez A. Thoracic manifestations of tropical parasitic infections: a pictorial review. *Radiographics*. January-February 2005;25(1):135-155.

Pedrosa I, Saíz A, Arrazola J, Ferreirós J, Pedrosa CS. Hydatid disease: radiologic and pathologic features and complications. *Radiographics*. May-June 2000;20(3):795-817.

Zylak CJ, Eyler WR, Spizarny DL, Stone CH. Developmental lung anomalies in the adult: radiologic-pathologic correlation. *Radiographics*. October 2002;22 Spec No:S25-S43.

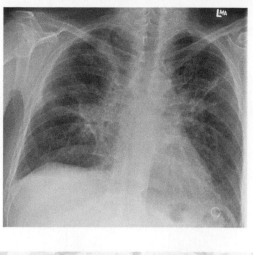
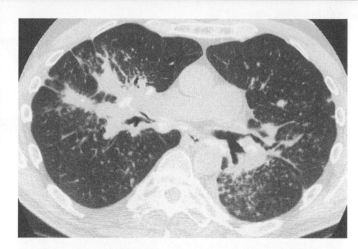
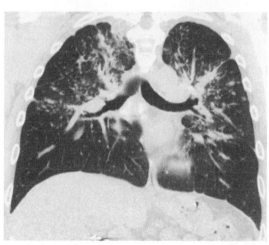
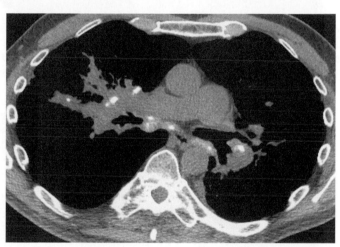

1. What are the chest radiographic findings?

2. What are the chest CT findings?

3. What is the differential diagnosis based on the overall imaging findings?

4. What is the differential diagnosis of calcified hilar lymph nodes?

5. What is the likely diagnosis in this presented case?

Case ranking/difficulty:

Category: Lungs

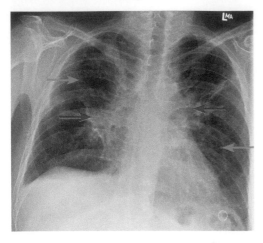

Bilateral irregular and confluent lung parenchymal opacities are present, in a perihilar distribution with extension into the upper and midlung zones (*red arrows*). A faint coarse reticulonodular background is seen (*green arrows*). The hila are elevated and mid upper lung volume loss is noted. A left nipple ring is seen.

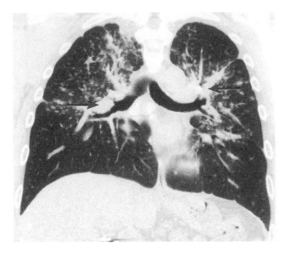

This is a coronal demonstration of the upper and midlung predominant peribronchovascular lung parenchymal abnormalities that radiate toward the periphery (*arrows*). The hila are elevated due to fibrosis.

Answers

1. The radiograph shows bilateral irregular perihilar lung parenchymal opacities in the upper and midlung zones, with hilar elevation and volume loss. A faint coarse reticulonodular background is also seen.

2. Bilateral upper and midlung peribronchovascular confluent irregular opacities are seen on CT and are associated with perilymphatic nodularity and fibrotic features. Heterogeneously calcified hilar and mediastinal lymph nodes are also present.

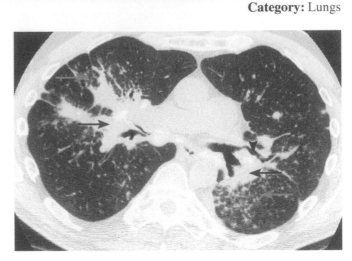

There are bilateral peribronchovascular confluent irregular opacities (*red arrows*). The abnormality is associated with surrounding perilymphatic nodularity (*green arrows*). In addition, associated traction bronchiectasis (*arrowhead*) and architectural distortion are present.

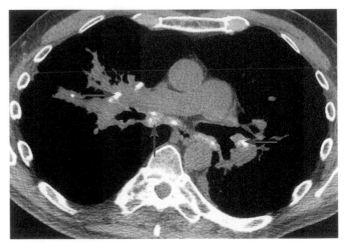

Heterogeneously calcified hilar and mediastinal lymph nodes are present (*arrows*).

3. The possible causes of a bilateral fibrotic upper lung parenchymal process include sarcoidosis, pneumoconiosis (such as silicosis, coal workers pneumoconiosis), infections (such as remote tuberculosis or fungal infections), hypersensitivity pneumonitis, radiation fibrosis, and ankylosing spondylitis.

4. The differential diagnosis of calcified hilar lymph nodes is mainly that of infections (such as remote tuberculosis or fungal infections), sarcoidosis, pneumoconiosis (such as silicosis, coal workers pneumoconiosis), and treated lymphoma (ie, after radiotherapy or chemotherapy).

5. Since perilymphatic nodularity is seen in this case, sarcoidosis should be the main diagnostic consideration.

Pearls

- Sarcoidosis is typically an upper lung parenchymal disease.
- Sarcoidosis is typically a bilateral and symmetric lung parenchymal disease.
- Sarcoidosis may manifest as perihilar parenchymal lung abnormalities that radiate peripherally.

Suggested Readings

Criado E, Sánchez M, Ramírez J, et al. Pulmonary sarcoidosis: typical and atypical manifestations at high-resolution CT with pathologic correlation. *Radiographics*. October 2010;30(6):1567-1586.

Kanne JP, Yandow DR, Haemel AK, Meyer CA. Beyond skin deep: thoracic manifestations of systemic disorders affecting the skin. *Radiographics*. October 2011;31(6):1651-1668.

Park HJ, Jung JI, Chung MH, Song SW, Kim HL, Baik JH, Han DH, Kim KJ, Lee KY. Typical and atypical manifestations of intrathoracic sarcoidosis. *Korean J Radiol*. November-December 2009;10(6):623-631.

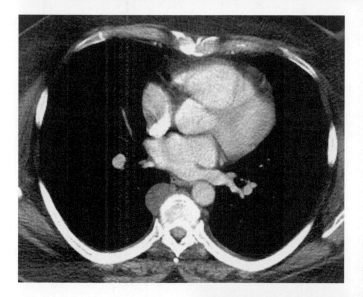

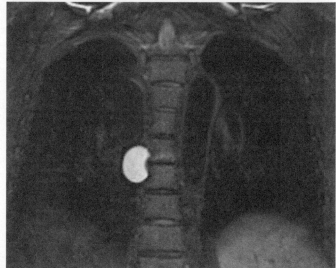

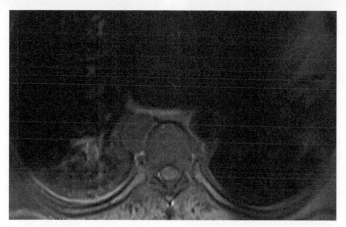

1. Where is the abnormality located?

2. What is the most likely composition of the lesion?

3. What is the differential diagnosis?

4. What are the biological properties of this lesion?

5. What are possible complications related to this entity?

Case ranking/difficulty:

Category: Mediastinum

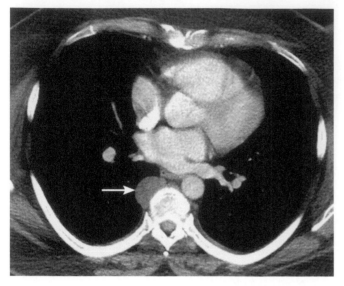

There is a well-defined, fluid-density right paravertebral lesion (*arrow*).

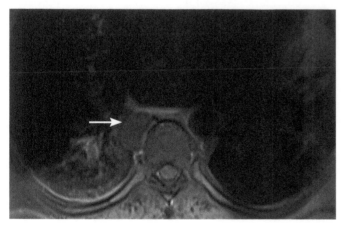

T1 Fat saturated post gadolinium axial MRI images show a well-defined, uniformly hypointense, nonenhancing right paravertebral lesion (*arrow*).

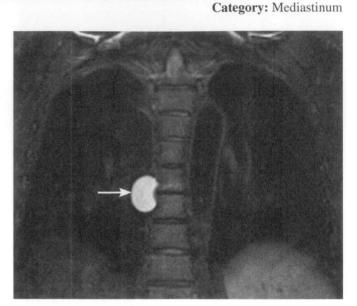

Coronal short tau inversion recovery (STIR) MRI image shows a well-defined, uniformly hyperintense right paravertebral lesion (*arrow*).

5. Possible complications associated with bronchogenic cysts include fistula formation with the bronchial tree, malignant transformation, cough, wheezing, stridor, dyspnea, cyanotic spells, and pneumonia.

Pearls

- Bronchopulmonary foregut malformations include bronchogenic cysts, enteric duplications cysts, and neurenteric cysts.
- Bronchogenic cysts do not communicate with airway.
- Bronchogenic cysts are typically mediastinal, most commonly residing in the subcarinal region.

Answers

1. The lesion is located in the posterior mediastinum.

2. The imaging findings on CT and MRI are consistent with fluid composition.

3. The differential diagnosis should include neurogenic tumors, bronchogenic cyst, foregut duplication cyst, and neurenteric cyst.

4. Pathogenesis of bronchogenic cysts is similar to neurenteric cysts. Initially, they do not communicate with tracheobronchial tree. Most are mediastinal, with subcarinal location being the most common. They are lined by ciliated columnar or cuboidal epithelium.

Suggested Reading

Berrocal T, Madrid C, Novo S, Gutiérrez J, Arjonilla A, Gómez-León N. Congenital anomalies of the tracheobronchial tree, lung, and mediastinum: embryology, radiology, and pathology. *Radiographics*. January-February 2004;24(1):e17.

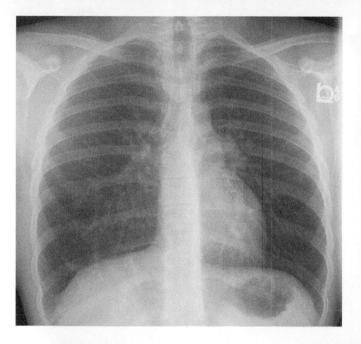

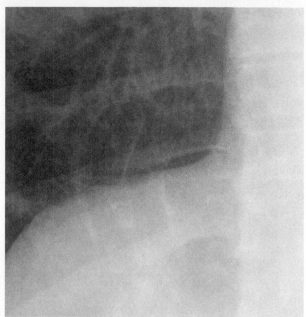

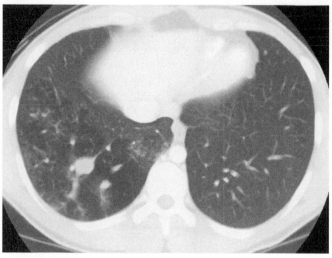

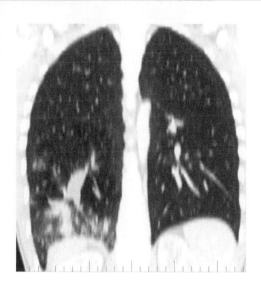

1. What are the findings?

2. What is the most likely diagnosis?

3. What should be included in the differential diagnosis?

4. What congenital pulmonary pathologies can be associated with the abnormality shown in the figures?

5. What is the clinical significance of bronchial atresia?

Case ranking/difficulty:

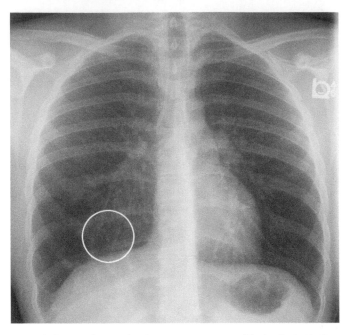

Frontal chest radiography demonstrates a gas-filled tubular lesion with thin walls and rounded superior edge at the right lung base (*circle*).

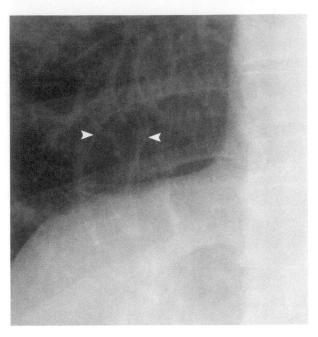

Magnification of the medial aspect of the right lung base better demonstrates the gas-filled tubular lesion with thin walls and rounded superior edge (*arrowheads*).

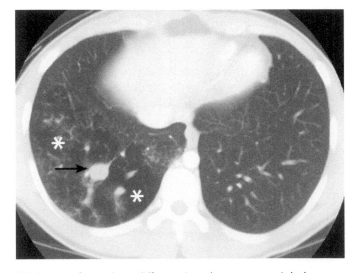

CT chest performed at a different time demonstrates right lower lobe impacted bronchi (*arrow*) and adjacent air trapping (*asterisks*).

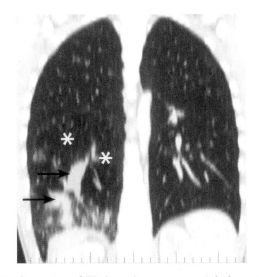

Coronal reformation of CT chest demonstrates right lower lobe dilated, impacted bronchi (*arrows*), and adjacent air trapping (*asterisks*).

Answers

1. Right lung base gas-filled tubular lesion with thin walls and rounded superior edge is demonstrated on chest radiograph. The CT obtained at a different time shows right lower lobe dilated impacted bronchi, which do not communicate with proximal airway. There is adjacent air trapping.

2. Bronchial atresia is the most likely diagnosis given lack of communication of the dilated bronchi with the airway.

3. The differential diagnosis should also include bronchiectasis, foreign body aspiration, allergic bronchopulmonary aspergillosis (ABPA), and endobronchial neoplasm.

4. Bronchial atresia can be associated with congenital lobar emphysema, extralobar and intralobar pulmonary sequestration, and congenital pulmonary airway malformation (CPAM).

5. Most individuals with bronchial atresia are asymptomatic. Dyspnea, recurrent pneumonia, and bronchial asthma can occur.

Pearls

- Classical findings of bronchial atresia (BA) on chest radiography are focal finger in glove opacity (representing dilated, mucous-filled bronchi, which do not communicate with the central airway) and adjacent air trapping appearing as hyperlucency.
- Other causes of focal bronchial dilatation such as foreign body aspiration, endobronchial lesion, ABPA, and bronchiectasis must be ruled out.
- Additional congenital pulmonary abnormalities, such as sequestration, congenital lobar emphysema, or CPAM can be associated with BA.

Suggested Readings

Berrocal T, Madrid C, Novo S, Gutiérrez J, Arjonilla A, Gómez-León N. Congenital anomalies of the tracheobronchial tree, lung, and mediastinum: embryology, radiology, and pathology. *Radiographics.* January-February 2004;24(1):e17.

Riedlinger WF, Vargas SO, Jennings RW, et al. Bronchial atresia is common to extralobar sequestration, intralobar sequestration, congenital cystic adenomatoid malformation, and lobar emphysema. *Pediatr Dev Pathol.* September-October 2006;9(5):361-373.

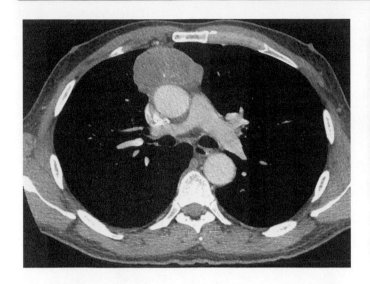 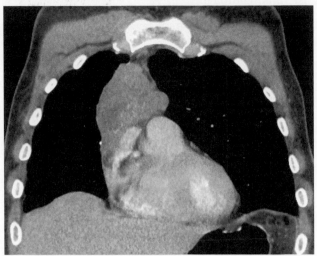

1. Where is the mass located?

2. What is the differential diagnosis?

3. What are the types of thymic epithelial tumors?

4. Which thymic tumor is the most aggressive?

5. What are potential differentiating features of thymic carcinoma?

Case ranking/difficulty:

Category: Mediastinum

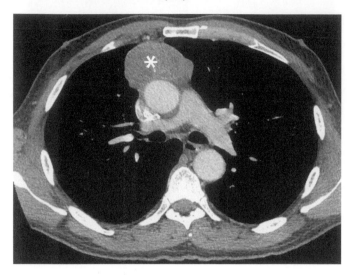

CT chest demonstrates a heterogenous, enhancing anterior mediastinal mass with smooth, lobulated borders (*asterisk*). It abuts the anterior wall of the ascending aorta with no obvious evidence of invasion.

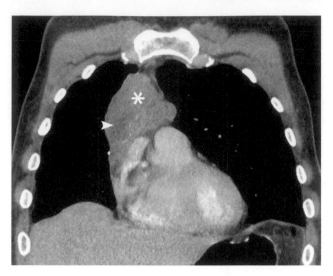

Coronal reformation of the CT chest demonstrates a heterogenous, enhancing anterior mediastinal mass with smooth, slightly lobulated borders (*asterisk*), and a small area of necrosis (*arrowhead*).

Answers

1. The mass localizes to the anterior mediastinum.

2. The differential diagnosis of the anterior mediastinal mass includes thymic lesions, lymphoma, germ cell tumor, thyroid tumor, and metastasis.

3. The different types of thymic epithelial tumors are thymoma, atypical thymoma, and thymic carcinoma.

4. Among the different types of thymic tumors, thymic carcinoma is the most aggressive.

5. Great vessel invasion, mediastinal lymphadenopathy, phrenic nerve palsy, and hematogenous metastases favor thymic carcinoma over (atypical) thymoma. Thymic carcinoma is rarely associated with paraneoplastic syndromes.

Pearls

- Thymic epithelial tumors comprise thymoma, atypical thymoma, and thymic carcinoma.
- The most common histologic type of thymic carcinoma is squamous cell.
- Great vessel invasion, mediastinal lymphadenopathy, phrenic nerve palsy, and hematogenous metastases favor thymic carcinoma over (atypical) thymoma.
- Paraneoplastic syndromes, such as myasthenia gravis, Lambert-Eaton myasthenic syndrome, pemphigus, subacute sensory neuronopathy, pure red cell aplasia, and immunodeficiency, often seen with thymomas, are rare in the context of thymic carcinoma.

Suggested Reading

Jung KJ, Lee KS, Han J, Kim J, Kim TS, Kim EA. Malignant thymic epithelial tumors: CT-pathologic correlation. *AJR Am J Roentgenol*. February 2001;176(2):433-439.

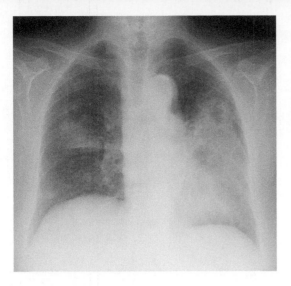 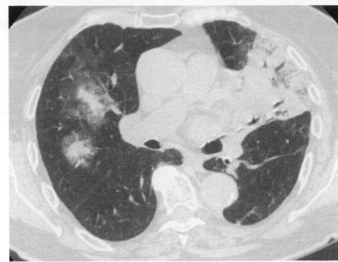

1. What are the findings?

2. What is the differential diagnosis of acute multifocal consolidations?

3. What is the differential diagnosis of chronic consolidations?

4. What type of lung cancer does bronchioloalveolar cell carcinoma (BAC) belong to?

5. What are the new terms for BAC?

Case ranking/difficulty:

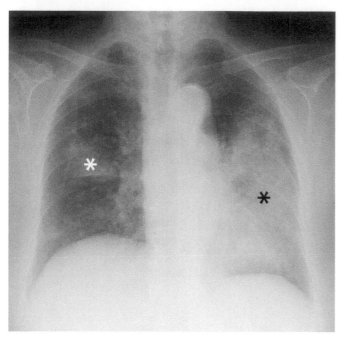

The frontal chest radiograph demonstrates a large left upper lobe and lingula consolidation (*black asterisk*) and a small parafissural consolidation in the right upper lobe (*white asterisk*).

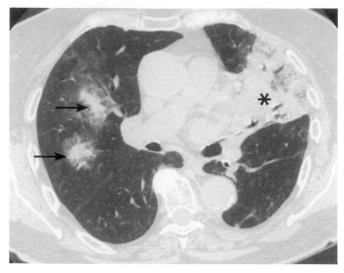

The CT shows a large left lower lobe consolidation with air bronchograms (*asterisk*) and two right upper lobe rounded consolidations with halo of ground glass (*arrows*).

Answers

1. Both chest radiograph and CT demonstrate bilateral consolidations with air bronchograms on the left.

2. The differential diagnosis of acute multifocal lung consolidations should include multifocal pneumonia, aspiration, pulmonary edema, pulmonary hemorrhage, vasculitis, acute eosinophilic pneumonia, pulmonary infarctions, and drug reaction.

3. The differential diagnosis of chronic lung consolidations should include bronchioloalveolar cell carcinoma (BAC), cryptogenic organizing pneumonia (COP), lipoid pneumonia, lymphoma, chronic eosinophilic pneumonia, sarcoidosis, pulmonary alveolar proteinosis, and atypical pneumonia.

4. BAC is a type of adenocarcinoma.

5. New terms for BAC are adenocarcinoma in situ (AIS) and minimally invasive adenocarcinoma (MIA).

Pearls

- According to the new nomenclature, bronchioloalveolar carcinoma (BAC) should now be referred to as adenocarcinoma in situ (AIS) and minimally invasive adenocarcinoma (MIA).
- BAC/AIS/MIA usually has a more indolent clinical course than other types of lung cancer.
- Smoking is not a risk factor for BAC/AIS/MIA.
- Chronic lung consolidation should prompt possible diagnosis of BAC/AIS/MIA.
- Bronchorrhea is a rare but classical clinical presentation of BAC/AIS/MIA.

Suggested Readings

Lee KS, Kim Y, Han J, Ko EJ, Park CK, Primack SL. Bronchioloalveolar carcinoma: clinical, histopathologic, and radiologic findings. *Radiographics*. Novemebr-December 1997;17(6):1345-1357.

Travis WD, Brambilla E, Noguchi M, et al. International Association for the Study of Lung Cancer/American Thoracic Society/European Respiratory Society International Multidisciplinary Classification of Lung Adenocarcinoma. *J Thorac Oncol*. February 2011;6(2): 244-285.doi: 10.097/JTO.b013e318206a221. Review.

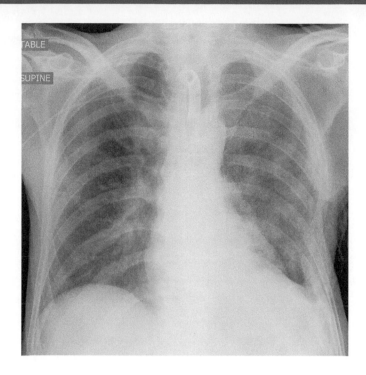

1. What are the findings?

2. What surgeries did this patient have?

3. What is the main indication for the kind of major body wall surgery this patient had?

4. List some causes of empyema.

5. What eponyms are used to describe this procedure?

Case ranking/difficulty:

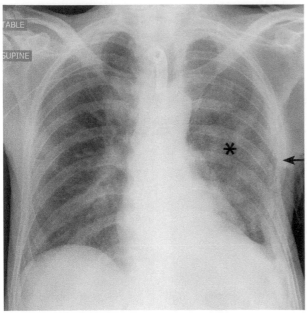

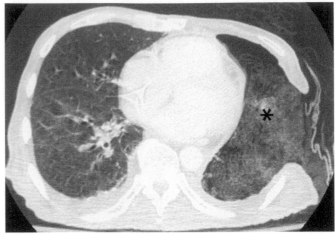

CT demonstrates status post left pneumonectomy, as well as left thoracoplasty and packing of the pneumonectomy bed (*asterisk*).

Frontal chest radiograph shows an abnormal left hemithorax, featuring diffuse reticulonodular densities, absent vascular markings (*asterisk*), deformity of the left lateral chest wall, and partial absence of the lateral ribs (*arrow*). There are also median sternotomy wires, mediastinal clips, a tracheostomy tube, and a right PICC in situ.

Pearls

- Open-window thoracostomy is an effective drainage method to control septic symptomatology in patients with empyema.
- This procedure is most commonly used in setting of post pulmonary resection empyemas or tuberculosis.
- Open-window thoracostomy is commonly referred to as Clagett window or Eloesser window, depending on the surgical technique used.

Answers

1. The chest radiographic findings include diffuse left hemithorax reticulonodular densities and absent vascular markings, left lateral chest wall deformity, and partially resected left lateral ribs. There are also median sternotomy wires, mediastinal clips, a tracheostomy tube, and a right PICC in situ.

2. The chest radiograph reveals sequela of previous median sternotomy, presumably for coronary artery bypass grafting (CABG), tracheostomy, left pneumonectomy, and left open-window thoracostomy.

3. The most common indication for an open-window thoracostomy is treatment of empyema following failure of closed drainage.

4. The most common causes of empyema are parapneumonic effusions followed by thoracic surgical procedures, trauma, esophageal perforation, cystic fibrosis, foreign body impaction, chest wall infections, tuberculosis, and subdiaphragmatic abscesses.

5. Open-window thoracostomy is also known as Clagett window or Eloesser window, depending on the surgical technique used.

Suggested Readings

García-Yuste M, Ramos G, Duque JL, et al. Open-window thoracostomy and thoracomyoplasty to manage chronic pleural empyema. *Ann Thorac Surg.* March 1998;65(3):818-822.

Madan R, Chick JF. Spectrum of radiologic appearances of surgical thoracostomy and thoracoplasty in the treatment of pleuroparenchymal infections. *AJR Am J Roentgenol.* February 2014;202(2):W123-W132.

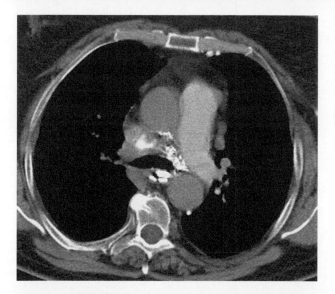
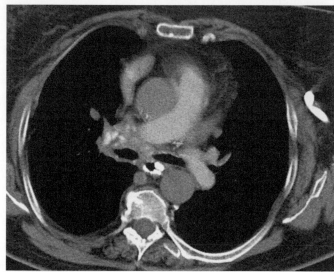
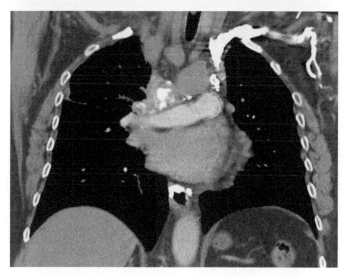
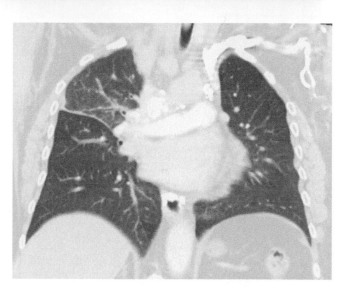

1. What are the findings in mediastinal windows?

2. What are the findings in lung windows?

3. What is the most likely etiology of the right upper lobe findings?

4. What is the most likely diagnosis?

5. What are likely etiologies of the entity shown?

Case ranking/difficulty: 🦴🦴

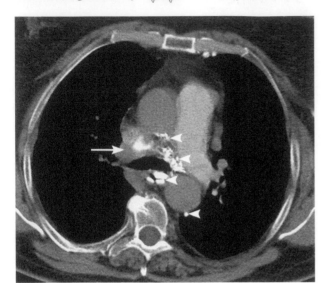

Contrast-enhanced CT demonstrates a right paratracheal calcified mass (*arrow*) and multiple mediastinal venous collaterals (*arrowheads*).

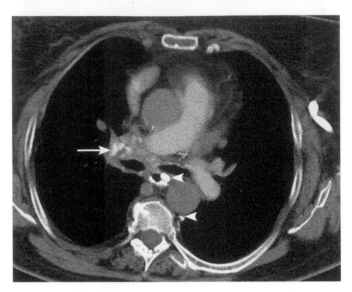

CT image at the level of carina demonstrates a right hilar calcified mass (*arrow*) and multiple mediastinal and chest wall venous collaterals (*arrowheads*).

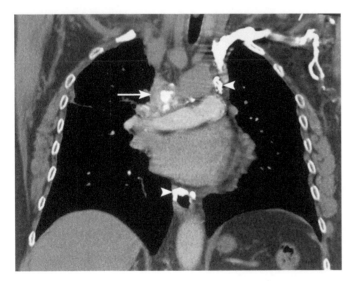

Coronal reformation shows a right paratracheal/hilar calcified mass (*arrow*) and multiple venous collaterals (*arrowheads*).

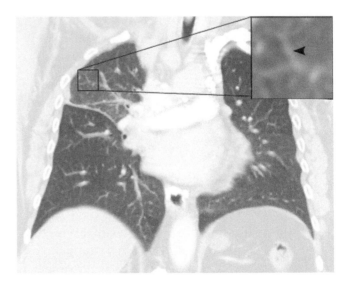

Coronal reformation in lung windows shows right upper lobe ground-glass opacities and septal thickening (*arrowhead in magnified image*).

Answers

1. CT images in mediastinal windows demonstrate a large calcified right mediastinal mass extending to the right hilum and multiple mediastinal venous collaterals.

2. The coronal image in lung windows shows right upper lobe ground-glass opacities and septal thickening.

3. The right upper lobe findings are suggestive of focal pulmonary edema and, together with the mediastinal findings, point to right upper lobe congestion due to pulmonary venous obstruction.

4. The most likely diagnosis is fibrosing mediastinitis.

5. Fibrosing mediastinitis can be idiopathic or secondary to a number of causes, which include histoplasmosis, tuberculosis, sarcoidosis, radiation therapy, and methysergide therapy.

Pearls

- Fibrosing mediastinitis (FM) represents benign proliferation of fibrous tissue in mediastinum, which can be focal of diffusely infiltrative.
- FM of focal type is likely secondary to histoplasmosis or tuberculosis, and commonly calcifies.
- The diffuse type FM is likely idiopathic, and usually does not calcify.
- Signs and symptoms relate to the mediastinal structure(s) involved.

Suggested Reading

Rossi SE, McAdams HP, Rosado-de-Christenson ML, Franks TJ, Galvin JR. Fibrosing mediastinitis. *Radiographics*. January 2010;21(3):737-757.

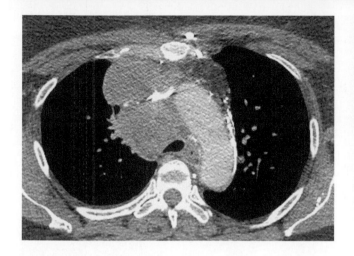
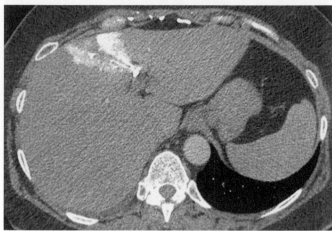

1. What are the chest findings?

2. What are the abdominal findings?

3. What might the liver abnormality be referred to in the light of the chest findings?

4. What is the significance of the liver abnormality?

5. What are the clinical manifestations of the patient's syndrome?

Case ranking/difficulty:

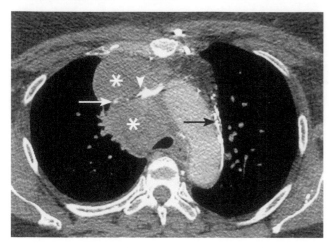

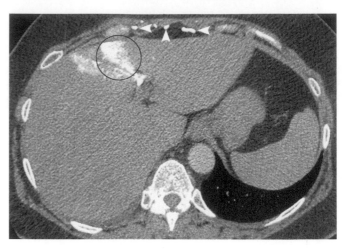

CT chest shows extensive mediastinal lymphadenopathy (*asterisks*) causing occlusion of the left brachiocephalic vein (*arrowhead*) and of the SVC (*white arrow*). There is also mass effect on the trachea. There are mediastinal collateral vessels (*black arrow*).

CT of the upper abdomen shows focal hyperenhancement in liver segment IVA (*circle*) and anterior abdominal wall collateral vessels (*arrowheads*).

Answers

1. CT chest shows extensive mediastinal lymphadenopathy causing occlusion of the left brachiocephalic vein and SVC. There is also mass effect on the trachea. Mediastinal collateral vessels are present.

2. The abdominal portion of the CT shows an area of hyperenhancement in liver segment IVA and dilated anterior abdominal wall collateral vessels.

3. In some cases of SVC obstruction, a focal area of hyperattenuation can be seen in liver segment IV during the arterial or early portal venous phases of contrast-enhanced CT. It is referred to as liver "hot spot" sign.

4. Focal area of hyperattenuation in liver segment IVA during the arterial or early portal venous phases, known as liver "hot spot" sign, suggests SVC obstruction and indicates the presence of collateral blood flow through paraumbilical veins.

5. Obstruction of the SVC results in impaired venous drainage of the head and neck and upper extremities, resulting in SVC syndrome. Clinical manifestations include facial and neck swelling, distended neck veins, headache, and dyspnea. The severity of symptoms depends on the level of obstruction (above or below the level of the azygos arch) and the development of collateral vessels.

Pearls

- Liver "hot spot" sign refers to focal hyperattenuation in liver segment IVA due to collateral blood flow.
- Liver "hot spot" sign should not be confused with a liver lesion and should prompt a search for SVC obstruction.
- Localization of the "hot spot" to liver segment IVA, characteristic enhancement pattern with wedge-shaped hyperattenuation in arterial and portal phases, isodensity in delayed phase, and presence of collateral vessels should help avoid potential pitfalls.

Suggested Readings

Joseph J, Narayanan H, Babu H, Praveen A. The focal hepatic 'hot spot' sign of superior vena cava obstruction in contrast-enhanced computed Tomography. *J HK Coll Radiol*. 2010;13:26-28.

Sheth S, Ebert MD, Fishman EK. Superior vena cava obstruction evaluation with MDCT. *AJR Am J Roentgenol*. April 2010;194(4):W336-W346.

Chest pain

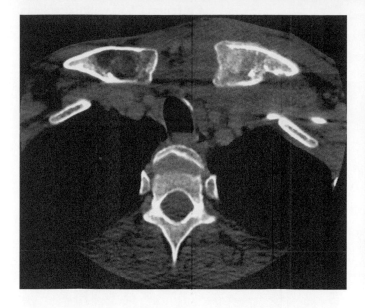 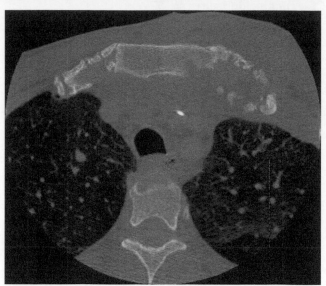

1. What are the findings?

2. What is the differential diagnosis?

3. What are the risk factors for this condition?

4. What is the most common pathogen responsible for this condition?

5. What are common complications of this condition?

Case ranking/difficulty:

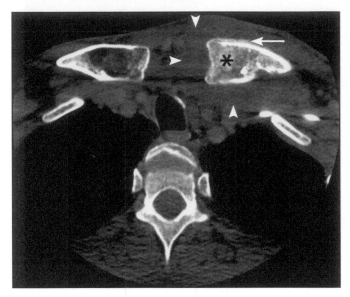

The left clavicular head demonstrates diffuse sclerosis (*asterisk*) and periosteal reaction (*arrow*). There is an abnormal soft tissue component around the left clavicle (*arrowheads*).

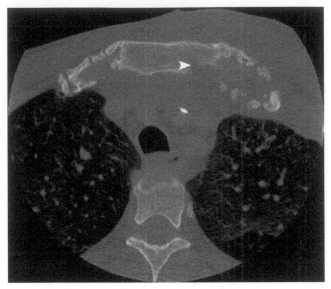

There is a lytic lesion in the manubrium (*arrowhead*).

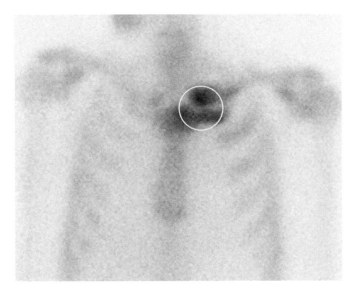

The bone scan shows markedly increased bone tracer uptake in the medial aspect of the left clavicle, left superolateral aspect of the manubrium, and the anteromedial portion of the left first rib (*circle*).

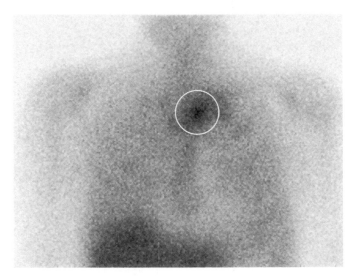

There is incongruent increased Gallium activity in the region of the left sternoclavicular joint (*circle*).

Answers

1. The proximal left clavicle demonstrates cortical irregularities and diffuse sclerosis. There is an abnormal soft tissue component surrounding the left clavicle and a lytic lesion on the left side of the manubrium.

2. The differential diagnosis includes septic arthritis and osteomyelitis, inflammatory arthritis including gout and pseudogout, rheumatoid arthritis, systemic lupus erythematosus, psoriasis, Still disease, reactive arthritis, trauma, SAPHO syndrome (which consists of synovitis, acne, pustulosis, hyperostosis, and osteitis), metastasis, and primary bone tumors.

3. The recognized risk factors for sternoclavicular joint septic arthritis are intravenous drug use, bacteremia, diabetes mellitus, chest wall trauma, and infected central venous line.

4. *Staphylococcus aureus* is the most common pathogen of sternoclavicular joint septic arthritis.

5. Common complications of sternoclavicular joint septic arthritis are osteomyelitis, chest wall abscess or phlegmon, and mediastinitis.

Pearls

- Sternoclavicular septic arthritis is uncommon in general population, but is relatively common in intravenous drug users.
- Additional risk factors for sternoclavicular septic arthritis are bacteremia, diabetes mellitus, trauma, and infected central lines.
- Associated osteomyelitis, chest wall abscess/ phlegmon, and mediastinitis are common.
- The radiological features favoring an infectious process over neoplasia include a joint centered process, bone involvement on either side of the joint, and presence of soft tissue abscesses.

Suggested Readings

Akkasilpa S, Osiri M, Ukritchon S, Junsirimongkol B, Deesomchok U. Clinical features of septic arthritis of sternoclavicular joint. *J Med Assoc Thai*. January 2001;84(1):63-68.

Ross JJ, Shamsuddin H. Sternoclavicular septic arthritis: review of 180 cases. *Medicine (Baltimore)*. May 2004;83(3):139-148.

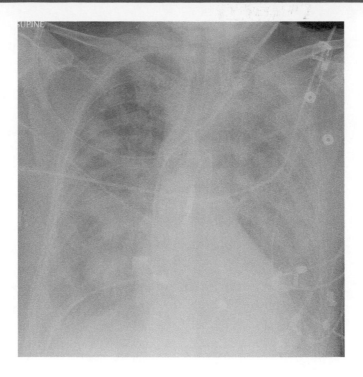

1. What are the findings?

2. What anatomical structures does the left heart device span?

3. What are the indications for this device use?

4. What could be alternative treatments to this device insertion?

5. What are clinical features of this device?

Case ranking/difficulty:

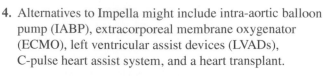

AP chest radiograph demonstrates bilateral alveolar pulmonary edema and pleural effusions. The patient is intubated. There are a nasogastric tube and left internal jugular vein Swan-Ganz catheter in place. There are multiple electrocardiography leads and extracorporeal tubes. The Impella cardiac assist device, inserted via femoral approach, has its distal tip in the left ventricle (*arrowhead*). Its ascending aorta component is indicated by *black arrows* and descending aorta portion by *white arrows*.

Answers

1. There is pulmonary edema. The patient is intubated. There is a nasogastric tube in situ and a left internal jugular vein Swan-Ganz catheter with distal tip in the right pulmonary artery. There is an Impella percutaneous cardiac assist device in good position.

2. Impella is usually inserted via femoral arterial approach; thus, its tubing spans the femoral and iliac arteries and the entire length of the aorta. Its intracardiac tip is positioned in the left ventricle and the pump components are located on either side of the aortic valve, aspirating blood in the left ventricle and ejecting it in the ascending aorta.

3. There are two types of Impella. One, LP 2.5, is principally used as a prophylactic measure in patients undergoing high-risk percutaneous coronary interventions. The other, LP 5.0, is principally used in the management of acute life-threatening left ventricular failure, either as a bridge to recovery or as a bridge to a surgically implanted left ventricular assist device or to heart transplantation.

4. Alternatives to Impella might include intra-aortic balloon pump (IABP), extracorporeal membrane oxygenator (ECMO), left ventricular assist devices (LVADs), C-pulse heart assist system, and a heart transplant.

5. Several studies have shown that Impella is more clinically effective than IABP or ECMO. It is also less traumatic and less expensive than other available ventricular assist devices. It is usually inserted percutaneously and does not require open heart surgery. Only mild hemolysis associated with the use of the device was reported.

Pearls

- Impella is a percutaneously inserted, minimally invasive cardiac assist device.
- It is used as a prophylactic measure in patients undergoing high-risk percutaneous coronary interventions or in acute heart failure.
- The Impella is usually introduced via a femoral arterial approach. Its distal J-shaped tip and the inflow part should be positioned in the left ventricle; the outflow part should be positioned in the ascending aorta.

Suggested Readings

Esfandiari S, Erickson L, McGregor M. The Impella® Percutaneous Ventricular Assist Device. Technology Assessment Unit of the McGill University Health Centre, Report Number 37, June 16, 2009. www.cgill.a/tau/.

Mohamed I, Lau CT, Bolen MA, El-Sherief AH, Azok JT, Karimov JH, Moazami N, Renapurkar RD. Building a bridge to save a failing ventricle: radiologic evaluation of short- and long-term cardiac assist devices. *Radiographics*. March-April 2015;35(2):327-356.

Cough and dyspnea

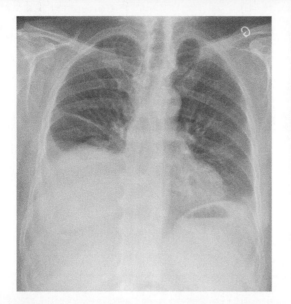
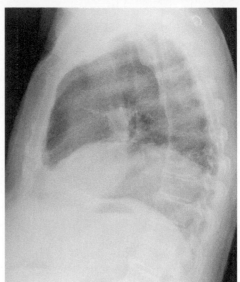

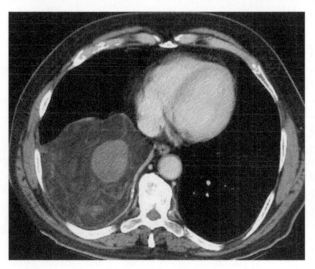
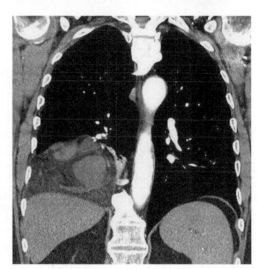

1. What are the findings on chest radiographs?

2. What is the differential diagnosis for the radiographic findings?

3. What are the CT findings?

4. What is the differential diagnosis for the CT findings?

5. What are the most common anatomical locations of this pathology in adults?

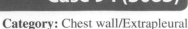
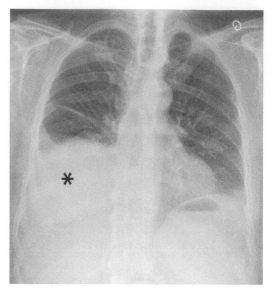

Frontal chest radiograph shows a large right lung base opacity (*asterisk*).

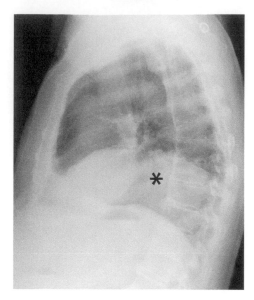

Lateral chest radiograph again shows a right lung base opacity (*asterisk*).

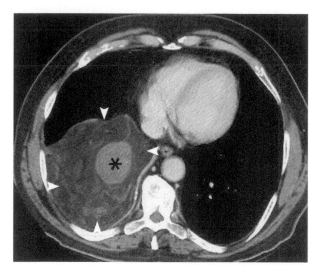

CT chest demonstrates a large right hemithoracic lesion of mixed fat (*arrowheads*) and soft tissue (*asterisk*) density.

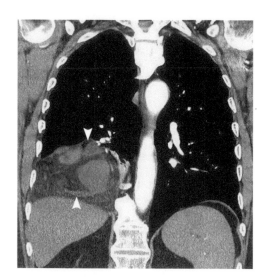

Coronal image shows the craniocaudal span of the large right hemithoracic fat and soft tissue density lesion (*arrowheads*).

Answers

1. Chest radiographs show a large right lung base opacity.

2. The differential diagnosis should include right hemidiaphragm paralysis, diaphragmatic hernia, diaphragmatic eventration, loculated pleural effusion, right lung base mass, and right lower lobe atelectasis.

3. CT shows a large right hemithoracic fat-containing mass with nodular solid components.

4. Differential diagnosis of an intrathoracic fat-containing lesion with solid components should include primary thoracic liposarcoma, metastasis from extrathoracic liposarcoma, thymolipoma, germ cell tumor, and herniated peritoneal fat. Lipoma is not considered here due to the presence of solid component.

5. Primary liposarcomas in adults commonly arise in the extremities and retroperitoneum. Intrathoracic liposarcomas are very rare.

Pearls

- Differential diagnosis of elevated hemidiaphragm should include causes of ipsilateral lung volume loss: atelectasis, lobectomy, pneumonectomy, pulmonary hypoplasia; diaphragmatic, pleural, and abdominal causes: phrenic nerve palsy, diaphragmatic eventration, abdominal mass, subphrenic abscess, distended stomach or colon, pleural effusion, diaphragmatic hernia or rupture, and pleural, pulmonary, or diaphragmatic tumors.
- Differential diagnosis of fat-containing thoracic lesions should include lipoma, hamartoma, lipoid pneumonia, mediastinal lipomatosis, thymolipoma, teratoma, lipoblastoma, liposarcoma, lipomatous hypertrophy of the interatrial septum (when confined to the septum), liposarcoma metastases, fat-containing neurogenic tumors, extramedullary hematopoiesis, epipericardial fat necrosis and diaphragmatic hernias containing intra-abdominal fat.
- Although liposarcomas are one of the commonest soft tissue sarcomas in extremities and retroperitoneum, primary intrathoracic liposarcomas are very rare, and most of the latter are mediastinal.
- Presence of solid components and local invasion are the radiological features that are used to distinguish liposarcomas from lipomas.

Suggested Readings

Barbetakis N, Samanidis G, Samanidou E, et al. Primary mediastinal liposarcoma: a case report. *J Med Case Rep*. December 2007;1(1):161.

Uchikov A, Poriazova E, Zaprianov Z, Markova D. Low-grade pulmonary myxoid liposarcoma. *Interact Cardiovasc Thorac Surg*. October 2005;4(5):402-403.

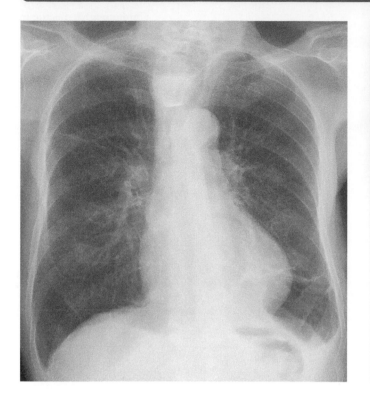

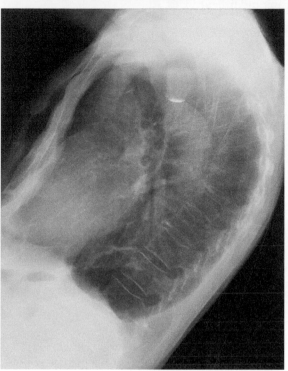

1. What are the findings?

2. What is the differential diagnosis?

3. What is the anatomical localization of this abnormality?

4. What are possible clinical presentations of this abnormality?

5. What are different types of esophageal pulsion diverticula?

Case ranking/difficulty:

Category: Mediastinum

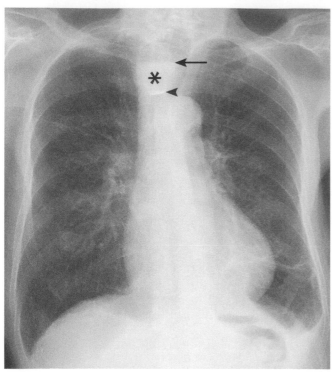

The frontal chest radiograph demonstrates a right paratracheal ovoid cystic lesion (*asterisk*) with an air-fluid level (*arrow*) and layering dense material (*arrowhead*), causing leftward tracheal deviation. There is a small left pleural effusion.

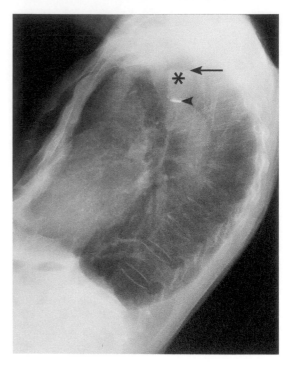

The lateral chest radiograph shows a retrotracheal cystic lesion (*asterisk*) with an air-fluid level (*arrow*) and layering dense material (*arrowhead*). Small left pleural effusion is again noted.

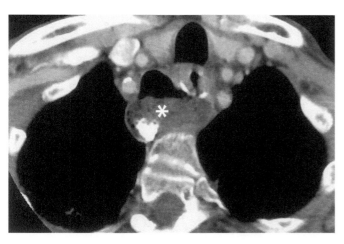

CT chest shows a large cystic lesion containing gas, food, and contrast (*asterisk*), posterior to and communicating with the esophagus.

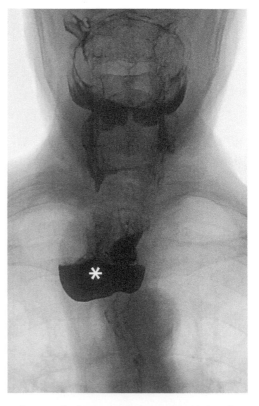

Barium swallow study demonstrating a large Zenker diverticulum (*asterisk*).

Answers

1. There is a retrotracheal lesion extending to the right of the midline, containing an air-fluid level and layering barium, causing leftward tracheal deviation. There is a small left pleural effusion.

2. The differential diagnosis includes Zenker diverticulum, Killian-Jamieson diverticulum, esophageal duplication cyst, infected bronchogenic cyst, and abscess.

3. Zenker diverticulum occurs between the circular and oblique fibers of the cricopharyngeus muscle, an area known as Killian dehiscence.

4. The clinical presentation of Zenker diverticulum can include dysphagia, regurgitation, aspiration, halitosis, or a mass or air-fluid level on neck and chest radiographs.

5. The esophageal pulsion diverticula are classified as Zenker, Killian-Jamieson, epiphrenic, midesophageal, and aortopulmonary recess diverticula.

Pearls

- Zenker diverticulum is the most common type of esophageal pulsion diverticulum.
- Zenker diverticulum occurs posteriorly in the midline through the dehiscence of Killian.
- Presence of air-fluid levels or contained gas collections in the upper mediastinum or abnormal densities in the retrotracheal space on chest radiography should suggest Zenker diverticulum.

Suggested Readings

Kanne JP, Rohrmann CA Jr, Lichtenstein JE. Eponyms in radiology of the digestive tract: historical perspectives and imaging appearances. Part 2. Liver, biliary system, pancreas, peritoneum, and systemic disease. *Radiographics*. March-April 2006;26(2):465-480.

Khan N, Ismail F, Van de Werke IE. Oesophageal pouches and diverticula: a pictorial review. *S Afr J Surg*. August 2012;50(3):71-75.

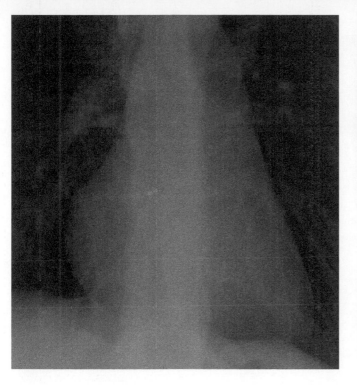 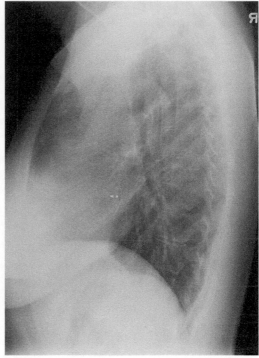

1. What is the finding?

2. What is the device used for?

3. What are contraindications to this device insertion?

4. What are potential complications related to this device insertion?

5. What are clinical properties of this device?

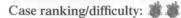
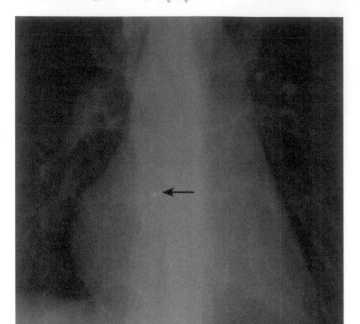

Magnified view of a frontal chest radiograph, centered on the heart, demonstrates typical appearance of the septal occluder device, seen as two side-by-side hyperdense dots projecting over the cardiac shadow (*arrow*).

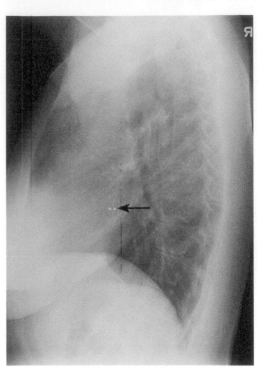

Lateral chest radiograph demonstrates typical appearance of the septal occluder device, seen as two side-by-side metallic mesh discs projecting over the cardiac shadow (*arrow*).

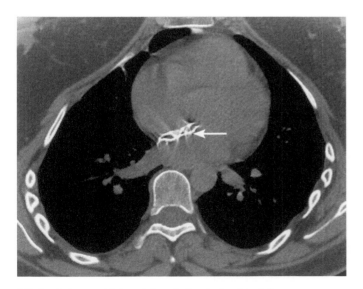

CT chest shows atrial septal occluder device (*arrow*).

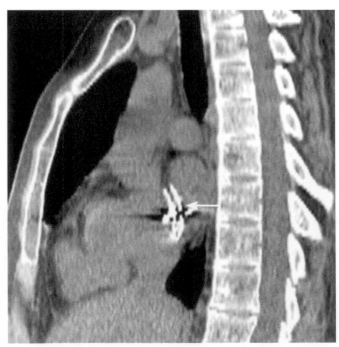

Sagittal reformation of CT chest shows atrial septal occluder device (*arrow*).

Answers

1. The images demonstrate typical appearance of a septal occluder device.

2. The device is intended for occlusion of secundum atrial septal defects (ASD).

3. The following are contraindications to septal occluder insertion: focal or generalized sepsis, any systemic infection, bleeding disorder, untreated ulcer or any other contraindications to aspirin therapy, intracardiac thrombi on echocardiography, margins of the defect <5 mm to the coronary sinus, atrioventricular valves and right superior pulmonary vein, inadequate safety margins from other vital structures (eg, aorta or inferior vena cava), and extensive congenital cardiac anomalies.

4. Potential complications of septal occluder placement include cardiac arrhythmias, device embolization, thrombus formation, delivery system failure, and allergic reaction to intravenous contrast used during procedure.

5. Septal occluder is MRI compatible. It is made of Nitinol alloy. The only alternative to it is an open heart surgery. The effectiveness of the ASD closure with an occluder device is similar to surgical repair. Treatment with this device has a lower complications rate than open heart surgery.

Pearls

- Septal occluder insertion is a minimally invasive effective alternative to surgical treatment of secundum ASD, showing similar effectiveness and lower complication rate compared to open heart surgery.
- Septal occluder devices may be difficult to visualize on frontal chest radiographs and could be recognized by noticing the two rounded dense metallic markers.
- Dedicated cardiac CT imaging is useful in evaluating the anatomical relationships of the cardiac defect before placement of a septal occluder device.

Suggested Readings

Quaife RA, Chen MY, Kim M, et al. Pre-procedural planning for percutaneous atrial septal defect closure: transesophageal echocardiography compared with cardiac computed tomographic angiography. *J Cardiovasc Comput Tomogr*. September-October 2010;4(5):330-338.

The AMPLATZER® Septal Occluder System. Summary of safety and effectiveness data (SSED). September, 6, 2001. http://www.fda.gov/ohrms/dockets/ac/01/briefing/3790b1_03_sponsorss&e.pdf

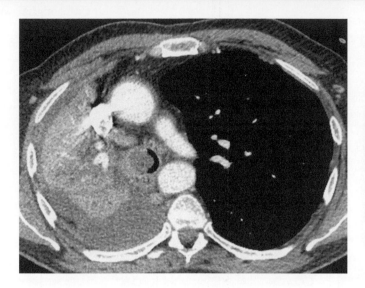 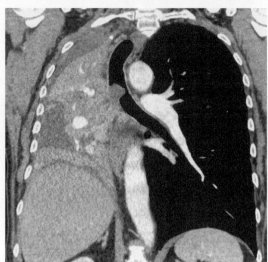

1. What is the differential diagnosis of a central airway endoluminal lesion?

2. What part of the airway is most frequently involved by mucoepidermoid carcinoma?

3. What is the prognosis associated with airway mucoepidermoid carinoma?

4. What type of organ tissue/cell type does mucoepidermoid carcinoma arise from?

5. What are possible risk factors for developing mucoepidermoid carcinoma of the airway?

Mucoepidermoid carcinoma of the main stem bronchus   Case 97 (2778)

Case ranking/difficulty:

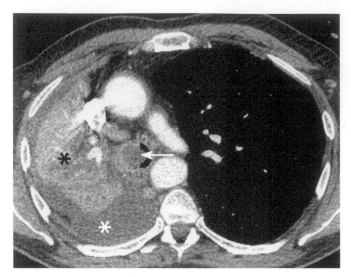

CT chest demonstrating a hypodense endoluminal lesion in the distal trachea (*arrow*), right lung atelectasis (*black asterisk*), and right pleural effusion (*white asterisk*).

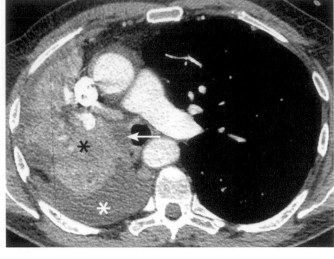

CT chest demonstrating a hypodense endoluminal lesion in the right main stem bronchus (*arrow*), right lung atelectasis (*black asterisk*), and right pleural effusion (*white asterisk*).

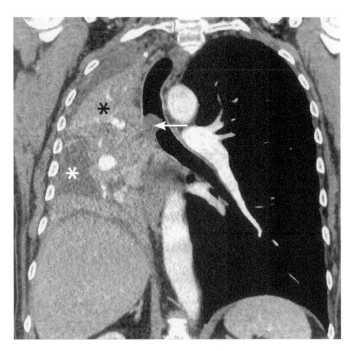

Coronal reformation of the CT chest demonstrating a hypodense lesion obliterating the lumen of the right main stem bronchus and projecting into the distal trachea (*arrow*). There is associated right lung atelectasis (*black asterisk*), and right pleural effusion (*white asterisk*).

Answers

1. The differential diagnosis of a central airway endoluminal lesion includes squamous cell carcinoma, carcinoid, aspirated material, adenoid cystic carcinoma, mucoepidermoid carcinoma, and hamartoma.

2. Most of the reported cases of airway mucoepidermoid carcinoma involved segmental bronchi.

3. Mucoepidermoid carcinomas are low grade, slowly growing tumors, rarely presenting with nodal metastases, and have excellent prognosis.

4. Mucoepidermoid carcinoma is a tumor of salivary glands, including the minor salivary glands of the airway.

5. Tobacco smoking was reported in 2/3 of cases of airway mucoepidermoid carcinoma patients.

Pearls

- Mucoepidermoid carcinoma is a rare minor salivary gland tumor of the airway.
- Mucoepidermoid carcinomas are low-grade tumors that are slow growing, do not metastasize, and have excellent prognosis.

Suggested Reading

Kim TS, Lee KS, Han J, et al. Mucoepidermoid carcinoma of the tracheobronchial tree: radiographic and CT findings in 12 patients. *Radiology*. September 1999;212(3):643-648.

Several years of minimally worsening shortness of breath

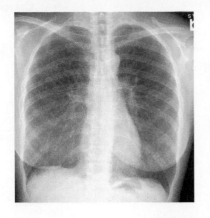
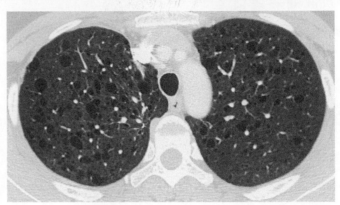

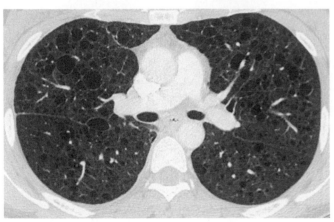
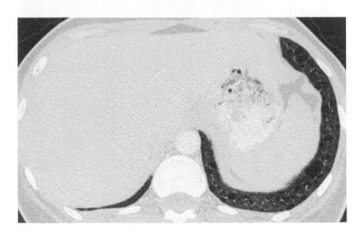

1. What are the radiographic findings?

2. What are the CT findings?

3. What is the differential diagnosis based on the CT appearance?

4. List two known complications of this condition.

5. What is Birt-Hogg-Dubé syndrome (BHDS)?

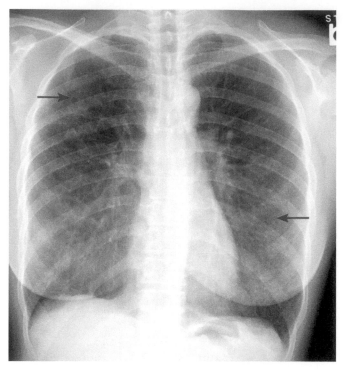

There are subtle, bilateral, smooth, reticular opacities (*red arrows*). The lung volumes are increased, as denoted by a diaphragmatic position that projects below the posterior 11th rib (*green arrow*). There is a surgical staple line from prior open lung biopsy (*blue arrow*).

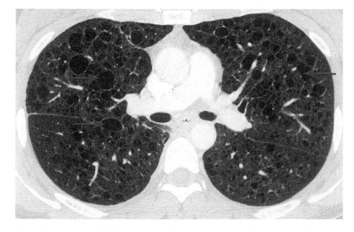

The bilateral and diffuse cystic lung disease is also seen in this lower lung image (*arrows*).

Answers

1. Subtle, bilateral, smooth, reticular opacities are seen on the radiograph. The lung volumes are increased, as denoted by a right hemidiaphragm that projects below the posterior 11th rib. There is a surgical staple line from prior open lung biopsy.

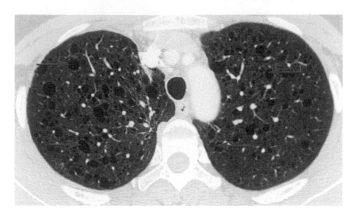

There are bilateral innumerable, diffusely distributed, variably sized, thin-walled lung parenchymal cysts (*arrows*).

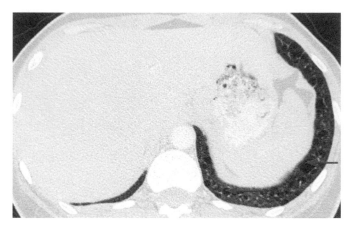

The costophrenic angles are also involved by the cystic lung changes (*arrows*).

2. The CT shows bilateral innumerable, diffusely distributed, variably sized, thin-walled lung parenchymal cysts. There are bilateral increased lung volumes.

3. The differential diagnosis of bilateral cystic lung disease includes lymphangioleiomyomatosis (LAM), tuberous sclerosis (TS), pulmonary Langerhans cell histiocytosis (PLCH), *Pneumocystis jiroveci* pneumonia (PJP), lymphocytic interstitial pneumonia (LIP), and Birt-Hogg-Dubé syndrome (BHD).

4. Spontaneous pneumothorax and chylothorax are two known complications of LAM.

5. BHDS is a rare inherited disease characterized by lung cysts, skin fibrofolliculomas, and renal tumors (ie, renal cell carcinoma and oncocytoma).

Pearls

- Establishing the diagnosis of LAM prior to childbearing is of utmost importance, since pregnancy can lead to fatal exacerbation of the disease.
- Pure LAM is seen exclusively in females.
- When pulmonary LAM is seen in a male patient, consider tuberous sclerosis.
- LAM may present in the form of recurrent spontaneous pneumothorax or chylous effusion.
- Finding of multiple renal angioleiomyomas may hint to the diagnosis of LAM.
- Diffuse cystic lung diseases, such as LAM, may appear as diffuse lung reticulations on chest radiography.

Suggested Readings

Avila NA, Dwyer AJ, Moss J. Imaging features of lymphangioleiomyomatosis: diagnostic pitfalls. *AJR Am J Roentgenol*. April 2011;196(4):982-986.

Raman SP, Pipavath SN, Raghu G, Schmidt RA, Godwin JD. Imaging of thoracic lymphatic diseases. *AJR Am J Roentgenol*. December 2009;193(6):1504-1513.

Toyoda K, Matsumoto K, Inoue H, et al. A pregnant woman with complications of lymphangioleiomyomatosis and idiopathic thrombocytopenic purpura. *Intern Med*. 2006;45(19):1097-1100.

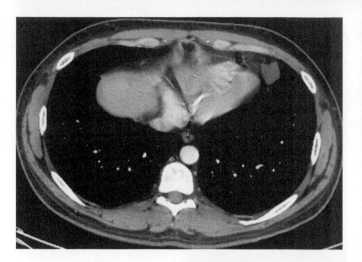 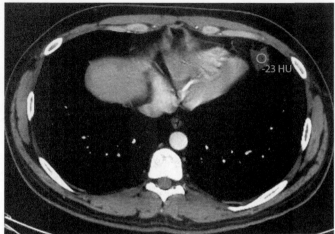

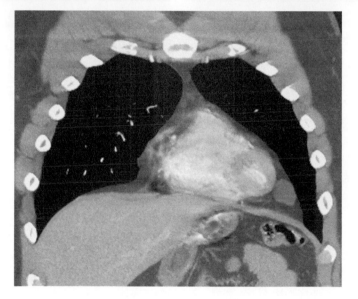

1. What abdominal pathologies are similar to the entity shown here?

2. What is the treatment for this entity?

3. Is this entity associated with other medical conditions?

4. What should be included in the differential diagnosis of a fat-containing anterior mediastinal lesion?

5. Why is it important to correctly diagnose this entity?

Case ranking/difficulty:

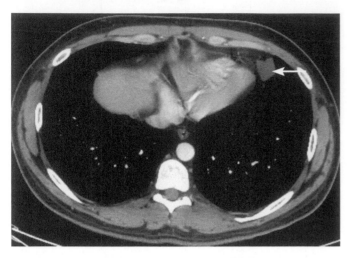

There is a rounded opacity in the epipericardial fat close to the cardiac apex (*arrow*).

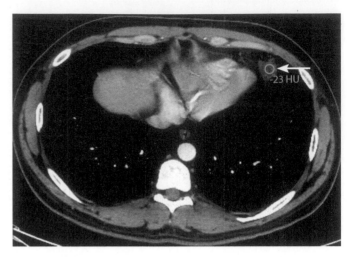

The internal density of the lesion (*arrow*) is -23 Hounsfield units.

4. Teratoma, Morgagni hernia, epipericardial fat necrosis, lipoma, liposarcoma, thymolipoma, and mediastinal lipomatosis should be included in the differential diagnosis of a fat-containing anterior mediastinal lesion.

5. Epipericardial fat necrosis is a benign and self-limiting condition with symptoms similar to ominous conditions, such as acute myocardial infarction, pulmonary embolism and aortic dissection. Making the correct diagnosis will avoid unnecessary and potentially detrimental interventions.

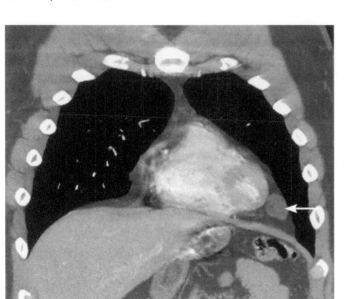

Coronal reformation maximal intensity projection image shows a rounded opacity in the epipericardial fat abutting the cardiac apex (*arrow*).

> **Pearls**
>
> - Epipericardial fat necrosis is a benign, self-limiting condition.
> - CT showing a fat-containing lesion in the pericardial fat establishes the diagnosis in the right clinical setting.
> - Epipericardial fat necrosis is the mediastinal equivalent of epiploic appendagitis.

Answers

1. Epipericardial fat necrosis, epiploic appendagitis, and omental infarct are similar pathologies due to idiopathic necrosis of the local fat, resulting in regional pain.

2. Epipericardial fat necrosis is a benign condition, requiring no intervention beyond pain control.

3. There arc no known associations between epipericardial fat necrosis and any other medical conditions.

Suggested Readings

Pineda V, Cáceres J, Andreu J, Vilar J, Domingo ML. Epipericardial fat necrosis: radiologic diagnosis and follow-up. *AJR Am J Roentgenol.* Nov 2005;185(5):1234-1236.

Runge T, Greganti MA. Epipericardial fat necrosis—a rare cause of pleuritic chest pain: case report and review of the literature. *Arch Med Sci.* Apr 2011;7(2):337-341.

Rule out pneumonia in a renal transplant patient

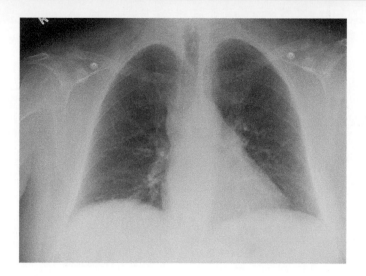

1. What are the findings?

2. What is the differential diagnosis when this abnormality is unilateral?

3. What is the differential diagnosis when this abnormality is bilateral?

4. What laboratory abnormalities are expected in this patient?

5. What are other common skeletal manifestations seen with this pathology?

Case ranking/difficulty: 🐞🐞

Category: Chest wall/Extrapleural

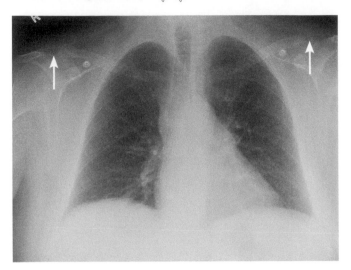

Chest radiograph demonstrates resorption of distal clavicles and widening of the acromioclavicular joint bilaterally (*arrows*).

Answers

1. The radiograph is essentially normal, except for resorption of the distal clavicles.

2. The differential diagnosis of unilateral resorption of the distal clavicle comprises posttraumatic osteolysis, osteomyelitis, myeloma, and metastasis.

3. Bilateral resorption of distal clavicles can be seen in hyperparathyroidism, rheumatoid arthritis, scleroderma, cleidocranial dysostosis, and pyknodysostosis.

4. Hyperparathyroidism results in elevated levels of plasma calcium and low levels of plasma phosphate.

5. Classical skeletal manifestations of hyperparathyroidism include subperiosteal bone resorption, which classically affects the radial aspects of the proximal and middle phalanges of the 2nd and 3rd fingers, terminal tuft erosion, rugger-jersey spine (more common in secondary and tertiary hyperparathyroidism), osteopenia, and brown tumors (more common in secondary and tertiary hyperparathyroidism).

Pearls

- Differential diagnosis of bilateral distal clavicular resorption includes hyperparathyroidism, rheumatoid arthritis, scleroderma, cleidocranial dysostosis, and pyknodysostosis.
- Differential diagnosis of unilateral distal clavicular resorption includes posttraumatic osteolysis, osteomyelitis, myeloma, and metastasis.
- "Rugger-jersey spine," a term used to describe prominent subendplate densities at multiple contiguous levels to produce an alternating dense-lucent-dense appearance of the spine, is another classical chest radiographic finding of hyperparathyroidism (more common in secondary and tertiary hyperparathyroidism).

Suggested Reading

Goswami P, Sarma PK, Sethi S, Hazarika S. Extensive skeletal manifestations in a case of primary hyperparathyroidism. *Indian J Radiol Imaging.* 2002;12(2):267-270.

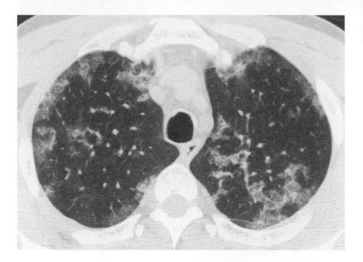
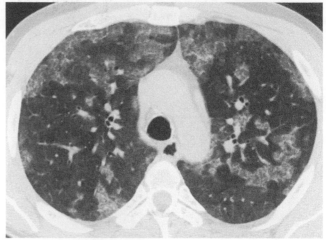
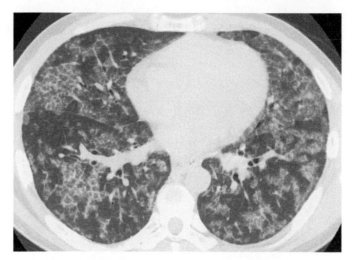

1. What are the CT findings?

2. What are the major differential considerations?

3. What are the types of pulmonary alveolar microlithiasis (PAP)?

4. What is the classic presentation for PAP?

5. What treatment options are available for PAP?

Case ranking/difficulty: Category: Lungs

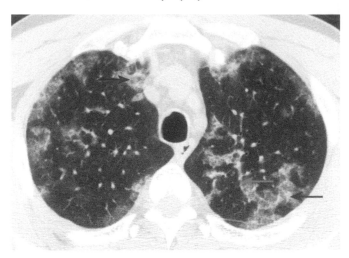

There is bilateral diffuse, multifocal, geographic, ground-glass lung attenuation (*red arrows*), with superimposed smooth inter- and intralobular septal thickening (*green arrow*), leading to a crazy-paving pattern.

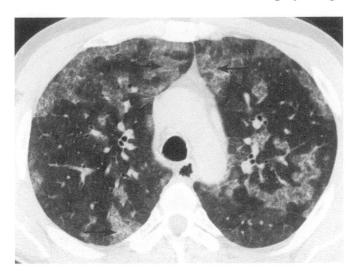

The same geographic abnormality is seen on this lower lung image (*red arrows*).

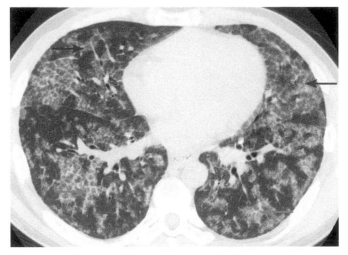

This more caudal image demonstrates the basal predominance of the abnormality (*arrows*).

Answers

1. Bilateral diffuse, multifocal, geographic areas of lung parenchymal ground-glass attenuation and superimposed smooth septal thickening are seen on CT, constituting a crazy-paving pattern. The abnormality has minimal basal predominance.

2. A crazy-paving pattern is classically described in the setting of pulmonary alveolar proteinosis (PAP), but can be seen in many other entities, a few of which are commoner than PAP. These other possibilities include pulmonary edema, pulmonary infection, pulmonary hemorrhage, diffuse alveolar damage, lipoid pneumonia, bronchoalveolar carcinoma/adenocarcinoma, organizing pneumonia, and nonspecific interstitial pneumonia.

3. PAP is classified according to etiology into primary (also known as idiopathic), secondary, and congenital types.

4. Insidious and slowly progressive dyspnea is the classic clinical presentation of PAP.

5. Bronchoalveolar lavage (BAL) is the treatment of choice for PAP, but supplemental granulocyte-macrophage colony-stimulating factor (GM-CSF) and lung transplantation are also known therapeutic options.

Pearls

- A crazy-paving pattern is typical of PAP, but can be seen in the setting of other much more common pathologies.
- Alveolar proteinosis is idiopathic (ie, primary) in 90% of the cases.
- Alveolar proteinosis may be secondary to inhalational exposure (eg, acute silicoproteinosis), hematological malignancies, and immunosuppression (eg, HIV and chemotherapy).
- PAP is among a few entities where the imaging findings can be extensive, while the patient is surprisingly asymptomatic or only mildly symptomatic (clinicoradiological discrepancy).

Suggested Readings

Frazier AA, Franks TJ, Cooke EO, Mohammed TL, Pugatch RD, Galvin JR. From the archives of the AFIP: pulmonary alveolar proteinosis. *Radiographics*. May-June 2008;28(3):883-899; quiz 915.

Rossi SE, Erasmus JJ, Volpacchio M, Franquet T, Castiglioni T, McAdams HP. "Crazy-paving" pattern at thin-section CT of the lungs: radiologic-pathologic overview. *Radiographics*. November-December 2003;23(6):1509-1519.

Mechanically ventilated patient

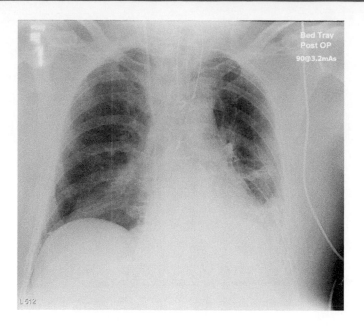

1. What is the most important finding on the provided radiograph?

2. What is the significance of such a finding?

3. What does the "double diaphragm sign" mean?

4. List other features of a pneumothorax on a supine patient's chest radiograph.

5. What are the two classic features of a pneumothorax on an erect chest radiograph?

Case ranking/difficulty: **Category:** Pleura

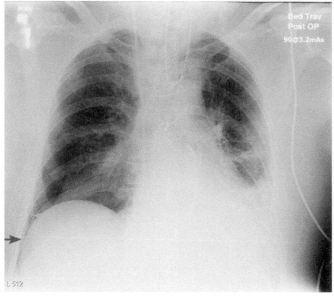

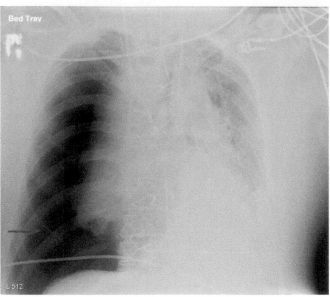

Support equipment and a left lower lung consolidation are seen, but the most important finding is the presence of a right-sided "deep sulcus sign" (*arrow*).

A radiograph obtained 3 hours after, showing a large right tension pneumothorax (*arrow*). The "deep sulcus sign" was missed on the initial radiograph, which resulted in an increase in the size of the pneumothorax in this mechanically ventilated patient.

Answers

1. The most important finding on the provided radiograph is the presence of a "deep sulcus sign."

2. The "deep sulcus sign" denotes the presence of a pneumothorax in a supine patient.

3. The "double-diaphragm sign" is another sign of pneumothorax in the supine patient. This results from air in the pleural space outlining the anterior costophrenic angle and air in the lung outlining the posterior diaphragmatic portions.

4. Pneumothorax in supine patients may also appear as a lucent hemithorax, increased sharpness of the cardiomediastinal border, or depressed hemidiaphragm.

5. The visceral pleural line and absence of the lung markings beyond that line are the two classic features of a pneumothorax on an erect chest radiograph.

Pearls

- Pneumothorax in a supine patient does not typically show the classic visceral pleural line and absence of lung marking beyond that line.
- Pneumothorax in a supine patient may present as a "deep sulcus sign."
- Positive pressure ventilation might convert a small pneumothorax into tension pneumothorax.

Suggested Readings

Kong A. The deep sulcus sign. *Radiology*. August 2003;228(2):415-416.

Woodside KJ, vanSonnenberg E, Chon KS, Loran DB, Tocino IM, Zwischenberger JB. Pneumothorax in patients with acute respiratory distress syndrome: pathophysiology, detection, and treatment. *J Intensive Care Med*. January-February 2003;18(1):9-20.

Incidentally discovered abnormality on a routine chest radiograph

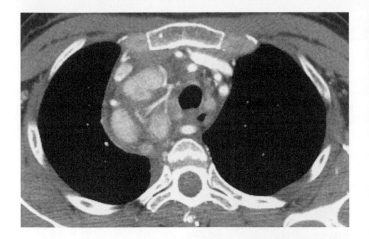

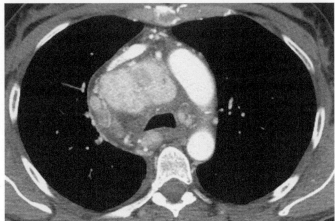

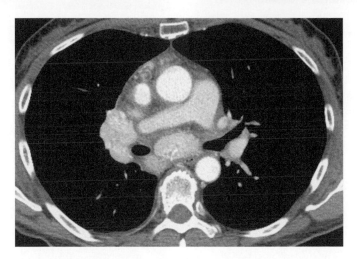

1. What are the imaging findings?

2. What is the differential diagnosis for a hypervascular mediastinal or hilar mass?

3. What is the likely diagnosis in this patient who has no known primary malignancy?

4. What are the types of Castleman disease?

5. What is the plasma cell type of Castleman disease associated with?

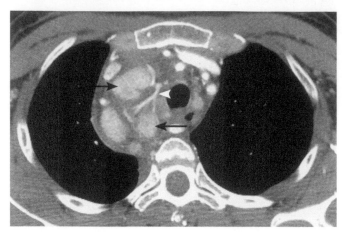

Multiple mediastinal hypervascular enlarged lymph nodes are seen (*arrows*), with perilesional tortuous vessels (*arrowhead*).

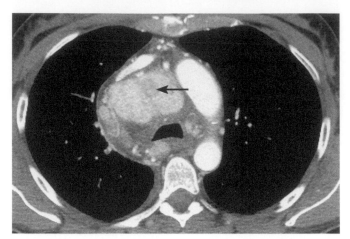

A few of the mediastinal hypervascular lesions show internal areas of hypoattenuation, suggesting necrosis or fibrosis (*arrow*).

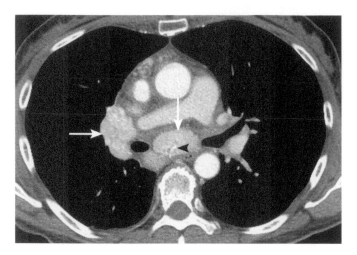

Multiple hilar and mediastinal hypervascular lesions are seen (*arrows*), with some lesions showing internal feeding vessels (*arrowhead*).

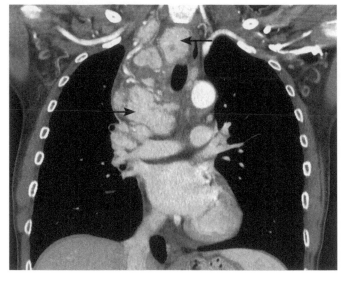

This coronal image demonstrates the well-defined and noninvasive nature of the hypervascular lesions (*arrows*).

Answers

1. Multiple hilar and mediastinal hypervascular lesions are seen, with intra- and perilesional tortuous vessels. Some lesions show internal areas of hypoattenuation, suggesting necrosis or fibrosis.

2. The differential diagnosis for a hypervascular mediastinal or hilar lesion is Castleman disease, hypervascular metastasis (classically from renal cell carcinoma), neuroendocrine tumors (carcinoid, pheochromocytoma, and paragangliomas), lymphoma, hemangioma, hemangiosarcoma, ectopic thyroid/parathyroid, and vascular aneurysm.

3. Castleman disease is the likely diagnosis in this case.

4. The two types of Castleman disease are *hyaline-vascular* and *plasma cell*.

5. The plasma cell type of Castleman disease is associated with human immunodeficiency virus (HIV), lymphocytic interstitial pneumonia (LIP), Sjögren syndrome, Kaposi sarcoma, and POEMS syndrome (polyneuropathy, organomegaly, endocrinopathy, monoclonal gammopathy, and skin changes).

Pearls

- The differential diagnosis for a hypervascular mediastinal or hilar lesion is Castleman disease, hypervascular metastasis (classically from renal cell carcinoma), neuroendocrine tumors (carcinoid, pheochromocytoma, and paragangliomas), lymphoma, hemangioma, hemangiosarcoma, ectopic thyroid/parathyroid, and vascular aneurysm.
- Always make sure that the hypervascular lesion is not an aneurysm!
- There are two different types of Castleman disease, with different clinical and imaging presentations: *hyaline-vascular* and *plasma cell* types.

Suggested Readings

Barrie JR, English JC, Müller N. Castleman's disease of the lung: radiographic, high-resolution CT, and pathologic findings. *AJR Am J Roentgenol*. May 1996;166(5):1055-1056.

Ko SF, Hsieh MJ, Ng SH, et al. Imaging spectrum of Castleman's disease. *AJR Am J Roentgenol*. March 2004;182(3):769-775.

Yuan ZG, Dun XY, Li YH, Hou J. Treatment of multicentric Castleman's disease accompanying multiple myeloma with bortezomib: a case report. *J Hematol Oncol*. 2009;2(2):19.

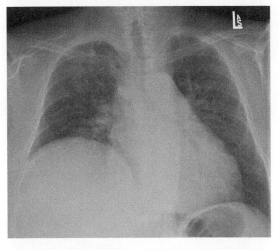

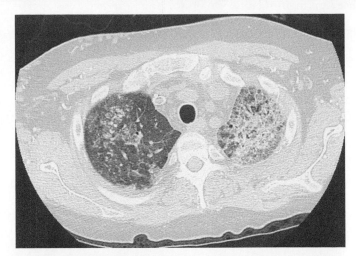

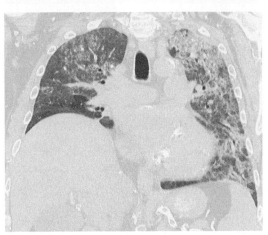

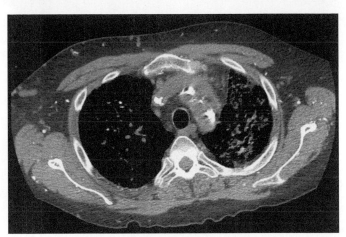

1. What are the radiographic findings?

2. What are the CT findings?

3. What is the likely diagnosis?

4. What is the general meaning of *metastatic calcification*?

5. What is the general meaning of *dystrophic calcification*?

Case ranking/difficulty: 🐾🐾🐾

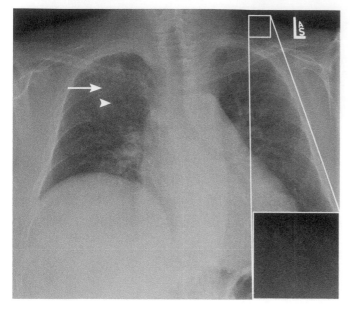

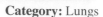

There are vague bilateral lung opacities, with a more confluent area of consolidation in the right upper lung zone (*arrow*). A few high-density nodules are seen, suggesting calcifications (*arrowhead*). A right brachiocephalic-SVC stent is seen as well. Note the soft tissue vascular calcifications (*magnified*). The patient also has an elevated right hemidiaphragm, which was persistent when compared to prior radiographs (not shown here). Cardiomegaly and central pulmonary arterial enlargement are also noted.

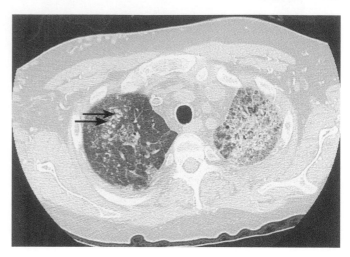

Bilateral patchy and diffuse areas of consolidation and ground-glass opacities are seen, being more pronounced in the left lung. There are nodular foci of high attenuation, in keeping with scattered calcifications (*arrows*). Scattered areas of interlobular septal thickening are also noted.

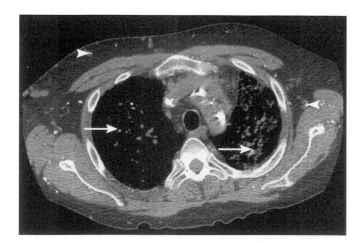

Scattered small calcified lung nodules are seen within the abnormal lung areas (*arrows*). There are extensive and diffuse vascular calcifications in the subcutaneous tissues (*arrowheads*).

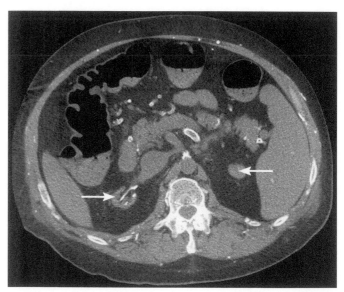

Note the atrophic kidneys (*arrows*), consistent with chronic renal failure. Vascular calcifications are also seen in the abdomen.

Answers

1. The radiograph shows vague bilateral lung opacities, with a more confluent area of consolidation in the right upper lung zone and a few high-density nodules, suggesting calcifications.

   There are soft tissue vascular calcifications, an elevated right hemidiaphragm, cardiomegaly, and central pulmonary arterial enlargement. A right brachiocephalic-SVC stent is also seen.

2. Bilateral patchy and diffuse consolidations and ground-glass opacities are seen on the CT. There are nodular foci of scattered calcifications. Scattered areas of interlobular septal thickening are also noted. There are extensive vascular calcifications in the subcutaneous tissues.

3. The likely diagnosis is metastatic pulmonary calcifications.

4. *Metastatic calcification* is defined as calcification of normal tissue due to hypercalcemia.

5. *Dystrophic calcification* is defined as calcification of abnormal tissue (eg, calcification of a tuberculous granuloma).

Pearls

• The appearance of metastatic pulmonary calcifications (MPC) on chest radiographs is not specific and might be mistaken for other acute or chronic airspace abnormalities.

• When MPC lung changes are seen in renal failure, extensive vascular calcifications are typically seen and can be a useful imaging hint to the correct diagnosis.

• The term *metastatic pulmonary calcifications* should not be confused with that of calcified lung metastasis from a distant primary malignancy (such as osteosarcoma metastasis).

Suggested Readings

Lingam RK, Teh J, Sharma A, Friedman E. Case report. Metastatic pulmonary calcification in renal failure: a new HRCT pattern. *Br J Radiol*. January 2002;75(889):74-77.

Marchiori E, Souza AS, Franquet T, Müller NL. Diffuse high-attenuation pulmonary abnormalities: a pattern-oriented diagnostic approach on high-resolution CT. *AJR Am J Roentgenol*. January 2005;184(1):273-282.

Rosenthal DI, Chandler HL, Azizi F, Schneider PB. Uptake of bone imaging agents by diffuse pulmonary metastatic calcification. *AJR Am J Roentgenol*. November 1977;129(5):871-874.

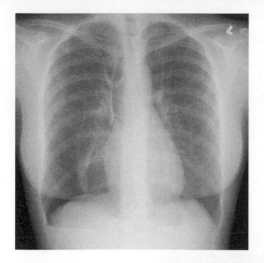
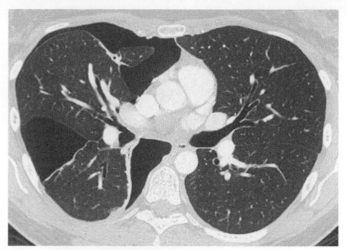

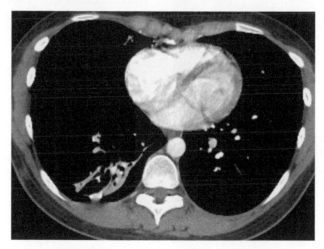

1. What are the radiographic findings?

2. What is the differential diagnostic list, if this radiographic abnormality developed spontaneously?

3. What are the CT findings?

4. What is the major diagnostic possibility, if the patient's symptoms were linked to the menstrual cycle?

5. What are the different thoracic presentations of catamenial syndrome?

Case ranking/difficulty: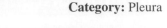

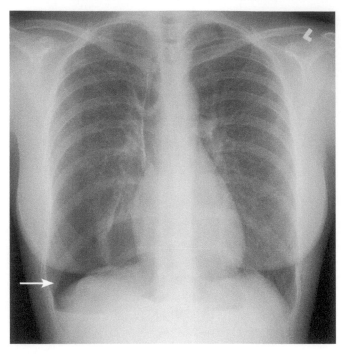

There is a right hydropneumothorax (*arrow*), with no airspace or interstitial opacities.

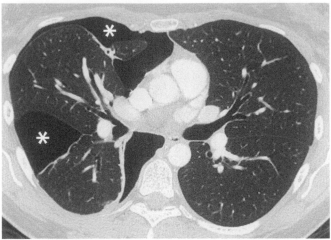

There is a sizable right pneumothorax (*asterisks*) and pleural adhesions. No ground-glass opacities, consolidations, cysts, or interstitial changes are noted.

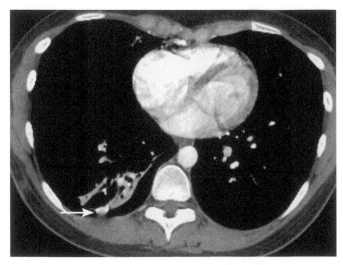

The right lower lung shows a questionable plaque-like area of visceral pleural enhancement, adjacent to a pleural adhesion (*arrow*).

Answers

1. The radiograph shows a right air-fluid level, denoting a hydropneumothorax.

2. When trauma, iatrogenic causes, or asthma are excluded, the following entities should be considered when a pneumothorax spontaneously develops in a young patient:

   bullous disease/blebs, lymphangioleiomyomatosis (LAM), tuberous sclerosis (TS), *Pneumocystis jiroveci* pneumonia (PJP), pulmonary Langerhans cell histiocytosis (PLCH), Birt-Hogg-Dubé syndrome (BHD), and catamenial pneumothorax.

3. The CT shows a sizable right pneumothorax and multiple pleural adhesions. The right lower lung shows a questionable plaque-like area of visceral pleural enhancement. No ground-glass opacities, consolidations, cysts, or interstitial changes are noted.

4. If the symptoms were linked to the menstrual cycle, catamenial pneumothorax would be the major diagnostic consideration.

5. Possible thoracic manifestations of catamenial syndrome are catamenial pneumothorax, catamenial hemothorax, catamenial hemoptysis, and lung nodules.

Pearls

- Consider catamenial syndrome when a female presents with menstruation-related cyclical chest symptoms.
- When spontaneous (nontraumatic) pneumothorax or hydropneumothorax occurs in a young female patient, consider the following: bullous disease/ blebs, lymphangioleiomyomatosis (LAM), tuberous sclerosis (TS), *Pneumocystis jiroveci* pneumonia (PJP), Birt-Hogg-Dubé syndrome (BHD), and catamenial pneumothorax.
- Thoracic or scapular pain during menses is highly suggestive of thoracic endometriosis and may precede the occurrence of pneumothorax.

Suggested Readings

Alifano M. Catamenial pneumothorax. *Curr Opin Pulm Med.* July 2010;16(4):381-386.

Kronauer CM. Images in clinical medicine. Catamenial pneumothorax. *N Engl J Med.* September 2006;355(10):e9.

Woodward PJ, Sohaey R, Mezzetti TP Jr. Endometriosis: radiologic-pathologic correlation. *Radiographics.* January-February 2001;21(1):193-216; questionnaire 288-294.

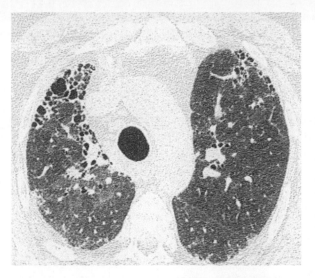
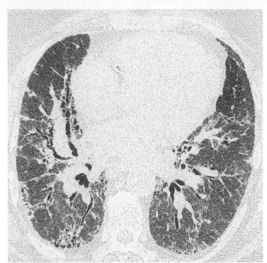
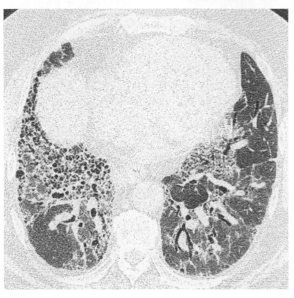
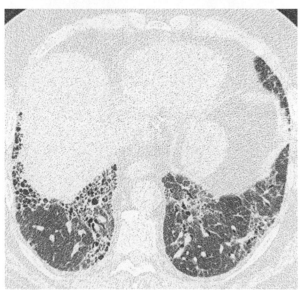

1. What are the CT findings?

2. What is the differential diagnosis based on the CT findings?

3. What is the likely diagnosis?

4. Why is the diagnosis of hypersensitivity pneumonitis (HP) favored over usual interstitial pneumonitis (UIP) and nonspecific pneumonitis (NSIP) in this case?

5. How is HP classified according to the radiology literature?

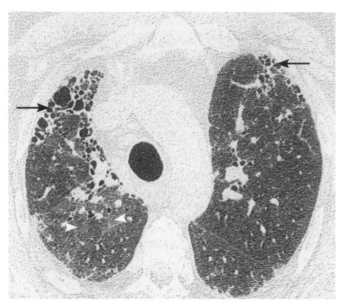

There is bilateral patchy pulmonary fibrosis with honeycombing (*arrows*). There is bilateral heterogeneous ground-glass lung density (*arrowheads*), resulting in mosaic attenuation.

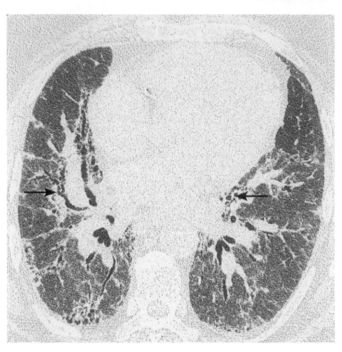

There are bilateral patchy peribronchovascular and subpleural reticulations, traction bronchiectasis, architectural distortion, and volume loss (*arrows*).

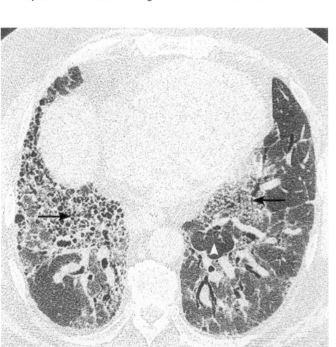

The heterogeneous fibrosis is also seen in the lower lung zones (*arrows*). Additionally, there is a lobular area of decreased lung attenuation and diminished pulmonary vessels calibers (*arrowhead*), possibly denoting air trapping from small airways involvement.

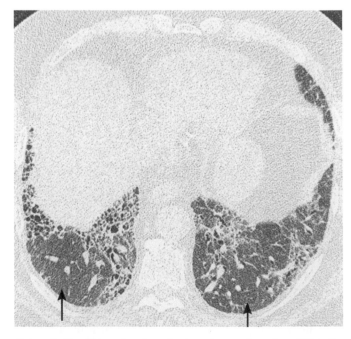

Although the disease involves the lung bases, there is sparing of the posterior costophrenic sulci (*arrows*).

Answers

1. The CT shows bilateral patchy pulmonary fibrosis with honeycombing. There is bilateral heterogeneous ground-glass lung density and mosaic attenuation that is probably a result of air trapping. There is peribronchovascular involvement and sparing of the posterior costophrenic sulci.

2. The differential diagnosis includes chronic hypersensitivity pneumonitis (HP), usual interstitial pneumonia (UIP), fibrotic nonspecific interstitial pneumonia (NSIP), drug reaction, and radiation fibrosis.

3. Chronic (fibrotic) hypersensitivity pneumonitis (HP) is the likely diagnosis.

4. The overall distribution of the parenchymal abnormalities (ie, peribronchovascular involvement and basal sparing) and the associated findings of airways involvement favor HP over UIP or NSIP.

5. HP is typically classified into acute, subacute, and chronic forms.

Pearls

- Basal sparing, air trapping, and centrilobular nodularity favor HP over UIP and NSIP.
- The presence of peribronchovascular involvement can occur in HP and NSIP, but not in UIP.
- Although HP is classically in the differential diagnosis list of upper lung fibrosis, it should be considered even when diffuse, patchy, or lower lung fibrosis is encountered.

Suggested Readings

Hirschmann JV, Pipavath SN, Godwin JD. Hypersensitivity pneumonitis: a historical, clinical, and radiologic review. *Radiographics*. November 2009;29(7):1921-1938.

Olson AL, Huie TJ, Groshong SD, et al. Acute exacerbations of fibrotic hypersensitivity pneumonitis: a case series. *Chest*. October 2008;134(4):844-850.

Trahan S, Hanak V, Ryu JH, Myers JL. Role of surgical lung biopsy in separating chronic hypersensitivity pneumonia from usual interstitial pneumonia/idiopathic pulmonary fibrosis: analysis of 31 biopsies from 15 patients. *Chest*. July 2008;134(1):126-132.

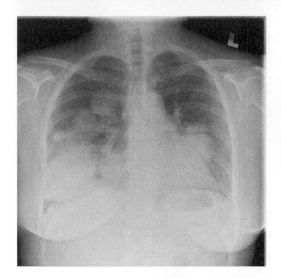 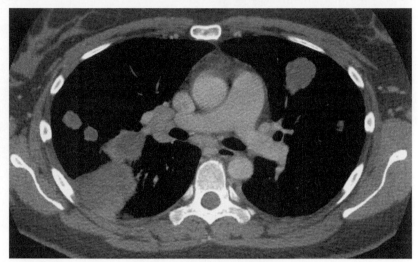

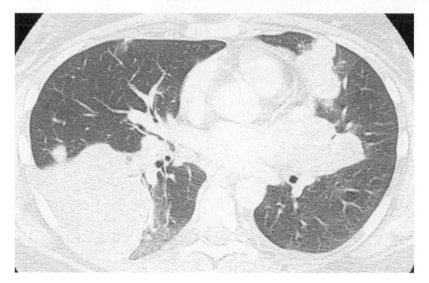

1. What are the radiographic findings?

2. What are the CT findings?

3. What is the differential diagnosis?

4. What are the types of *Cryptococcus*?

5. How does pulmonary cryptococcosis usually present on chest radiographs of immunocompetent patients?

Case ranking/difficulty: 🦴🦴🦴

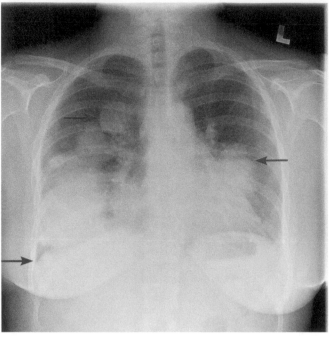

Multiple bilateral large, well-defined, and rounded opacities are seen (*red arrows*), with no obvious cavitations or calcifications. A small right pleural effusion is questioned, due to minimal blunting of the right costophrenic angle (*blue arrow*).

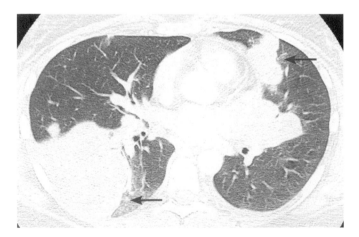

The lung windows show that a few of the lesions are surrounded by focal ground-glass attenuation (*arrows*).

Answers

1. Multiple bilateral rounded opacities are seen, with no obvious cavitations or calcifications. A small right pleural effusion is questioned.

2. Multiple bilateral well-defined and hypodense masses and nodules are seen, with no cavitations or calcifications. Enlarged right hilar and subcarinal lymph nodes are noted as well.

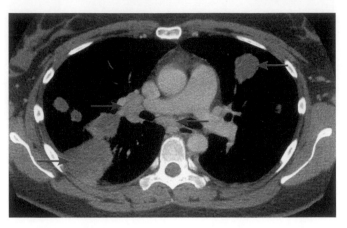

Multiple bilateral variably sized masses and nodules are seen (*red arrows*). These lesions have a well-defined rim and internal areas of low attenuation, but no cavitations or calcifications. Several enlarged hilar and mediastinal lymph nodes are seen (*blue arrows*).

3. The differential diagnosis for multiple bilateral lung masses (>3 cm): metastases is the first consideration (from lung, breast, colon, renal, and many other primary malignancies). Infection can also be considered in the absence of a primary malignancy (typically fungal infections, but mycobacterial and parasitic infections can be considered as unusual possible causes). Rare causes include parenchymal lymphoma, multiple large hamartomas, collagen vascular diseases (such as necrobiotic nodules in rheumatoid arthritis), and vasculitis (such as Wegener granulomatosis).

4. The two variants of *Cryptococcus* are: *neoformans* and *gattii*.

5. Pulmonary nodules, masses, consolidation, and diffuse nodular or reticulonodular patterns have been described in the immunocompetent patients. Note that cavitations, pleural effusions, lymphadenopathy, miliary pattern, and disseminated disease are usually seen in the immunocompromised patients.

Pearls

- Fungal infections can be included in the differential diagnosis of multiple nodules in an asymptomatic patient with no history of primary malignancy.
- Unlike cryptococcal infection of the immunocompetent hosts, immunocompromised patients commonly show cavitations, pleural effusions, lymphadenopathy, miliary pattern, and disseminated disease.

Suggested Readings

McAdams HP, Rosado-de-Christenson ML, Lesar M, Templeton PA, Moran CA. Thoracic mycoses from endemic fungi: radiologic-pathologic correlation. *Radiographics*. March 1995;15(2):255-270.

McAdams HP, Rosado-de-Christenson ML, Templeton PA, Lesar M, Moran CA. Thoracic mycoses from opportunistic fungi: radiologic-pathologic correlation. *Radiographics*. March 1995;15(2):271-286.

Sider L, Gabriel H, Curry DR, Pham MS. Pattern recognition of the pulmonary manifestations of AIDS on CT scans. *Radiographics*. July 1993;13(4):771-784; discussion 785-786.

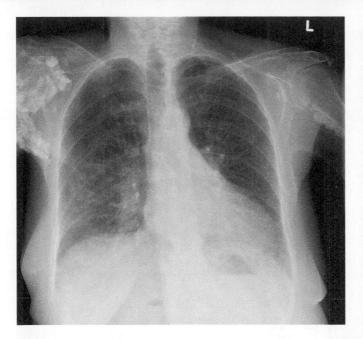

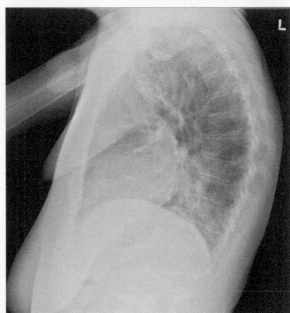

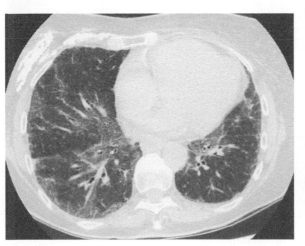

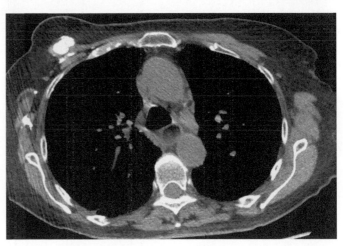

1. What are the radiographic findings?

2. What are the CT findings?

3. What is the most likely diagnosis?

4. What is the most common pattern of lung involvement in the presented entity?

5. What is CREST syndrome?

Case ranking/difficulty:

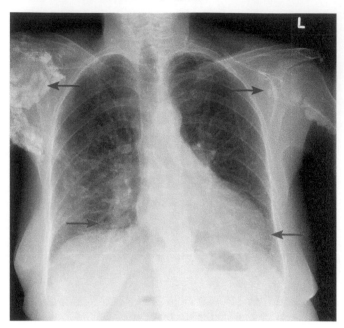

There are bilateral peripheral, lower lung predominant, fine reticular opacities (*red arrows*), with no obvious volume loss. Note the extensive bilateral soft tissue calcific changes around the shoulders (*blue arrows*).

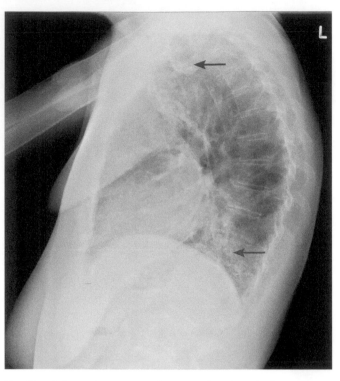

The fibrotic lung changes are also appreciated on the lateral view, being more pronounced at the lung bases (*red arrow*). The soft tissue calcifications project over the upper lung zone (*blue arrow*).

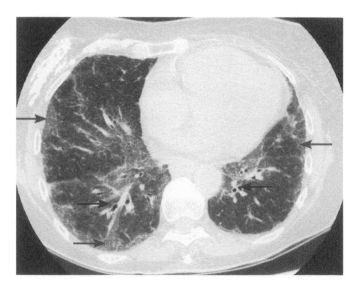

Bilateral peripheral reticulations and superimposed ground-glass opacities are seen (*red arrows*), along with minimal traction bronchiectasis and bronchiolectasis (*blue arrows*). The abnormality is in keeping with a nonspecific interstitial pneumonia pattern.

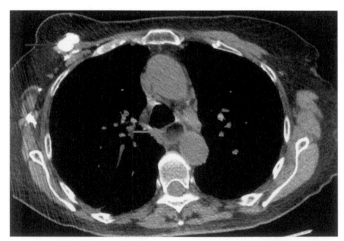

The esophagus is dilated and shows an internal air-debris level (*green arrow*). Extensive deep soft tissue calcifications are seen in the anterior and anterolateral chest wall (*blue arrows*).

Answers

1. Bilateral peripheral fine reticular opacities are seen on the radiographs, with predominance at the lung bases. No obvious volume loss is noted. Note the extensive bilateral soft tissue calcific changes around the shoulders.

2. Bilateral peripheral reticulations and superimposed ground-glass opacities are seen on CT, along with minimal traction bronchiectasis and bronchiolectasis. The esophagus is dilated and shows an internal air-debris level. Extensive deep soft tissue calcifications are seen in the anterior and anterolateral chest wall.

3. Progressive systemic sclerosis (PSS), ie, (scleroderma) is the likely diagnosis.

4. Nonspecific interstitial pneumonia is the most common pattern of lung involvement in PSS patients.

5. CREST syndrome (calcinosis, Raynaud phenomenon, esophageal dysmotility, sclerodactyly, telangiectasias) is a form of PSS.

Pearls

- The presence of a dilated esophagus in a case of fibrotic lung disease is a hint for the diagnosis of PSS.
- Assessing for the presence of pulmonary arterial hypertension (PHTN) and the extent of lung fibrosis is paramount, since they have important prognostic implications in PSS.
- A normal diameter of the central pulmonary arteries in the context of PSS does *not* exclude the diagnosis of PHTN.

Suggested Readings

Kim EA, Lee KS, Johkoh T, Kim TS, Suh GY, Kwon OJ, Han J. Interstitial lung diseases associated with collagen vascular diseases: radiologic and histopathologic findings. *Radiographics*. October 2002;22 Spec No:S151-S165.

Lynch DA. Lung disease related to collagen vascular disease. *J Thorac Imaging*. November 2009;24(4):299-309.

Mayberry JP, Primack SL, Müller NL. Thoracic manifestations of systemic autoimmune diseases: radiographic and high-resolution CT findings. *Radiographics*. November-December 2000;20(6):1623-1635.

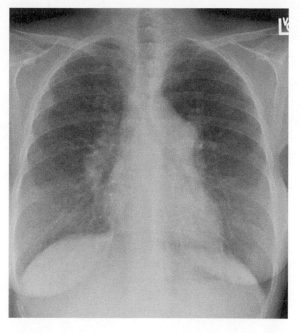
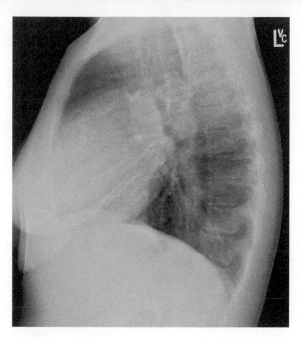

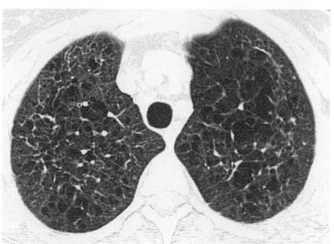
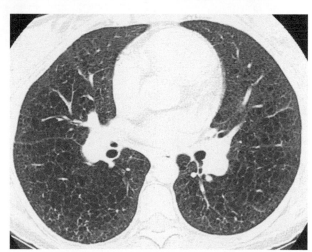

1. What are the radiographic findings?

2. What would be the differential diagnosis based on the radiographic features?

3. What are the CT findings?

4. What would be the differential diagnosis based on the CT features?

5. What is the recommended treatment of the presented entity?

Case ranking/difficulty: **Category:** Lungs

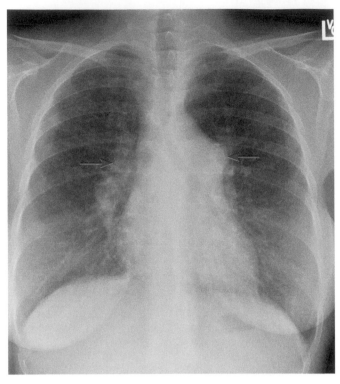

There is a bilateral diffuse coarse reticular pattern, with normal to increased lung volumes. There is central pulmonary arterial enlargement as well (*arrows*).

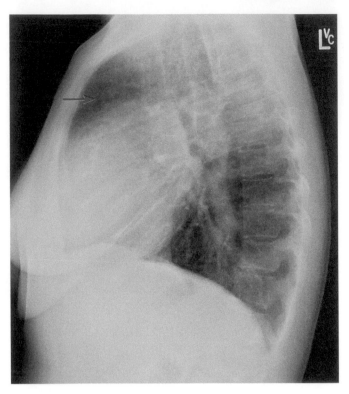

The lateral radiograph demonstrates the same subtle interstitial pattern (*arrow*), with relative sparing of the lower lung zones. The hemidiaphragms are minimally flattened and the anteroposterior thoracic diameter is increased, features suggesting mild hyperinflation.

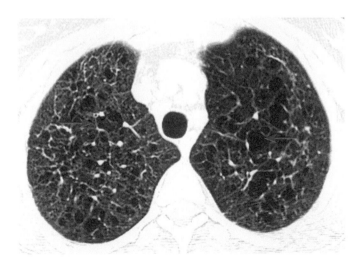

Numerous lung lucencies are seen and most show discernible thin walls, in keeping with cysts (*arrows*). The cysts have variable sizes and shapes, with some coalescing to form "bizarre" configurations.

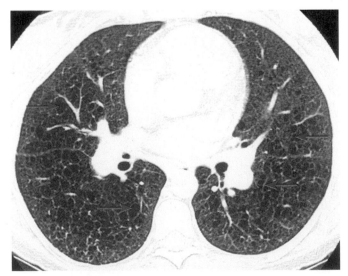

This midlung image shows the diffuse nature of the abnormality (*arrows*), but with less pronounced involvement when compared to the upper lungs.

Answers

1. The radiographs show a bilateral diffuse coarse reticular pattern, with relative sparing of the lower lung zones. There are normal to increased lung volumes. There is enlargement of the central pulmonary arteries.

2. The differential diagnosis of a diffuse interstitial lung pattern on chest radiography in the presence of normal or increased lung volumes includes lymphangioleiomyomatosis (LAM), tuberous sclerosis (TS), pulmonary Langerhans cell histiocytosis (PLCH), sarcoidosis, and fibrosis on a background of severe emphysema. Of note, lymphangitic carcinomatosis can present with a diffuse interstitial pattern with relatively preserved lung volumes. If such a pattern is seen acutely, interstitial pulmonary edema and interstitial pneumonia (eg, viral pneumonia) should be considered.

3. Numerous thin-walled lung cysts are present. The cysts have variable sizes and shapes, with some coalescing to form "bizarre" configurations. The pulmonary arterial trunk is enlarged.

4. The differential diagnosis of a predominantly cystic lung pattern includes LAM, TS, PLCH, and *Pneumocystis jiroveci* pneumonia (PJP).

5. Smoking cessation is recommended in adult smokers presenting with PLCH.

Pearls

- The differential diagnosis of a diffuse interstitial lung pattern on chest radiographs in the presence of normal or increased lung volumes includes LAM, TS, PLCH, sarcoidosis, and fibrosis on a background of severe emphysema. Of note, lymphangitic carcinomatosis can present with a diffuse interstitial pattern and relatively preserved lung volumes. If this pattern is acute, pulmonary edema and interstitial pneumonia should be considered.
- The differential diagnosis of upper lung fibrosis includes infection (from tuberculosis or histoplasmosis), pneumoconiosis (such as silicosis), sarcoidosis, hypersensitivity pneumonitis, pulmonary Langerhans cell histiocytosis, radiation, and rarely ankylosing spondylitis.
- Features that favor PLCH over other cystic lung diseases include history of smoking, upper lung predominance, irregular nodules, and "bizarre" cysts.

Suggested Readings

Abbott GF, Rosado-de-Christenson ML, Franks TJ, Frazier AA, Galvin JR. From the archives of the AFIP: pulmonary Langerhans cell histiocytosis. *Radiographics*. May-June 2004;24(3):821-841.

Attili AK, Kazerooni EA, Gross BH, Flaherty KR, Myers JL, Martinez FJ. Smoking-related interstitial lung disease: radiologic-clinical-pathologic correlation. *Radiographics*. September-October 2008;28(5):1383-1396; discussion 1396-1398.

Leatherwood DL, Heitkamp DE, Emerson RE. Best cases from the AFIP: Pulmonary Langerhans cell histiocytosis. *Radiographics*. January-February 2007;27(1):265-268.

Known case of prostate cancer, with a few months of progressive dry cough and shortness of breath

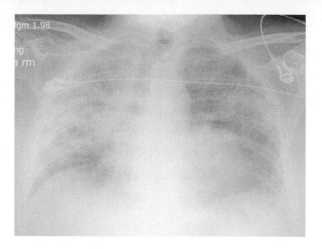
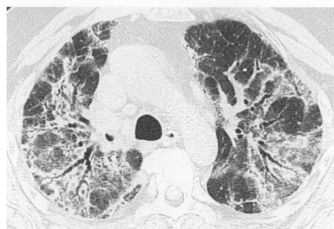
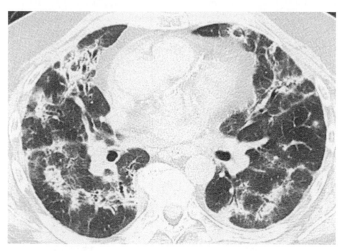
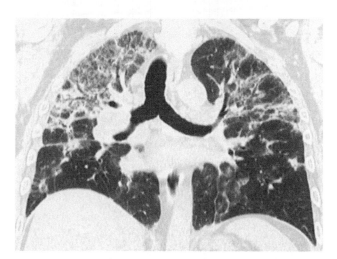

1. Describe the radiographic findings.

2. What is the differential diagnosis based on the chest radiograph appearance?

3. Describe the CT findings.

4. What is the differential diagnosis based on the chest CT appearance?

5. What is nitrofurantoin commonly used for?

Case ranking/difficulty:

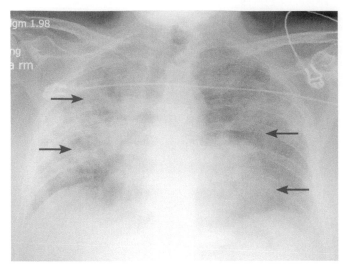

This bedside chest radiograph shows diffuse bilateral heterogeneous consolidations (*arrows*), with relative basal sparing and a background of reduced lung volumes.

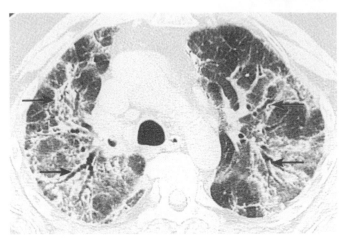

The lung parenchymal opacities have a band-like configuration that involves the edges of multiple secondary pulmonary lobules, leading to the so-called perilobular distribution (*red arrows*). This perilobular pattern has been associated with organizing pneumonia.

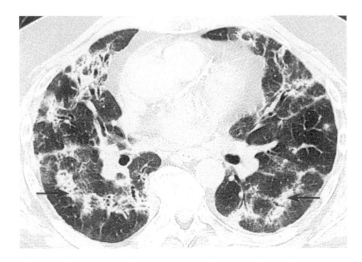

More perilobular opacities are seen in the lower lungs (*arrows*).

Answers

1. The radiograph shows diffuse bilateral heterogeneous consolidations, with relative basal sparing and reduced lung volumes.

2. The radiographic picture is that of bilateral diffuse airspace opacities. If the presentation was acute, the differential diagnosis would include infection, cardiogenic and noncardiogenic pulmonary edema, pulmonary hemorrhage, aspiration pneumonitis, drug reaction, and acute respiratory distress syndrome. If the presentation was chronic, the differential diagnosis would include organizing pneumonia, eosinophilic pneumonia, adenocarcinoma, lymphoma, alveolar

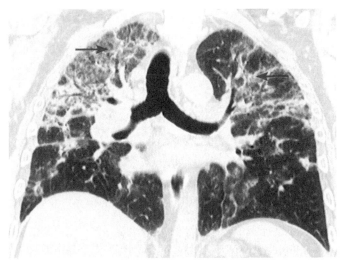

This coronal image shows upper lung predominance of the lung parenchymal abnormalities (*arrows*).

proteinosis, sarcoidosis, drug reaction, and atypical infections (tuberculous or fungal).

3. The CT shows heterogeneous consolidations and ground-glass opacities, in peribronchovascular and perilobular distributions. The involved areas show features of fibrosis. There is upper lung predominance of the lung parenchymal abnormalities.

4. The main diagnostic possibilities given the CT pattern are drug reaction, connective tissue diseases, infection, radiation, and hypersensitivity pneumonitis.

5. Nitrofurantoin is commonly used to treat recurrent urinary tract infections.

Pearls

- Pulmonary drug toxicity is commonly underdiagnosed and should be considered when bilateral and diffuse lung findings are seen, in the appropriate clinical context.
- When a mixed pattern of organizing pneumonia and nonspecific interstitial pneumonia is encountered, drug reaction and connective tissue disorders should be considered.
- Many drugs can cause lung toxicity and the list includes amiodarone, methotrexate, nitrofurantoin, cyclophosphamide, busulfan, bleomycin, and penicillamine.

Suggested Readings

Polverosi R, Maffesanti M, Dalpiaz G. Organizing pneumonia: typical and atypical HRCT patterns. *Radiol Med*. March 2006;111(2):202-212.

Rossi SE, Erasmus JJ, McAdams HP, Sporn TA, Goodman PC. Pulmonary drug toxicity: radiologic and pathologic manifestations. *Radiographics*. September-October 2000;20(5):1245-1259.

Vahid B, Marik PE. Pulmonary complications of novel antineoplastic agents for solid tumors. *Chest*. February 2008;133(2):528-538.

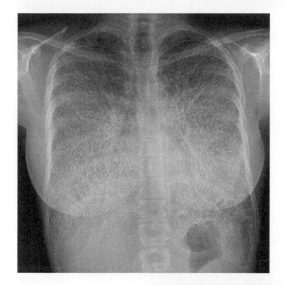

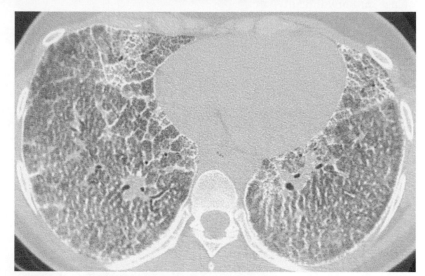

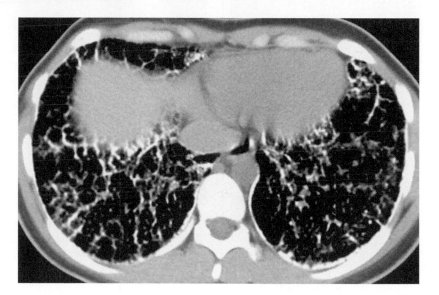

1. What are the radiographic findings?

2. What are the CT findings?

3. What is the diagnosis based on the CT appearance?

4. What are *calcospherites*?

5. What is the *black pleura line*?

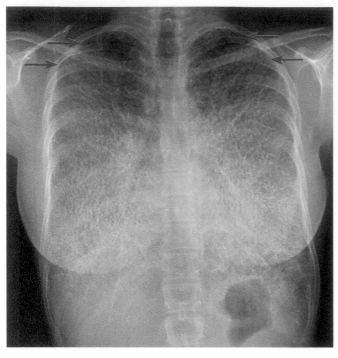

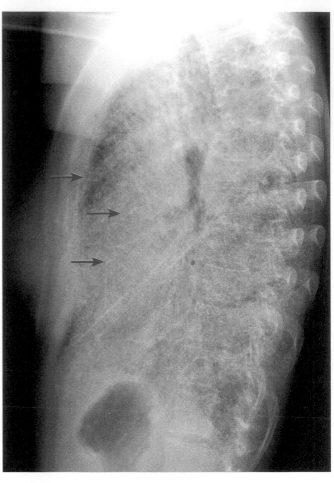

There is a bilateral diffuse lower lung–predominant calcific micronodular pattern, giving the so-called "sandstorm" appearance. The lung interface with the lateral osseous thorax shows thin linear lucencies at the apices, referred to as the *black pleura line* (*arrows*).

The lateral radiograph shows the same pattern seen on the PA film. However, the retrosternal area shows a more linear distribution of the calcific micronodules (*arrows*), suggesting an interlobular septal–based abnormality.

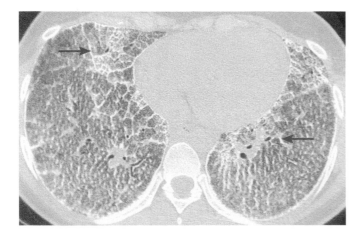

There is a bilateral diffuse calcific micronodular pattern (*arrows*). The nodules concentrate at the pleural surfaces and have an interlobular septal distribution. The innumerable tiny nodules give rise to diffuse ground-glass attenuation. No fibrotic changes are noted.

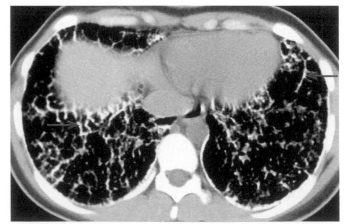

This soft tissue window shows that the micronodular abnormality is calcified (*arrows*).

Answers

1. The radiographs show a bilateral diffuse lower lung–predominant calcific micronodular pattern, giving the so-called "sandstorm" appearance. The lung interface with the lateral osseous thorax shows thin linear lucencies at the apices, referred to as the *black pleura line*.

2. The CT shows a bilateral diffuse calcific micronodular pattern, with lower lung predominance. The nodules concentrate at the pleural surfaces and have an interlobular septal distribution. The innumerable tiny nodules give rise to diffuse ground-glass attenuation. No fibrotic changes are noted.

3. The diagnosis is pulmonary alveolar microlithiasis (PAM).

4. Calcospherites are calcium phosphate deposits.

5. The *black pleura line* is a sign of PAM, which is postulated to be due to tiny subpleural cysts, creating a thin linear lucency between dense lung and lateral osseous thorax.

Pearls

- PAM is a rare entity caused by intra-alveolar calcium phosphate (calcospherites) deposition.
- Patients with PAM have normal serum calcium and phosphate.
- A "sandstorm" appearance and the *black pleura line* are classic signs for PAM.
- Patients with PAM may be relatively asymptomatic despite a strikingly abnormal imaging appearance (ie, clinicoradiological discrepancy).

Suggested Readings

Abdalla G, Marchiori E, Zanetti G, et al. Pulmonary alveolar microlithiasis: a case report with emphasis on imaging findings. *Case Rep Med*. 2010;2010:819242.

Marchiori E, Souza AS, Franquet T, Müller NL. Diffuse high-attenuation pulmonary abnormalities: a pattern-oriented diagnostic approach on high-resolution CT. *AJR Am J Roentgenol*. January 2005;184(1):273-282.

Shah M, Joshi JM. Bone scintigraphy in pulmonary alveolar microlithiasis. *Indian J Chest Dis Allied Sci*. July 2012;53(4):221-223.

Prior coronary arterial bypass graft (CABG) patient with 6 months of progressive shortness of breath and hypoxia

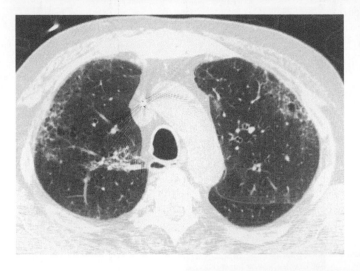
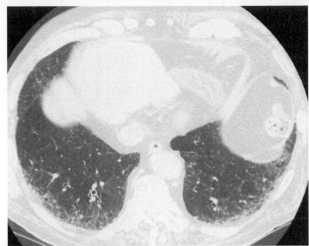
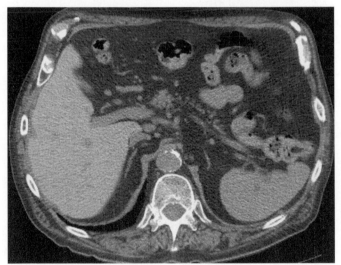

1. What are the imaging findings?

2. Based on the CT findings, which pattern of interstitial lung disease is most likely?

3. What is the most likely diagnosis?

4. List a few known patterns of pulmonary drug reaction.

5. What are the treatment options for amiodarone pulmonary toxicity?

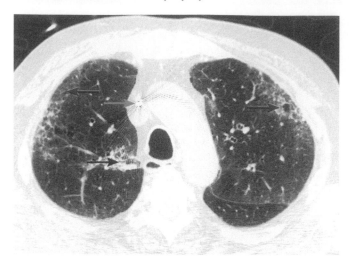

There are biapical patchy subpleural reticulations (*red arrows*), with mild superimposed ground-glass attenuation, mild traction bronchiectasis, and minimal architectural distortion. A right upper lobe focal consolidation is also seen (*blue arrow*). Note the presence of an implantable cardioverter defibrillator (ICD) (*green arrow*).

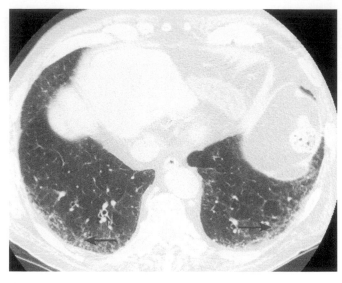

There are bilateral subpleural reticulations (*arrows*), with bibasilar predominance, mild superimposed ground-glass attenuation, mild traction bronchiectasis, and minimal architectural distortion.

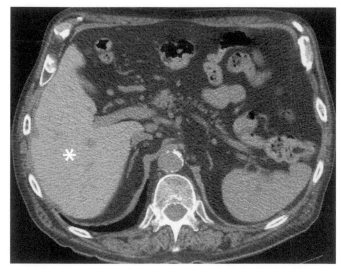

The liver appears hyperdense on this nonenhanced upper abdominal image (*asterisk*).

Answers

1. There are bilateral subpleural reticulations, with bibasilar predominance, mild superimposed ground-glass attenuation, mild traction bronchiectasis, and minimal architectural distortion. The liver appears hyperdense on the nonenhanced upper abdominal image.

2. The most likely pattern is that of nonspecific interstitial pneumonia (NSIP).

3. Amiodarone lung toxicity is the most likely diagnosis.

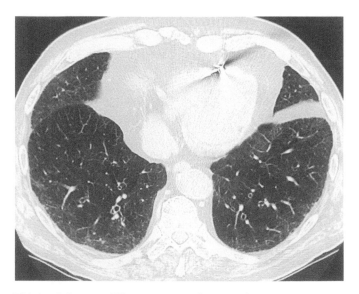

This is a follow-up CT image, 1 year after amiodarone was discontinued. The overall picture has improved, with interval resolution of the peripheral ground-glass opacities. However, the fibrotic lung changes (mainly seen in the form of reticulations) have not substantially changed.

4. Patterns of pulmonary drug reaction include NSIP usual interstitial pneumonia (UIP), organizing pneumonia (OP), diffuse alveolar damage (DAD)/acute respiratory distress syndrome (ARDS), eosinophilic pneumonia (EP), hypersensitivity pneumonitis (HP), pulmonary hemorrhage (PH), and desquamative interstitial pneumonia (DIP).

5. Most patients with a pulmonary drug reaction will improve and will have a good prognosis with discontinuation of the drug. Corticosteroid administration and supportive treatment might be needed in severe cases.

Pearls

- Like with many other drugs, amiodarone lung toxicity can present in acute or chronic forms.
- NSIP is the most common manifestation of amiodarone lung toxicity.
- Hyperdense liver and hyperdense pulmonary consolidation on nonenhanced CT are considered a classic radiological appearance of amiodarone lung toxicity. However, amiodarone toxicity can present in several other forms, often in the absence of these typical findings.

Suggested Readings

Papiris SA, Triantafillidou C, Kolilekas L, Markoulaki D, Manali ED. Amiodarone: review of pulmonary effects and toxicity. *Drug Saf.* July 2010;33(7):539-558.

Rossi SE, Erasmus JJ, McAdams HP, Sporn TA, Goodman PC. Pulmonary drug toxicity: radiologic and pathologic manifestations. *Radiographics.* September-October 2000;20(5):1245-1259.

Intravenous drug abuser with septicemia

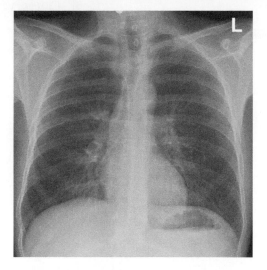 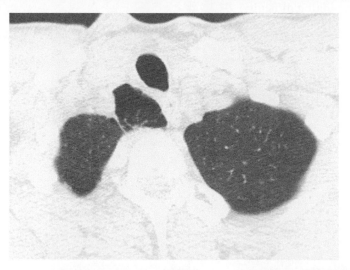

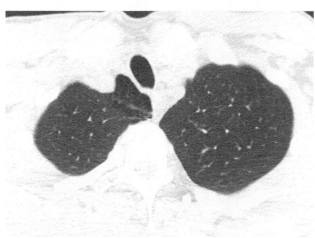 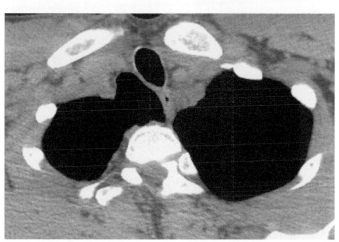

1. What are the radiographic findings?

2. What are the CT findings?

3. What is the differential diagnosis?

4. What is Sibson facia?

5. On which side is apical lung hernia more common?

Case ranking/difficulty:

Category: Lungs

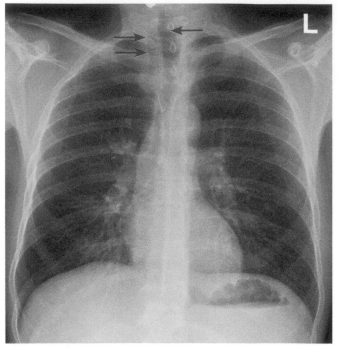

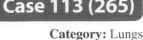

An elongated subtle area of well-defined lucency projects over the upper tracheal region, slightly off to the right side of the midline (*arrows*). Note that this abnormality can be easily missed if attention was not paid to the central radiographic structures.

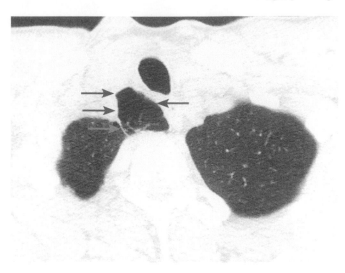

There is right apical lung herniation (*red arrows*), with minimal retrotracheal extension. The herniated lung shows an internal septated appearance, which is probably a result of focal emphysema. A linear apical opacity is seen, possibly representing Sibson facia (*green arrow*).

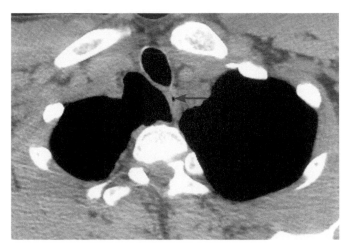

The esophagus is minimally displaced to the left side (*arrow*) by the retrotracheal extension of the right apical lung hernia.

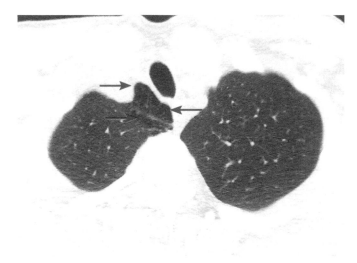

This more caudal image shows the continuity of the apical hernia with the intrathoracic lung (*arrows*).

Answers

1. An elongated well-defined lucency projects over the upper tracheal region.

2. There is right apical lung tissue herniation, with minimal retrotracheal extension. The esophagus is minimally displaced to the left side by this abnormality.

3. The differential diagnosis of a contained air lucency beside the trachea is tracheal diverticulum, Zenker diverticulum, Killian-Jamieson diverticulum, laryngocele, pharyngocele, and apical lung herniation.

4. Sibson facia is a continuation of the endothoracic facia along the lung apex.

5. Apical lung herniation is more common on the right side.

Pearls

- Apical lung hernia can be easily missed on chest radiographs.
- Apical lung hernia may be invisible on an expiratory chest radiograph or CT.
- Central venous line insertion in a patient with apical lung herniation could be complicated by lung injury and pneumothorax.

Suggested Readings

Bhalla M, Leitman BS, Forcade C, Stern E, Naidich DP, McCauley DI. Lung hernia: radiographic features. *AJR Am J Roentgenol*. January 1990;154(1):51-53.

Evans AS, Nassif RG, Ah-See KW. Spontaneous apical lung herniation presenting as a neck lump in a patient with Ehlers-Danlos syndrome. *Surgeon*. February 2005;3(1):49-51.

McAdams HP, Gordon DS, White CS. Apical lung hernia: radiologic findings in six cases. *AJR Am J Roentgenol*. October 1996;167(4):927-930.

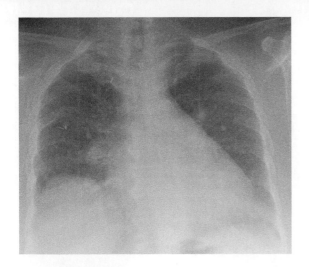

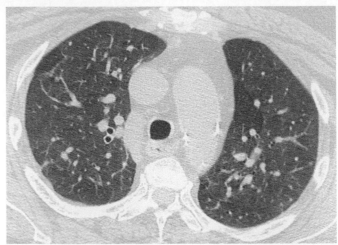

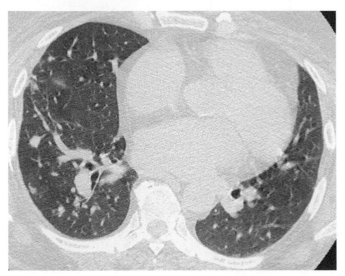

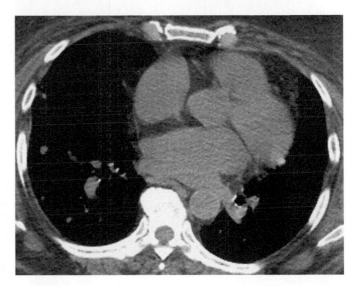

1. What are the radiographic findings?

2. What are the CT findings?

3. What is the differential diagnosis?

4. What is the likely diagnosis?

5. What is a neuroendocrine tumorlet?

Diffuse idiopathic pulmonary neuroendocrine cell hyperplasia (DIPNECH)

Case ranking/difficulty:

Category: Lungs

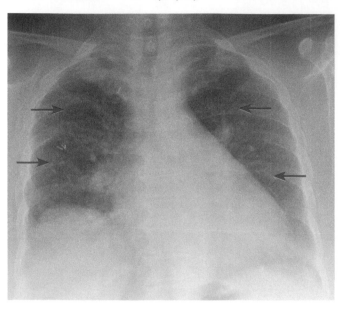

There are bilateral diffuse small nodular opacities (*arrows*). Right hemithoracic surgical clips from prior lung resection are noted. There is unrelated cardiomegaly.

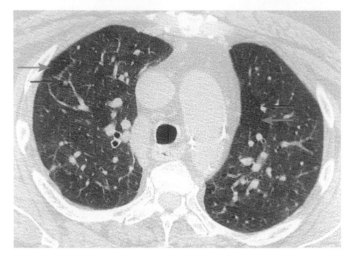

There are variably sized, well-defined, and mostly rounded nodules (*red arrows*), scattered throughout the lung parenchyma. The nodules show no cavitation. In addition, there are bilateral geographic areas of hypoattenuation with internal small caliber pulmonary vasculature (*green arrows*). This appearance suggests small airways-related mosaic attenuations.

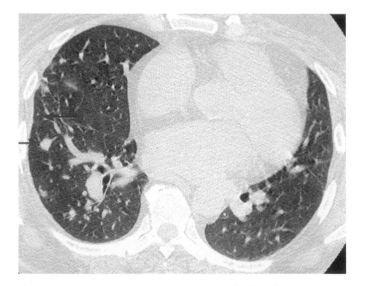

The nodular abnormalities are also seen at the lung bases (*arrows*). In addition, air trapping is suspected, as denoted by diffuse mosaic lung attenuation.

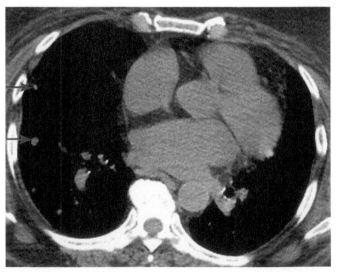

The nodules are of soft tissue attenuation and have no internal fat or calcification (*arrows*).

Bilateral geographic parenchymal hyperlucency is also seen, in keeping with mosaic attenuation due to small airways disease.

Answers

1. Bilateral diffuse small nodular opacities are seen on the radiograph.

2. The CT shows variably sized, well-defined, and mostly rounded nodules, with no cavitation, fat, or calcification.

3. The differential diagnosis of multiple bilateral small lung nodules includes metastases, infection (mycobacterial or fungal), primary pulmonary neoplasms (such as lymphoma, Kaposi sarcoma, and bronchoalveolar

carcinoma), sarcoidosis, vasculitis (such as Wegener granulomatosis), pneumoconiosis (such as silicosis), multiple arteriovenous malformations, connective tissue diseases (such as necrobiotic rheumatoid nodules), and amyloidosis.

The differential diagnosis of mosaic attenuation due to air trapping includes hypersensitivity pneumonitis, infectious bronchiolitis, inhalation injury, obliterative bronchiolitis, and age-related lung changes.

4. The combination of bilateral lung nodules and air trapping raises the possibility of diffuse idiopathic pulmonary neuroendocrine cell hyperplasia (DIPNECH).

5. A tumorlet is a lesion that results from focal proliferation of neuroendocrine cells, extending beyond the basement membrane of the involved airway and measuring less than 5 mm.

Suggested Readings

Johney EC, Pfannschmidt J, Rieker RJ, Schnabel PA, Mechtersheimer G, Dienemann H. Diffuse idiopathic pulmonary neuroendocrine cell hyperplasia and a typical carcinoid tumor. *J Thorac Cardiovasc Surg*. May 2006;131(5):1207-1208.

Koo CW, Baliff JP, Torigian DA, Litzky LA, Gefter WB, Akers SR. Spectrum of pulmonary neuroendocrine cell proliferation: diffuse idiopathic pulmonary neuroendocrine cell hyperplasia, tumorlet, and carcinoids. *AJR Am J Roentgenol*. September 2010;195(3):661-668.

Warth A, Herpel E, Schmähl A, Storz K, Schnabel PA. Diffuse idiopathic pulmonary neuroendocrine cell hyperplasia (DIPNECH) in association with an adenocarcinoma: a case report. *J Med Case Rep*. 2008;2(2):21.

Pearls

- DIPNECH is diffuse neuroendocrine cellular hyperplasia that is confined to the mucosa of the airways.
- DIPNECH should be considered when both bilateral scattered lung nodules and air trapping are seen.
- DIPNECH requires continuous surveillance due to its preneoplastic nature.
- If the neuroendocrine cellular hyperplasia extends beyond the basement membrane of the involved airway, it is referred to as a tumorlet (ie, size of less than 5 mm) or a carcinoid tumor (ie, size of 5 mm or larger).

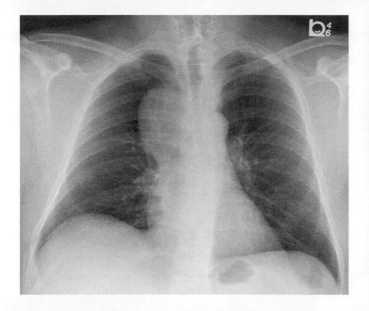
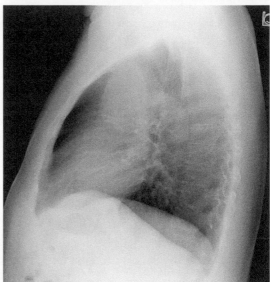
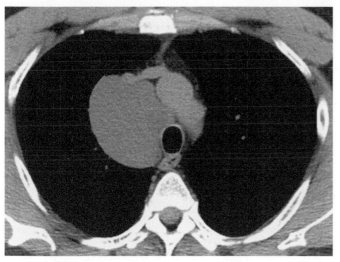
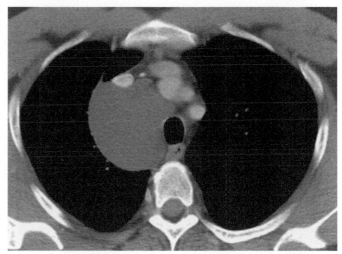

1. What is the radiographic abnormality?

2. What is the CT abnormality?

3. What is the differential diagnosis?

4. What are the different histological types of this entity?

5. List two characteristic features of this entity.

Case ranking/difficulty: 🐾🐾🐾

Category: Mediastinum

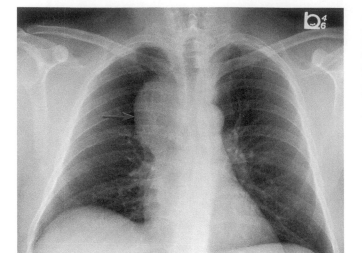

There is a well-defined and homogenous right paratracheal lesion (*arrow*), with no calcification or obvious mass effect on the adjacent tracheal air column. No hilar abnormalities or pleural effusions are seen.

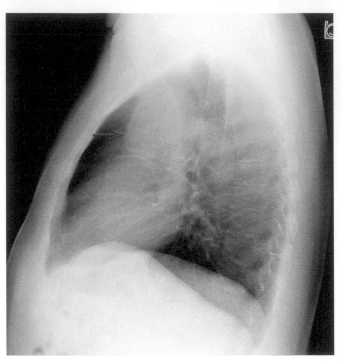

The abnormality has an anterior mediastinal location on the lateral radiograph (*arrow*).

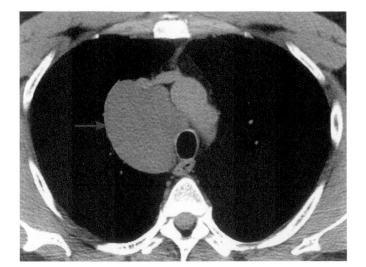

There is a large and well-defined low-attenuation right paratracheal lesion (*arrow*), with no invasive features. The lesion displaces the superior vena cava anteriorly and abuts the trachea and major mediastinal vessels. The lesion is homogenous, with no internal fat, calcification, or soft tissue components.

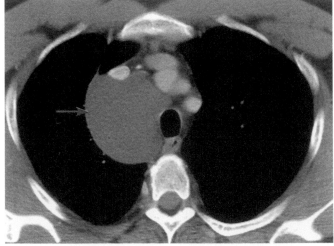

The abnormality shows no change in density on this contrast-enhanced image (*arrow*), in keeping with its cystic nature.

Answers

1. The radiographs show a well-defined and homogenous right paratracheal lesion.

2. The CT shows a large, well-defined, homogenous, fluid density, and nonenhancing right paratracheal lesion, with no invasive features. The lesion displaces the superior vena cava anteriorly and abuts the trachea and major mediastinal vessels.

3. The differential diagnosis of a fluid-density mediastinal lesion includes: foregut duplication cyst, lymphangioma, pericardial cyst, cystic teratoma, cystic thymoma, and thymic cyst.

4. The different histological types of lymphangioma are cystic, cavernous, and capillary.

5. Insinuation in-between structures and internal thin septations are features highly suggestive of lymphangioma.

Pearls

- Isolated mediastinal lymphangiomas are rare in adults.
- An insinuating multicompartmental cystic lesion, with thin and enhancing internal septations, is highly suggestive of lymphangioma.
- The histologic types of lymphangioma are cystic (hygroma), cavernous, and capillary.

Suggested Readings

Correia FM, Seabra B, Rego A, Duarte R, Miranda J. Cystic lymphangioma of the mediastinum. *J Bras Pneumol.* November 2008;34(11):982-984.

Jeung MY, Gasser B, Gangi A, et al. Imaging of cystic masses of the mediastinum. *Radiographics.* October 2002;22 Spec No:S79-S93.

Melo IA, Camargo Jde J, Gomes Bde M, Cabrera GA, Machuca TN. [Isolated mediastinal cystic lymphangioma]. *Rev Port Pneumol.* 2011;15(4):697-703.

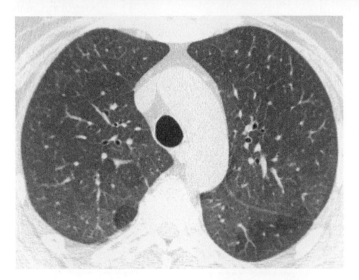
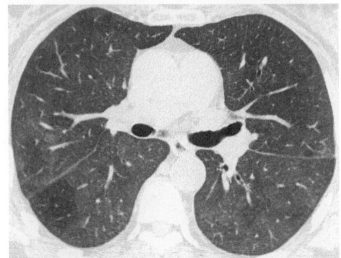
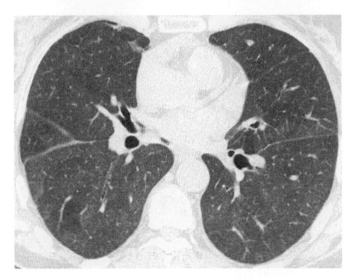

1. What are the CT findings?

2. What is the differential diagnosis?

3. What is the differential diagnosis of thin-walled pulmonary cysts in a Sjögren syndrome patient?

4. What is the taxonomic classification of *Pneumocystis jiroveci*?

5. What is the biological sample of choice for the microbiological diagnosis of *Pneumocystis jiroveci* pneumonia?

Case ranking/difficulty: 🐾🐾🐾

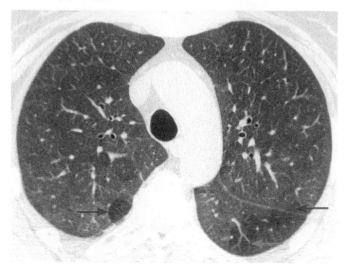

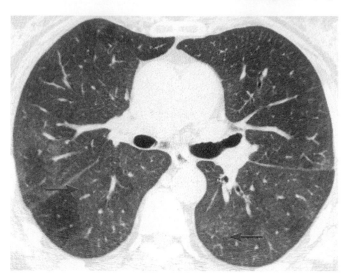

There is bilateral diffuse lung parenchymal ground-glass attenuation. The abnormality is heterogeneous, with areas of focal low attenuation (*red arrows*). However, the areas of low attenuation show normal internal pulmonary vascular caliber (*green arrow*).

The diffuse bilateral ground-glass abnormality (*arrows*) is seen on this midlung image, with no centrilobular nodules or cysts.

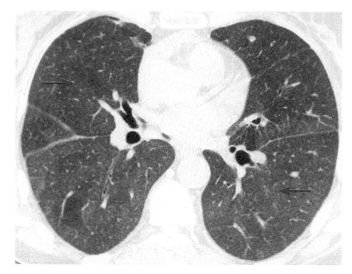

The same abnormality (*arrows*) is seen on this lower lung image.

respiratory bronchiolitis-associated interstitial lung disease and desquamative interstitial pneumonia), other chronic interstitial pneumonias (eg, nonspecific interstitial pneumonia, lymphocytic interstitial pneumonia, and organizing pneumonia), drug toxicity, pulmonary edema (from cardiogenic and noncardiogenic causes), sarcoidosis, and adenocarcinoma spectrum (formerly known as bronchoalveolar carcinoma).

3. Lymphocytic interstitial pneumonia (LIP) and *Pneumocystis jiroveci* pneumonia (PJP) should be considered, if thin-walled pulmonary cysts are seen in a Sjögren syndrome patient.

4. *Pneumocystis jiroveci* is a yeast-like fungus of the genus *Pneumocystis*.

5. Bronchoalveolar lavage (BAL) is the biological sample of choice for the microbiological diagnosis of *PJP*.

Answers

1. The CT shows bilateral diffuse and heterogeneous lung parenchymal ground-glass attenuation. The areas of focal low attenuation show normal internal pulmonary vascular caliber.

2. The differential diagnosis of diffuse bilateral ground-glass attenuation includes infection (eg, *Pneumocystis jiroveci* pneumonia, viral pneumonia such as cytomegalovirus, and atypical pneumonia such as *Mycoplasma* and *Chlamydia*), hypersensitivity pneumonitis, smoking-related lung diseases (eg,

Pearls

- When compared to immunocompromised HIV patients, *PJP* in non-HIV immunocompromised patients is more severe, has worse prognosis, and is more difficult to diagnose.
- A high index of suspicion for PJP should be maintained when reading CT scans of non-HIV immunocompromised patients.
- Sulfamethoxazole-trimethoprim is the drug of choice for treating PJP.

Suggested Readings

Shah RM, Kaji AV, Ostrum BJ, Friedman AC. Interpretation of chest radiographs in AIDS patients: usefulness of CD4 lymphocyte counts. *Radiographics*. January-February 1997;17(1):47-58; discussion 59-61.

Sider L, Gabriel H, Curry DR, Pham MS. Pattern recognition of the pulmonary manifestations of AIDS on CT scans. *Radiographics*. July 1993;13(4):771-784; discussion 785-786.

Tasaka S, Tokuda H, Sakai F, et al. Comparison of clinical and radiological features of pneumocystis pneumonia between malignancy cases and acquired immunodeficiency syndrome cases: a multicenter study. *Intern Med*. 2010;49(4):273-281.

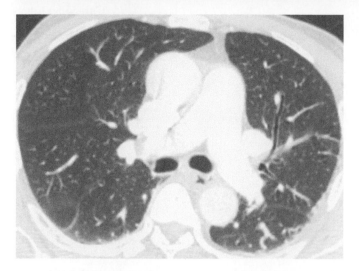
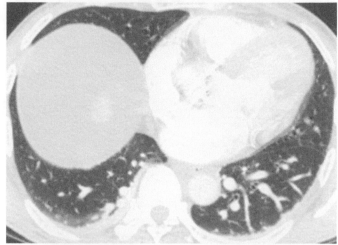

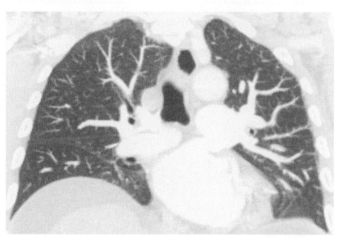
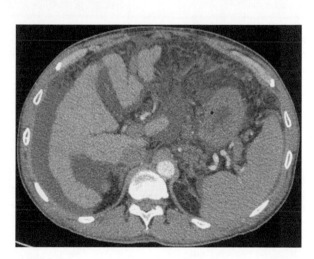

1. What are the CT findings?

2. What are the pulmonary manifestations of chronic liver diseases?

3. What is platypnea?

4. What is orthodeoxia?

5. What is portopulmonary hypertension?

Case ranking/difficulty:

Category: Lungs

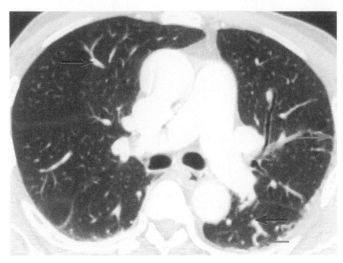

Bilateral diffuse enlargement of the peripheral pulmonary arterial branches is seen (*red arrows*). Note that several vessels demonstrate contact with the pleural surfaces (*green arrows*).

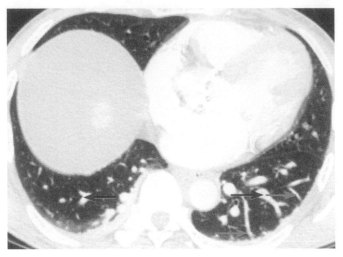

There are peripherally enlarged pulmonary arterial branches in the lower lungs as well (*red arrows*) and several vessels are in contact with the pleura (*green arrows*).

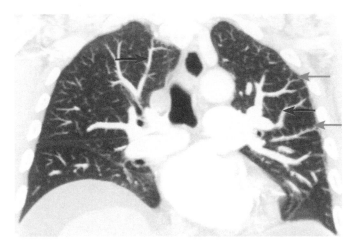

The enlarged pulmonary arterial branches (*red arrows*) and their pleural contact (*green arrows*) are noted on this coronal image.

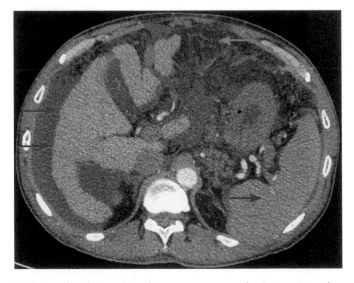

Features of end-stage liver disease are seen on this image: irregular liver surface due to cirrhosis (*red arrows*), splenomegaly (*blue arrow*), numerous venous collaterals (*green arrows*), and ascites.

Answers

1. Bilateral diffuse enlargement of the peripheral pulmonary arterial branches is seen, with several vessels contacting the pleural surfaces. In addition, irregular liver surface due to cirrhosis, splenomegaly, numerous venous collaterals, and ascites are noted.

2. Pulmonary manifestations of chronic liver diseases include hepatopulmonary syndrome, portopulmonary hypertension, intrathoracic portosystemic collaterals, hepatic hydrothorax, acute respiratory distress syndrome (in the context of acute hepatic failure), infection (due to impaired immunity), intrathoracic metastases (from hepatocellular carcinoma), and drug reactions.

3. Platypnea is shortness of breath exaggerated by sitting or standing, but relieved by lying flat.

4. Orthodeoxia is reduced oxygen saturation that is exaggerated by sitting or standing, but relieved by lying flat.

5. Portopulmonary hypertension is the development of pulmonary hypertension in the setting of portal hypertension, usually in the context of chronic liver disease. This entity is not to be confused with hepatopulmonary syndrome.

Pearls

- On a normal chest CT, pulmonary arterioles should not touch the pleura.
- In hepatopulmonary syndrome, circulating toxic substances may induce pulmonary arterial vasodilatation, resulting in right-to-left shunting of blood.
- The peripheral pulmonary arteries may be dilated and touching the pleura on chest CT examinations of patients with chronic liver disease (ie, due to hepatopulmonary syndrome).
- Portopulmonary hypertension is a different entity that should not to be confused with hepatopulmonary syndrome.

Suggested Readings

Kim YK, Kim Y, Shim SS. Thoracic complications of liver cirrhosis: radiologic findings. *Radiographics*. May-June 2009;29(3):825-837.

Martinez-Jimenez S, Heyneman LE, McAdams HP, et al. Nonsurgical extracardiac vascular shunts in the thorax: clinical and imaging characteristics. *Radiographics*. September 2010;30(5):e41.

Meyer CA, White CS, Sherman KE. Diseases of the hepatopulmonary axis. *Radiographics*. May-June 2000;20(3):687-698.

Fever and hemoptysis

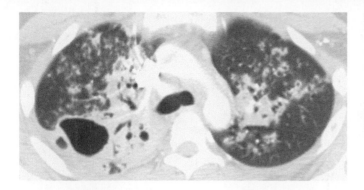
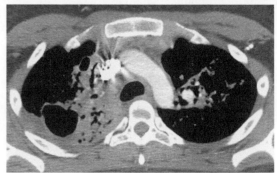
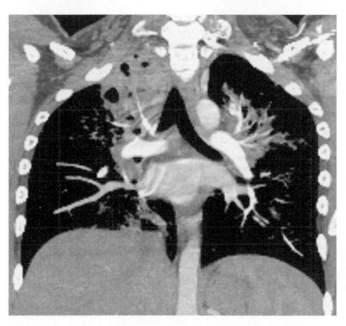
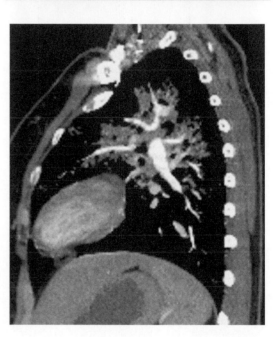

1. What are the CT features?

2. What is the major diagnosis based on the parenchymal lung abnormalities?

3. What potentially fatal complication is depicted on the provided CT images?

4. How is this complication treated?

5. List the possible causes of pulmonary arterial aneurysms.

Case ranking/difficulty:

Category: Lungs

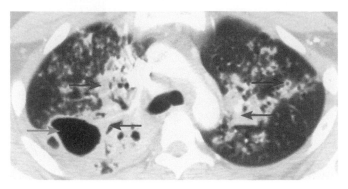

There are extensive bilateral consolidations (*red arrows*), predominantly in the peribronchovascular regions. There is associated bronchial wall thickening and bronchial dilatation (*blue arrows*). A right upper lobe cavity is also seen (*green arrow*). There are tree-in-bud nodules as well.

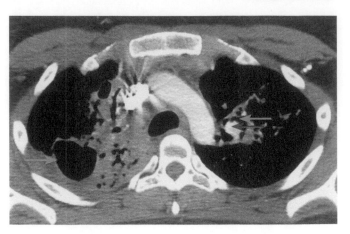

Cavitations are seen in the upper lobes (*green arrows*), with a small segmental left upper pulmonary arterial intracavitary aneurysm (*red arrow*).

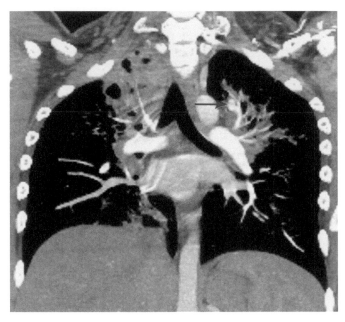

The left upper lobe segmental pulmonary artery aneurysm is well depicted on this coronal image (*arrow*).

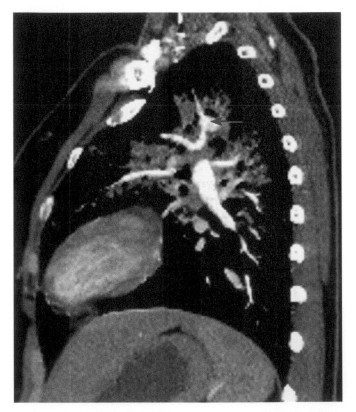

The left upper lobe segmental pulmonary artery aneurysm is well depicted on this sagittal image (*arrow*).

Answers

1. There are extensive bilateral consolidations, predominantly in the peribronchovascular regions. There is associated bronchial wall thickening and bronchial dilatation. Bilateral upper lobar lung cavities are also seen. A small pulmonary arterial aneurysm resides in a left upper lobe cavity. There are tree-in-bud nodules as well.

2. Cavitary pneumonia is the major diagnostic consideration, with tuberculosis being the most likely diagnosis.

3. The potentially fatal complication depicted on the provided CT is that of a Rasmussen aneurysm.

4. Rasmussen aneurysm may be treated by coil angioembolization or surgical exploration, in addition to appropriately managing any active tuberculosis.

5. Causes of pulmonary arterial aneurysms can be congenital or acquired. Congenital causes include cardiac shunts and vascular stenosis. Acquired causes include chronic and severe pulmonary arterial hypertension, vasculitis (Behçet or Hughes-Stovin syndromes), mycotic (tuberculosis, fungal pneumonia, necrotizing bacterial pneumonia, or septic embolism), trauma, iatrogenic (Swan-Ganz catheters, pulmonary catheter angiography, or chest tube insertion), invading neoplasm (lung cancer or metastasis), and connective tissue abnormalities (Marfan or Ehlers-Danlos syndromes).

Pearls

- Bronchial arteries are the origin of hemoptysis in most cases, but nonbronchial systemic and pulmonary arteries can also be the site of bleeding in some cases.
- Pulmonary arterial aneurysms can result from congenital or acquired causes.
- The presence of tuberculous parenchymal lung lesions and an associated intracavitary pulmonary artery aneurysm is a classic appearance for Rasmussen aneurysm.
- Rasmussen aneurysm can lead to fatal hemoptysis.

Suggested Readings

Bruzzi JF, Rémy-Jardin M, Delhaye D, Teisseire A, Khalil C, Rémy J. Multi-detector row CT of hemoptysis. *Radiographics*. January-February 2006;26(1):3-22.

Nguyen ET, Silva CI, Seely JM, Chong S, Lee KS, Müller NL. Pulmonary artery aneurysms and pseudoaneurysms in adults: findings at CT and radiography. *AJR Am J Roentgenol*. February 2007;188(2):W126-W134.

Santelli ED, Katz DS, Goldschmidt AM, Thomas HA. Embolization of multiple Rasmussen aneurysms as a treatment of hemoptysis. *Radiology*. November 1994;193(2):396-398.

Shortness of breath in an intravenous drug user

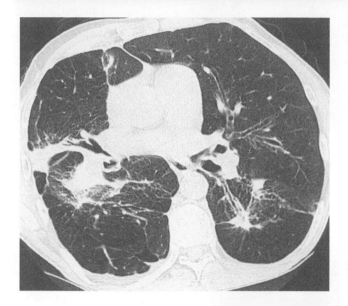
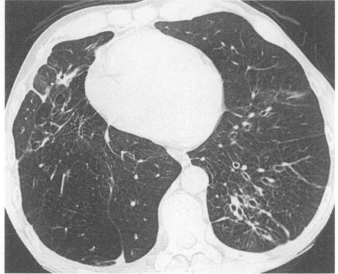
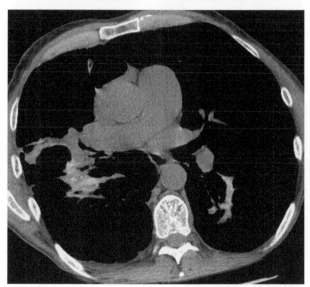

1. What are the CT findings?

2. How is this entity acquired?

3. What is the lesion size cutoff beyond which progressive massive fibrosis (PMF) can be called?

4. What is the differential diagnosis for PMF?

5. What is the differential diagnosis for bilateral basilar panlobular emphysema?

Case ranking/difficulty: **Category:** Lungs

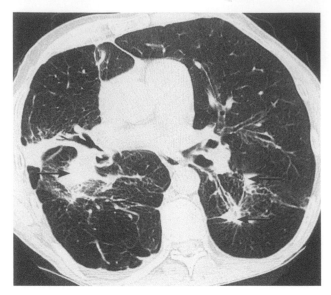

There are bilateral parahilar conglomerate, irregular, mass-like opacities, with architectural distortion (*arrows*), consistent with progressive massive fibrosis. An emphysematous background is seen.

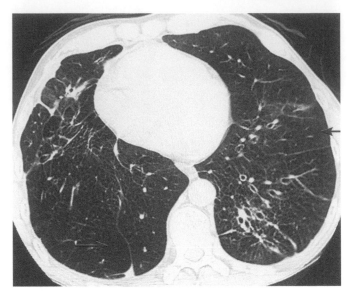

Diffuse emphysematous changes are seen, which are more pronounced at the lung bases and have a panlobular pattern (*arrows*).

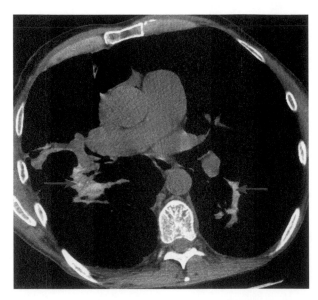

The parahilar opacities have a characteristic high attenuation despite the absence of calcification on this nonenhanced CT image (*arrows*).

Answers

1. There are bilateral parahilar conglomerate, irregular, mass-like opacities, with architectural distortion. Despite the absence of obvious calcifications, the parahilar opacities have a characteristic high attenuation on this nonenhanced CT image, consistent with progressive massive fibrosis in the context of talcosis. An emphysematous background is seen, which is more pronounced at the lung bases and has a panlobular pattern.

2. Talcosis is acquired by intravenous or inhalational routes.

3. The mass-like opacity should be larger than 1 cm before it can be called PMF.

4. The differential diagnosis for PMF is that of pneumoconiosis (eg, silicosis, coal worker pneumoconiosis, talcosis, berylliosis, and hard metal pneumoconiosis) and sarcoidosis.

5. The main differential diagnosis for bilateral basilar panlobular emphysema is alpha-1-antitrypsin deficiency and IV Ritalin injection.

Pearls

- The differential diagnosis for PMF is pneumoconiosis (silicosis, coal worker pneumoconiosis, talcosis, berylliosis, and hard metal pneumoconiosis) and sarcoidosis.
- PMF in talcosis may appear hyperattenuated despite absence of calcifications.
- The main differential diagnosis for bibasilar panacinar emphysema is alpha-1-antitrypsin deficiency and IV Ritalin injection.

Suggested Readings

Chong S, Lee KS, Chung MJ, Han J, Kwon OJ, Kim TS. Pneumoconiosis: comparison of imaging and pathologic findings. *Radiographics*. January-February 2006;26(1): 59-77.

Restrepo CS, Carrillo JA, Martínez S, Ojeda P, Rivera AL, Hatta A. Pulmonary complications from cocaine and cocaine-based substances: imaging manifestations. *Radiographics*. July-August 2007;27(4):941-956.

Ward S, Heyneman LE, Reittner P, Kazerooni EA, Godwin JD, Müller NL. Talcosis associated with IV abuse of oral medications: CT findings. *AJR Am J Roentgenol*. March 2000;174(3):789-793.

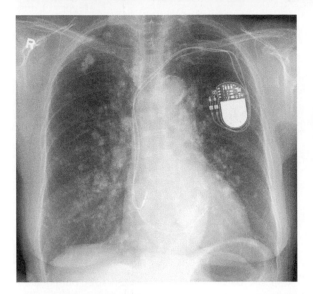
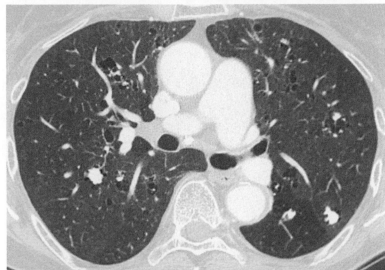
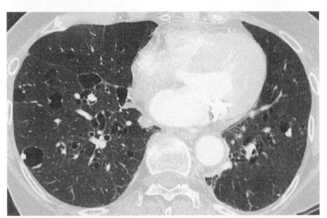
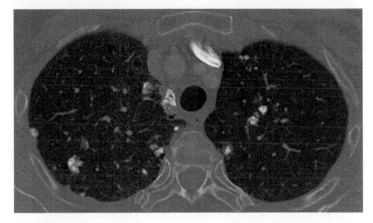

1. What are the radiographic findings?

2. What are the CT findings?

3. What is the differential diagnosis?

4. What are the different types of amyloidosis?

5. List a few amyloid-associated conditions.

Case ranking/difficulty:

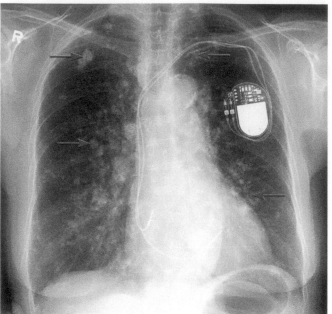

Multiple, bilateral, well-defined, nodular opacities are scattered throughout the lung parenchyma (*arrows*), with most nodules showing high density. Cardiomegaly, a dual-chamber pacemaker, and atherosclerotic aorta are also noted.

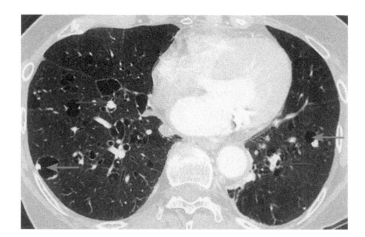

The nodules (*red arrows*) and cysts (*green arrows*) are intimately related and are scattered throughout both lungs.

Answers

1. There are bilateral, multiple, scattered, well-defined, nodular lung opacities, with most nodules showing high density suggesting calcifications.

2. The CT shows bilateral, multiple, scattered, variably sized pulmonary nodules and cysts. The nodules are lobulated and well defined, with most showing high attenuation. The cysts are round or irregular, with thin walls.

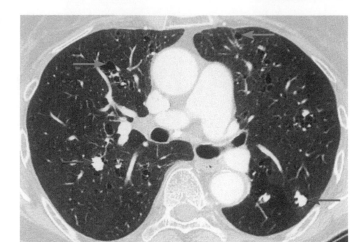

There are bilateral, multiple, scattered, variably sized pulmonary nodules (*red arrows*) and cysts (*green arrows*). The nodules are lobulated and well defined, with most showing high attenuation.

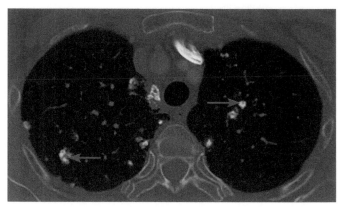

On bone window, the nodules are clearly calcified (*arrows*).

3. The differential diagnosis of multiple bilateral large calcified nodular opacities includes: metastases (ie, bone-forming or mucin-producing neoplasms), infection (ie, tuberculosis and histoplasmosis), progressive massive fibrosis in pneumoconiosis (ie, silicosis and coal worker pneumoconiosis), metastatic pulmonary calcification in renal failure, amyloidosis, sarcoidosis, and hyalinizing granuloma. However, the concomitant presence of cystic lung disease raises the possibility of amyloidosis.

4. The main types of amyloidosis are primary (AL), secondary (AA), and hereditary.

5. A few amyloid-associated conditions are multiple myeloma, macroglobulinemia, rheumatoid arthritis, Sjögren syndrome, tuberculosis, and familial Mediterranean fever.

Pearls

- Amyloid is a nonsoluble protein that deposits in the extracellular spaces and is characterized by exhibiting apple-green birefringence when stained by Congo red and viewed under polarized light.
- Amyloidosis can be simply classified into primary (AL), secondary (AA), and hereditary types.
- Amyloidosis should be considered when encountering atypical imaging features in patients with hematological or chronic inflammatory conditions (especially in patients with multiple myeloma).
- Cystic lung disease with calcified or noncalcified lung nodules raises the possibility of amyloidosis.

Suggested Readings

Colombat M, Stern M, Groussard O, et al. Pulmonary cystic disorder related to light chain deposition disease. *Am J Respir Crit Care Med*. April 2006;173(7):777-780.

Ohdama S, Akagawa S, Matsubara O, Yoshizawa Y. Primary diffuse alveolar septal amyloidosis with multiple cysts and calcification. *Eur Respir J*. July 1996;9(7):1569-1571.

Seaman DM, Meyer CA, Gilman MD, McCormack FX. Diffuse cystic lung disease at high-resolution CT. *AJR Am J Roentgenol*. June 2011;196(6):1305-1311.

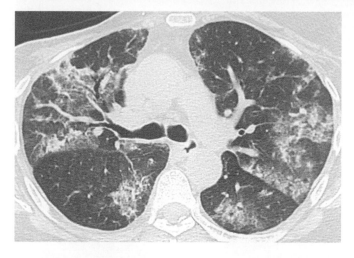
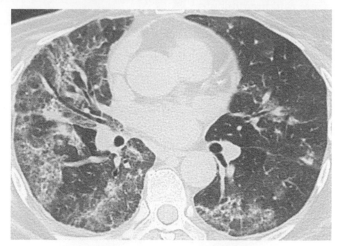
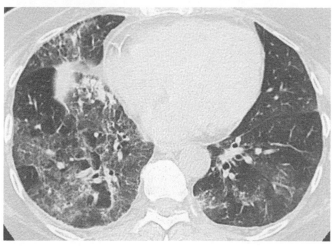
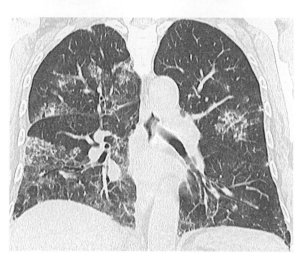

1. What are the CT findings?

2. What is the differential diagnosis?

3. What is the clinical definition of diffuse alveolar hemorrhage (DAH)?

4. What is the differential diagnosis for diffuse alveolar hemorrhage (DAH)?

5. What is the difference between microscopic polyangiitis (MPA) and polyarteritis nodosa (PAN)?

Case ranking/difficulty: 🌢🌢🌢

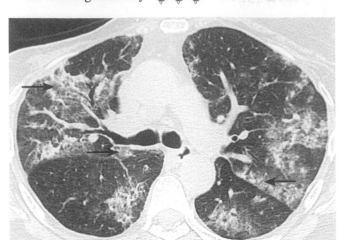

There are bilateral patchy areas of ground-glass opacification and septal thickening (*arrows*).

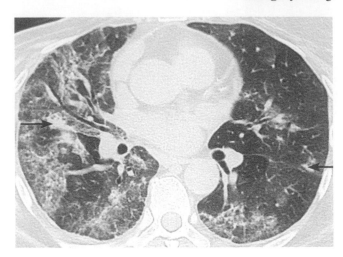

This lower lung image shows additional areas of consolidation (*red arrows*) and mild smooth cylindrical bronchial dilatation (*green arrow*).

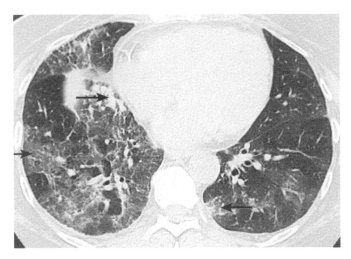

Multifocal ground-glass opacities (*red arrows*), consolidation (*blue arrow*), and septal thickening (*green arrow*) are noted at the lung base as well.

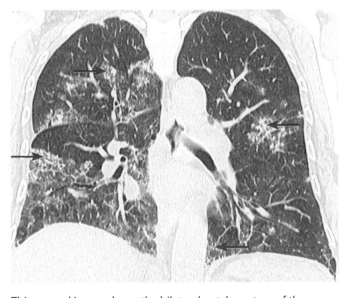

This coronal image shows the bilateral patchy nature of the abnormality (*arrows*).

Answers

1. There are bilateral patchy areas of ground-glass opacification, septal thickening, multifocal consolidation, and bronchial dilatation.

2. The major categories to consider for acute airspace opacities are infection (bacterial, mycobacterial, fungal, and viral), pulmonary edema (cardiogenic and noncardiogenic), pulmonary hemorrhage, diffuse aspiration pneumonitis, drug reaction, and vasculitis.

3. DAH is defined by the presence of hemoptysis, diffuse alveolar opacities, and decreasing hemoglobin count.

4. DAH causes can be divided into pulmonary-renal syndromes and those without renal involvement. Pulmonary-renal syndromes include microscopic polyangiitis, Wegener granulomatosis, Goodpasture syndrome, systemic lupus erythematosus/lupus anticoagulants, and a few other rare entities. DAH without renal involvement is seen with bone marrow transplant, anticoagulants, drug-induced thrombocytopenia, connective tissue disorders, and idiopathic pulmonary hemorrhage.

5. MPA is an ANCA-positive pulmonary-renal syndrome in the category of small vessel vasculitis. PAN, on the other hand, although affecting the kidneys, only rarely involves the pulmonary system, and is considered a medium-vessel vasculitis.

Pearls

- MPA is the most common cause of pulmonary-renal syndrome and commonly results in DAH.
- Hemoptysis and/or radiographic abnormalities can be absent even when anemia or CT abnormalities are present in some cases of DAH.
- P-ANCA is usually positive in MPA, but a negative p-ANCA serology does not exclude the diagnosis.

Suggested Readings

Castañer E, Alguersuari A, Gallardo X, et al. When to suspect pulmonary vasculitis: radiologic and clinical clues. *Radiographics*. January 2010;30(1):33-53.

Chung MP, Yi CA, Lee HY, Han J, Lee KS. Imaging of pulmonary vasculitis. *Radiology*. May 2010;255(2):322-341.

Marten K, Schnyder P, Schirg E, Prokop M, Rummeny EJ, Engelke C. Pattern-based differential diagnosis in pulmonary vasculitis using volumetric CT. *AJR Am J Roentgenol*. March 2005;184(3):720-733.

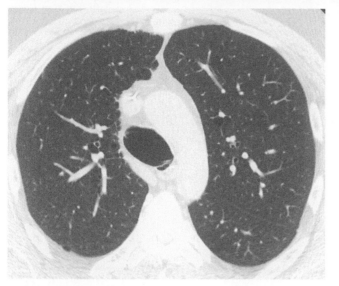 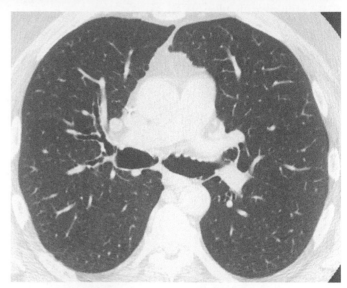

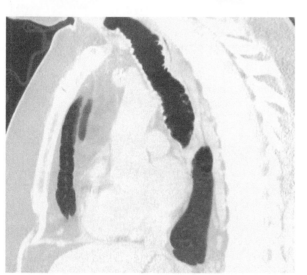 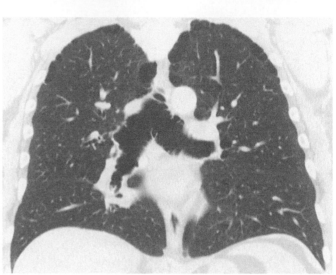

1. What are the CT findings?

2. What is considered a normal coronal tracheal diameter?

3. What is considered a normal sagittal tracheal diameter?

4. Which bronchial order is affected by bronchiectasis in Mounier-Kuhn syndrome?

5. Is there a way to differentiate William-Campbell syndrome from Mounier-Kuhn syndrome based on imaging?

Case ranking/difficulty: **Category:** Airways

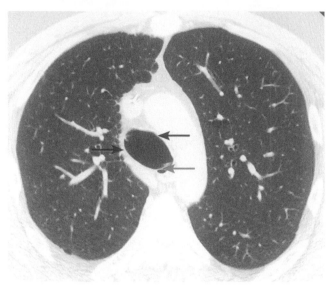

Marked dilatation of the trachea is seen (*red arrows*). Note the partially visualized tracheal diverticulum (*green arrow*).

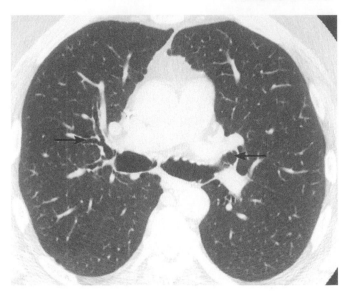

The main bronchi and central airways show dilatation (*arrows*), which spares the peripheral airways.

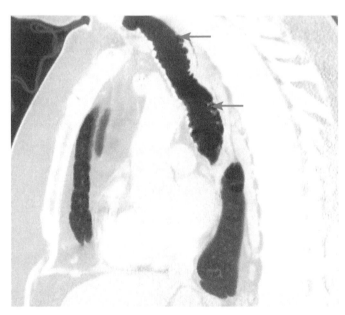

This sagittal image demonstrates diverticula bulging in between cartilaginous tracheal rings (*arrows*), resulting in a "corrugated" appearance.

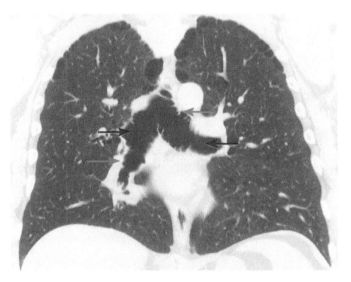

The carina and main bronchi are markedly dilated (*red arrows*) and airway diverticula are seen (*green arrows*).

Answers

1. Marked dilatation of the trachea, main bronchi, and lobar bronchi is seen. There is sparing of the peripheral airways. Diverticula bulging in between cartilaginous rings are seen throughout the central airways, resulting in a "corrugated" appearance.

2. The normal coronal tracheal diameter is 13 to 25 mm in males and 13 to 21 mm in females.

3. The normal sagittal tracheal diameter is 13 to 27 mm in males and 10 to 23 mm in females.

4. The trachea, main bronchi, and bronchi down to the fourth order are involved in Mounier-Kuhn syndrome.

5. In contrast to Mounier-Kuhn syndrome, airway ectasia in William-Campbell syndrome involves the fourth- to sixth-order bronchi, while the trachea and central airways are spared.

Pearls

- Mounier-Kuhn syndrome is diagnosed when tracheal diameter is larger than 3 cm and main bronchial diameter is larger than 2.4 cm.
- In contrast to William-Campbell syndrome, bronchiectasis in Mounier-Kuhn syndrome does not extend distal to the fourth-order bronchi.
- A "corrugated" tracheal appearance is typical of Mounier-Kuhn syndrome.

Suggested Readings

Chung JH, Kanne JP, Gilman MD. CT of diffuse tracheal diseases. *AJR Am J Roentgenol*. March 2011;196(3):W240-W246.

Falconer M, Collins DR, Feeney J, Torreggiani WC. Mounier-Kuhn syndrome in an older patient. *Age Ageing*. January 2008;37(1):115-116.

Menon B, Aggarwal B, Iqbal A. Mounier-Kuhn syndrome: report of 8 cases of tracheobronchomegaly with associated complications. *South Med J*. January 2008;101(1):83-87.

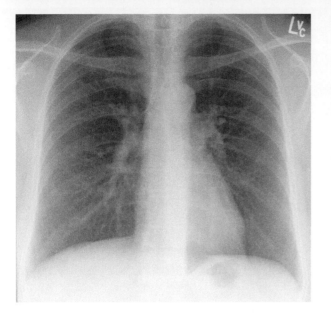
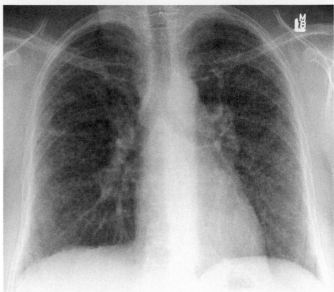

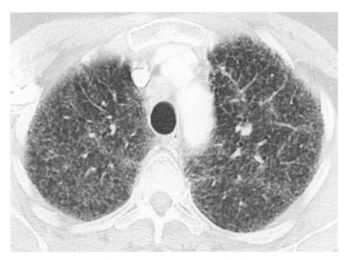
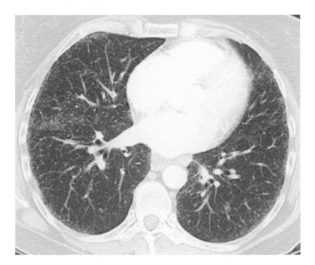

1. Describe the interval change occurring on the 18 months' follow-up radiograph (Top-right figure) when compared to the initial image (Top-left figure).

2. What are the CT findings?

3. What are the components of a micronodular perilymphatic distribution?

4. What is the differential diagnosis for this case?

5. What is the most likely diagnosis in the presented case?

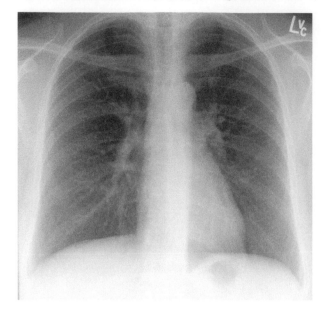

An initial normal chest radiograph, at the time of first diagnosing the patient with localized pelvic lymphoma.

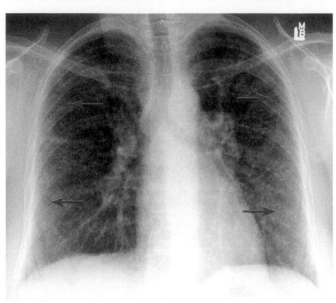

This 18 months' follow-up chest radiograph demonstrates new bilateral, diffuse, nodular opacities (*arrows*).

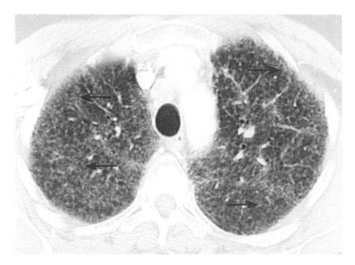

The follow-up CT demonstrates new bilateral, innumerable, tiny nodules involving both upper lungs (*arrows*).

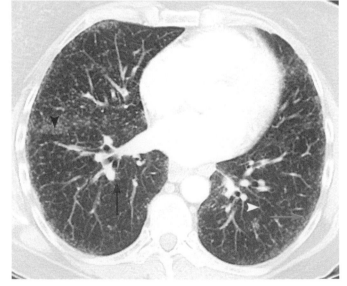

The abnormality is less pronounced in the lower lungs, where it is easier to determine the exact nodular pattern. The nodules assume a peribronchovascular (*red arrow*), perifissural (*blue arrowhead*), subpleural (*green arrow*), and septal (*white arrowhead*) locations, denoting an overall perilymphatic pattern.

Answers

1. The follow-up chest radiograph demonstrates new bilateral, diffuse, nodular opacities.

2. A perilymphatic nodular pattern is noted, with upper lung predominance.

3. Peribronchovascular, perifissural, subpleural, and septal distributions are all part of the perilymphatic pattern.

4. A perilymphatic nodular pattern is typically due to sarcoidosis, pneumoconiosis, and lymphangitic carcinomatosis. Less frequently, this pattern can be seen with lymphoma and amyloidosis.

5. Since the patient is asymptomatic, had lymphoma, and no prior sarcoidosis, a sarcoid-like reaction is favored. However, pulmonary lymphoma is also possible. The lack of septal thickening, despite extensive nodularity, would argue against lymphangitic carcinomatosis. Noncaseating granulomata were seen on an open surgical lung biopsy, consistent with the clinical diagnosis of sarcoid-like reaction.

Pearls

- Sarcoid-like reaction has been seen in association with various malignancies (eg, lymphoma, testicular carcinoma, breast carcinoma, and head and neck malignancies).
- Sarcoid-like reaction appears similar to sarcoidosis on biopsy, demonstrating noncaseating granulomata.
- Sarcoid-like reaction might be mistaken for lymphoma or metastatic disease on imaging.

Suggested Readings

Hunsaker AR, Munden RF, Pugatch RD, Mentzer SJ. Sarcoidlike reaction in patients with malignancy. *Radiology*. July 1996;200(1):255-261.

Risbano MG, Groshong SD, Schwarz MI. Lung nodules in a woman with a history of breast cancer. Diagnosis: a sarcoid-like reaction in metastatic breast cancer. *Chest*. November 2007;132(5):1697-1701.

Yao M, Funk GF, Goldstein DP, DeYoung BR, Graham MM. Benign lesions in cancer patients: Case 1.Sarcoidosis after chemoradiation for head and neck cancer. *J Clin Oncol*. January 2005;23(3):640-641.

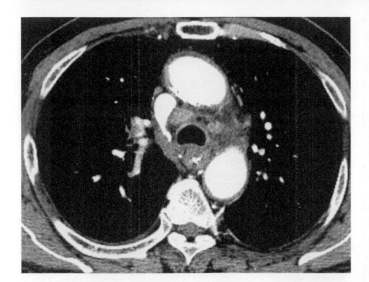

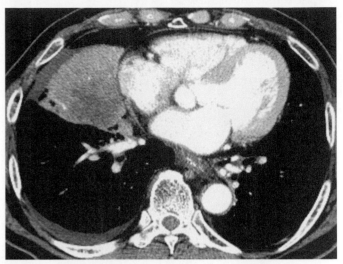

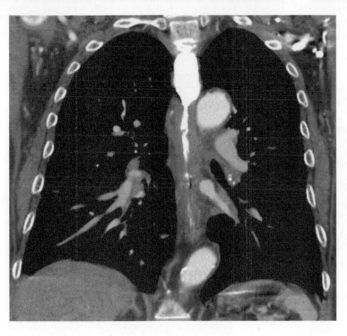

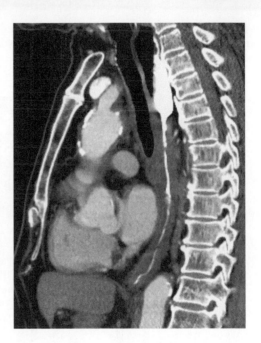

1. What are the imaging findings?

2. What is the differential diagnosis based on these findings?

3. List a few tumors that have been reported to metastasize to the esophagus.

4. What is the most common tumor to metastasize to the esophagus?

5. Which layer of the esophagus is usually not involved by metastatic disease?

Case ranking/difficulty: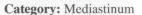

Category: Mediastinum

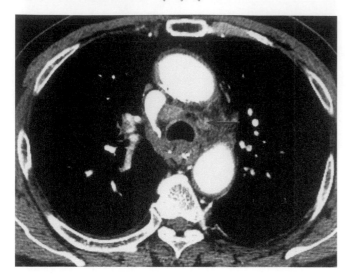

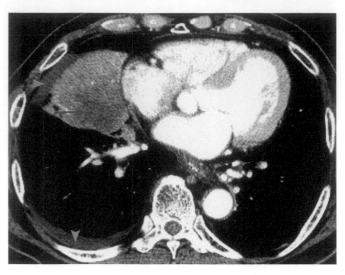

There is circumferential mural thickening of the thoracic esophagus, with luminal narrowing (*arrowhead*). Mediastinal lymph node enlargement is noted (*arrow*).

There is a right middle lobe heterogeneous consolidation with volume loss (*arrow*), where a mass lesion is possible. A small right pleural effusion is seen as well (*arrowheads*).

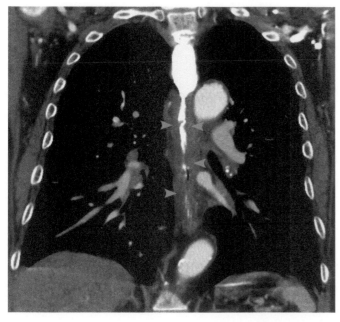

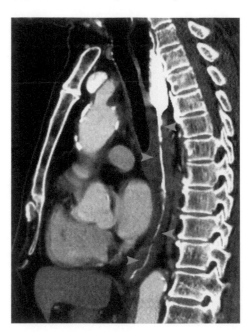

This coronal image demonstrates diffuse mural thickening of the lower two-thirds of the esophagus (*arrowheads*).

This sagittal image demonstrates the same abnormality (*arrowheads*) and shows esophageal luminal narrowing, but no occlusion.

Answers

1. There is circumferential mural thickening of the lower two-thirds of the esophagus, with luminal narrowing, but no occlusion. Additionally, there is right middle lobe heterogeneous consolidation with volume loss, where a mass lesion is possible. A small right pleural effusion is also present.

2. The differential diagnosis for long segment esophageal mural thickening includes carcinoma, lymphoma, metastasis, and esophagitis (ie, from infection, gastric reflux, radiation, and eosinophilia). Esophageal varices may mimic mural thickening on unenhanced CT.

3. Lung, breast, gastrointestinal, renal, and thyroid cancers are among the tumors that have been reported to metastasize to the esophagus.

4. Lung cancer is thought to be the most common tumor to metastasize to the esophagus.

5. Metastatic esophageal involvement usually spares the mucosa.

Pearls

- Metastasis to the esophagus is extremely rare.
- Metastasis to the esophagus spares the mucosa, which can lead to false-negative endoscopic results.
- Metastasis to the esophagus may mimic esophageal carcinoma on imaging.

Suggested Readings

Luedtke P, Levine MS, Rubesin SE, Weinstein DS, Laufer I. Radiologic diagnosis of benign esophageal strictures: a pattern approach. *Radiographics*. July-August 2003;23(4):897-909.

Mizobuchi S, Tachimori Y, Kato H, Watanabe H, Nakanishi Y, Ochiai A. Metastatic esophageal tumors from distant primary lesions: report of three esophagectomies and study of 1835 autopsy cases. *Jpn J Clin Oncol*. December 1997;27(6):410-414.

Noh HM, Fishman EK, Forastiere AA, Bliss DF, Calhoun PS. CT of the esophagus: spectrum of disease with emphasis on esophageal carcinoma. *Radiographics*. September 1995;15(5):1113-1134.

Hemoptysis

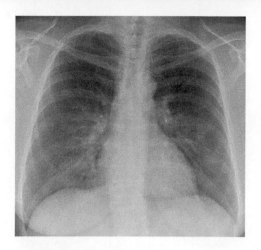
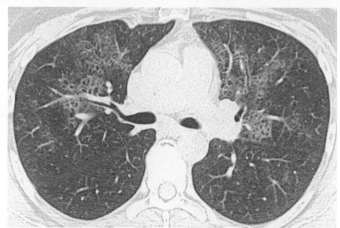
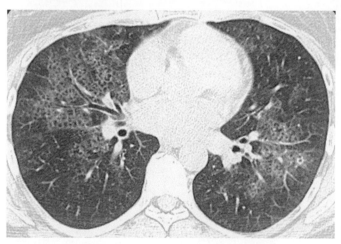
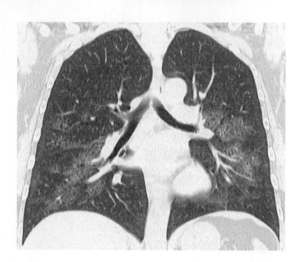

1. What are the radiographic findings?

2. What is the differential diagnosis based on the radiographic findings?

3. What are the CT findings?

4. What is the differential diagnosis based on the CT findings?

5. Which antibody is typically found in the serum of Goodpasture syndrome patients?

Case ranking/difficulty:

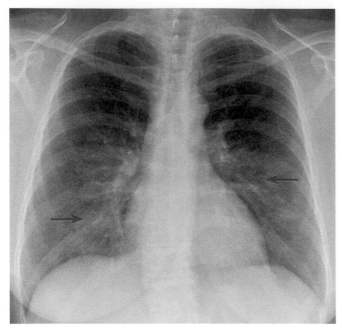

Bilateral faint lung opacification is noted, with central and bibasilar predominance (*arrows*).

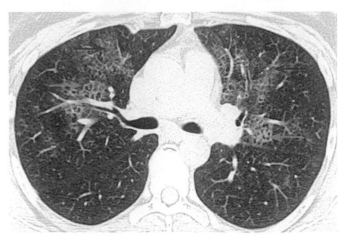

There are bilateral patchy areas of ground-glass attenuation (*red arrows*) and superimposed smooth interlobular septal thickening (*green arrows*), resulting in a crazy-paving appearance.

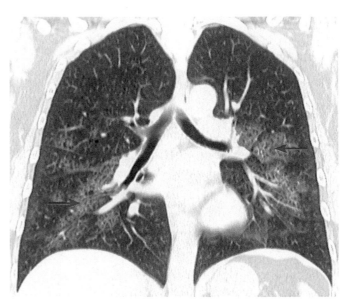

The abnormality shows relative peripheral sparing and an overall central predominance (*arrows*).

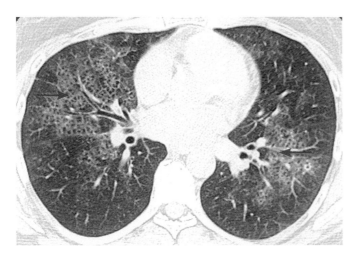

The bilateral crazy-paving pattern is also seen on this more caudal image (*arrows*).

Answers

1. Bilateral faint lung opacification is noted, with central and bibasilar predominance.

2. The major categories to consider for differential diagnosis of subtle central acute airspace opacities are atypical pneumonia (eg, *Pneumocystis jiroveci*, *Chlamydia*, *Mycoplasma*, and viruses), pulmonary edema (cardiogenic or noncardiogenic), pulmonary hemorrhage, aspiration pneumonitis, drug reaction, vasculitis, and subacute hypersensitivity pneumonitis.

3. There are bilateral patchy areas of ground-glass attenuation and superimposed smooth interlobular septal thickening, resulting in a crazy-paving appearance. The abnormality shows central predominance.

4. When central crazy paving is seen, the major considerations are atypical pneumonia (eg, *Pneumocystis jiroveci*, *Chlamydia*, *Mycoplasma*, and viruses), pulmonary edema, pulmonary hemorrhage, and drug reactions. If the process is long-standing, alveolar proteinosis, lipoid pneumonia, nonspecific interstitial pneumonia, and organizing pneumonia might be considered.

5. Antiglomerular basement membrane antibody (anti-GBMA) is the antibody that is typically found in the serum of Goodpasture syndrome patients.

Pearls

- The main differential diagnosis of central (ie, perihilar) crazy paving is atypical pneumonia, pulmonary edema, pulmonary hemorrhage, and drug reactions.
- The main differential diagnosis of long-standing crazy paving is alveolar proteinosis, lipoid pneumonia, nonspecific interstitial pneumonia, and organizing pneumonia.
- When pulmonary hemorrhage is confirmed, the differential diagnostic list can be further limited based on the presence or absence of renal involvement and of specific serologic findings (ie, ANCA or anti-GBMA).
- On imaging, features of pulmonary edema typically resolve quicker than those of pulmonary hemorrhage.

Suggested Readings

Malho A, Santos V, Cabrita A, et al. Severe Relapsing Goodpasture's Disease Successfully Treated with Mycophenolate Mofetil. *Int J Nephrol.* 2010 Aug 16;2010:383548.

Marten K, Schnyder P, Schirg E, Prokop M, Rummeny EJ, Engelke C. Pattern-based differential diagnosis in pulmonary vasculitis using volumetric CT. *AJR Am J Roentgenol.* March 2005;184(3):720-733.

Poddar B, Singhal S, Azim A, Gulati S, Baronia A. Goodpasture's syndrome in children. *Saudi J Kidney Dis Transpl.* September 2010;21(5):935-939.

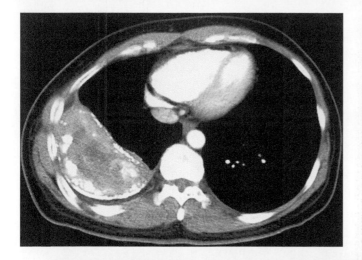
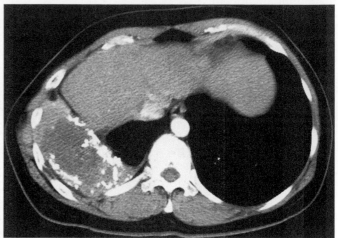
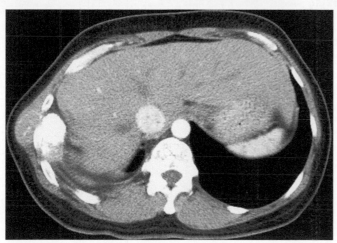
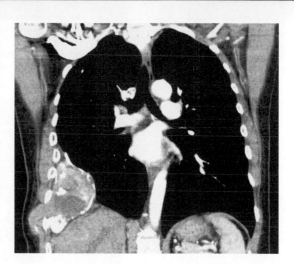

1. What are the CT findings?

2. What is the name of the presented entity?

3. What is the etiology of this lesion?

4. What should this lesion be differentiated from?

5. Is actinomycosis a bacterial or fungal infection?

Case ranking/difficulty:

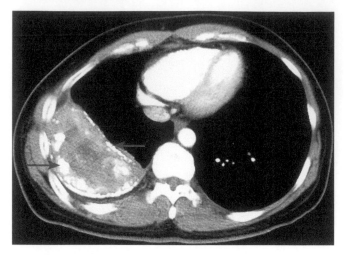

There is a large right lower hemithoracic pleural-based heterogeneous lesion, with peripheral rim-like and central dense calcifications (*arrows*).

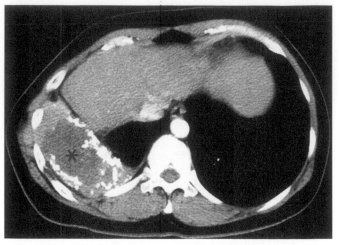

The center of the lesion is of fluid attenuation (*asterisk*).

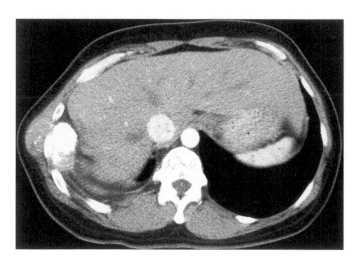

Part of the lesion shows extension into the chest wall and leads to a small subcutaneous component (*arrowhead*).

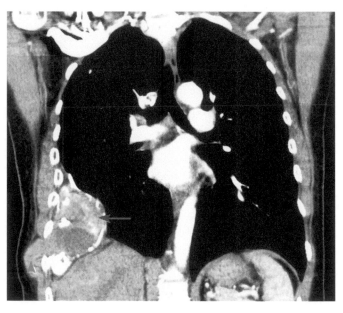

This coronal image demonstrates the intrathoracic lesion (*arrow*) and its smaller subcutaneous extension (*arrowhead*).

Answers

1. The CT shows a large right lower hemithoracic pleural-based lesion, with fluid, soft tissue, and calcific components. The lesion demonstrates transpleural extension into the chest wall, leading to a small subcutaneous component.

2. This condition is known as empyema necessitatis (also known as empyema necessitans), which is defined as a pleural empyema that involves the chest wall and forms a subcutaneous abscess.

3. Tuberculosis is the most common cause of empyema necessitatis, but other bacterial (eg, *Streptococcus* and

Actinomycosis) and fungal (eg, *Blastomycosis* and *Mucormycosis*) infections have been reported as well.

4. Empyema necessitatis should be differentiated from neoplastic process, such as mesothelioma, lymphoma, sarcoma, squamous cell carcinoma, and metastasis.

5. Actinomycosis is an infection by *Actinomyces*, a filamentous gram-positive bacterium. Due to the misleading term -*mycosis* as part of its name, many mistake actinomycosis for a fungal infection.

Pearls

- When a pleural empyema is seen, meticulous evaluation for possible osseous and chest wall involvement should be performed.
- Although the most common cause for empyema necessitatis is TB, other bacterial and fungal infections should be considered.
- Empyema necessitatis should be differentiated from neoplasms that may involve the chest wall.

Suggested Readings

Kim HY, Song KS, Goo JM, Lee JS, Lee KS, Lim TH. Thoracic sequelae and complications of tuberculosis. *Radiographics*. July-August 2001;21(4):839-858; discussion 859-860.

Senent C, Betlloch I, Chiner E, Llombart M, Moragón M. Tuberculous empyema necessitatis. A rare cause of cutaneous abscess in the XXI century. *Dermatol Online J*. 2008;14(3):11.

Ueda T, Andreas C, Itami J, et al. Pyothorax-associated lymphoma: imaging findings. *AJR Am J Roentgenol*. January 2010;194(1):76-84.

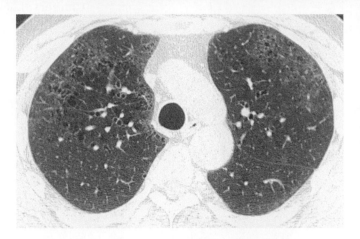
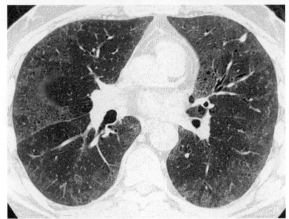

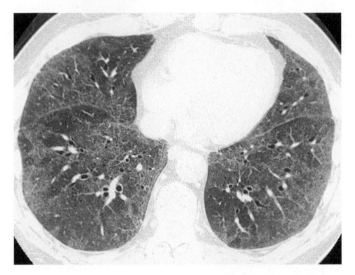

1. What are the CT findings?

2. What is the differential diagnosis based on the CT findings?

3. List a few smoking-related lung diseases.

4. What is the difference between respiratory bronchiolitis-interstitial lung disease (RB-ILD) and desquamative interstitial pneumonia (DIP)?

5. Among the variable imaging manifestations of DIP, what is considered the most typical?

Desquamative interstitial pneumonia (DIP) Case 127 (541)

Case ranking/difficulty: **Category:** Lungs

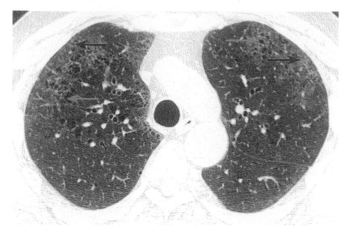

Bilateral peripheral ground-glass lung parenchymal attenuation (*red arrows*) and centrilobular emphysematous changes (*green arrows*) are seen.

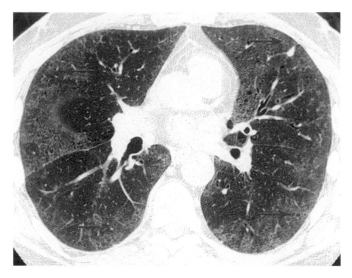

The peripheral distribution of the ground-glass abnormality is clearly seen on this image (*arrows*).

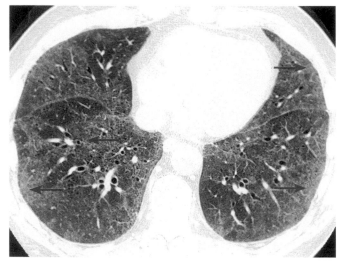

The ground-glass abnormality is more pronounced at the lung bases (*arrows*).

Answers

1. Bilateral peripheral ground-glass lung parenchymal attenuation with bibasilar predominance is seen on CT. A background of centrilobular emphysema is also noted.

2. The differential diagnosis of bibasilar and peripheral ground-glass attenuation incudes nonspecific interstitial pneumonia (NSIP), organizing pneumonia (OP), lymphocytic interstitial pneumonia (LIP), and desquamative interstitial pneumonia (DIP).

3. Smoking-related lung diseases include emphysema, chronic bronchitis, lung cancer, pulmonary Langerhans cell histiocytosis (PLCH), respiratory bronchiolitis (RB),

respiratory bronchiolitis-interstitial lung disease (RB-ILD), and desquamative interstitial pneumonia (DIP). Idiopathic pulmonary fibrosis (IPF) is commonly seen in chronic smokers and acute eosinophilic pneumonia (AEP) is commonly seen in new-onset smokers.

4. Both RB-ILD and DIP are symptomatic entities with substantial overlap in clinical presentation. The distinction between both entities depends on histological findings. The major finding of pigmented macrophages deposits is bronchocentric in RB-ILD and more diffuse in the alveolar spaces in DIP. Bilateral upper lung centrilobular ground-glass nodularity is considered typical of RB-ILD, but overlap in imaging features with DIP is common.

5. Bilateral peripheral ground-glass attenuation with bibasilar predominance is the most typical appearance of DIP.

Pearls

- Both RB-ILD and DIP are symptomatic smoking-related conditions, but differ on histological analysis and in chest imaging findings.
- Consider DIP in symptomatic smokers with ground-glass attenuation on chest CT.
- Smoking cessation is the main treatment in DIP.

436

Suggested Readings

Attili AK, Kazerooni EA, Gross BH, Flaherty KR, Myers JL, Martinez FJ. Smoking-related interstitial lung disease: radiologic-clinical-pathologic correlation. *Radiographics.* September-October 2008;28(5):1383-1396; discussion 1396-1398.

Miller WT, Shah RM. Isolated diffuse ground-glass opacity in thoracic CT: causes and clinical presentations. *AJR Am J Roentgenol.* February 2005;184(2):613-622.

Mueller-Mang C, Grosse C, Schmid K, Stiebellehner L, Bankier AA. What every radiologist should know about idiopathic interstitial pneumonias. *Radiographics.* May-June 2007;27(3):595-615.

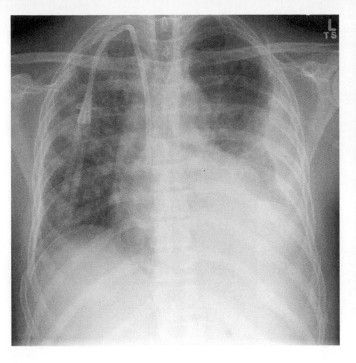
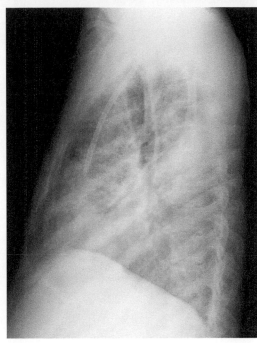

1. What is the most important radiographic finding?

2. What are the other radiographic findings?

3. In practice, what should you do immediately after reading this examination?

4. If the referring clinician doubts your salient finding, what should be the next step?

5. List a few complications that can be encountered with a central venous catheter (CVC).

Case ranking/difficulty:

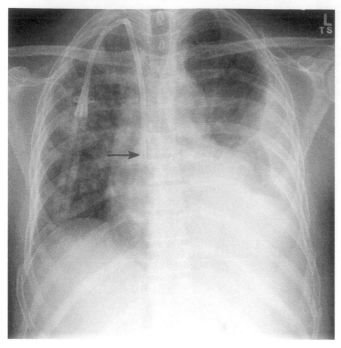

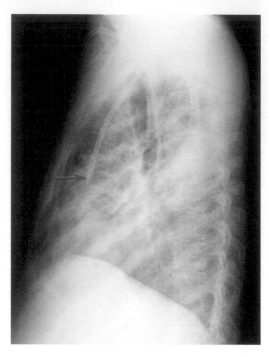

There is a double-lumen right internal jugular tunneled dialysis catheter, with a tip that "projects" over the expected superior cavoatrial region (*arrow*). Features of cardiogenic pulmonary edema, left loculated pleural effusion, and bilateral lower rib fractures are also noted.

The lateral chest radiograph shows that the course of the dialysis catheter is unusual and is curving anteriorly (*arrow*), instead of the normally expected straighter and more posterior course.

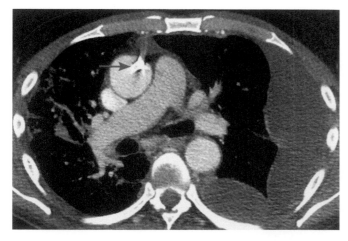

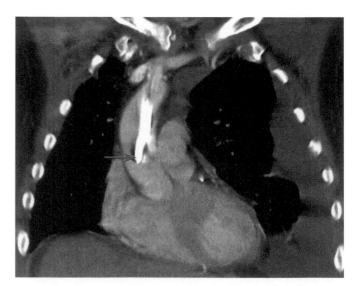

This transverse CT image shows the abnormal arterial location of the dialysis catheter in the ascending aorta (*arrow*).

This coronal CT image shows the abnormal arterial location of the dialysis catheter in the ascending aorta (*arrow*).

Answers

1. Although the dialysis catheter projects over the superior cavoatrial region on the frontal radiograph, it has an unusual anteriorly curving course on the lateral projection, suggesting an arterial location.

2. Features of cardiogenic pulmonary edema, left loculated pleural effusion, and bilateral lower rib fractures are also noted. Visualization of such findings might lead to satisfaction of search and the important lateral radiographic finding of an abnormal dialysis catheter course might go unrecognized.

3. Notify the referring clinician promptly regarding the likely malpositioned dialysis catheter.

4. The abnormal position can be confirmed by performing an arterial blood gas analysis or even performing a CT examination.

5. Potential complications of CVC insertion include pneumothorax, malpositioning, infection, perforation, hemorrhage, thrombosis, and arrhythmia.

Pearls

- Checking integrity, course, and position of CVC is a priority when interpreting chest radiographs, and the clinician should be immediately notified of malpositioned CVCs.
- Remember to make use of the lateral chest radiograph for assessment of CVC position. If the lateral projection is not available, comment on the tip's "projection" instead of its "exact" location.
- In problematic cases where CVC tip position is questioned, blood gas testing should be performed.

Suggested Readings

Hunter TB, Taljanovic M. Overview of medical devices. *Curr Probl Diagn Radiol.* July-August 2001;30(4):94-139.

Stonelake PA, Bodenham AR. The carina as a radiological landmark for central venous catheter tip position. *Br J Anaesth.* March 2006;96(3):335-340.

Vesely TM. Central venous catheter tip position: a continuing controversy. *J Vasc Interv Radiol.* May 2003;14(5):527-534.

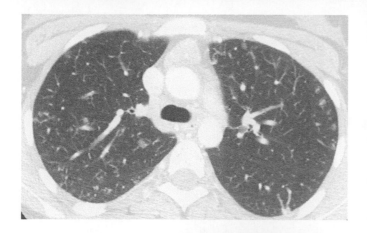

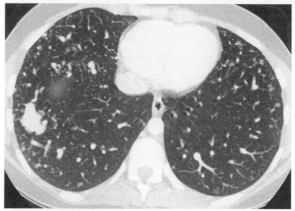

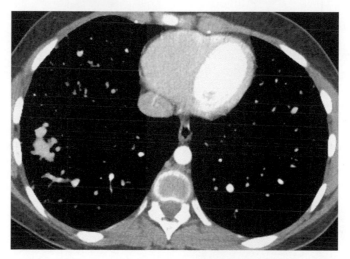

1. What are the CT findings?

2. What is the diagnosis?

3. What defines a "simple" pulmonary arteriovenous malformation (AVM)?

4. What are the major complications of a pulmonary AVM?

5. What is the mode of inheritance of hereditary hemorrhagic telangiectasia (HHT)?

Case ranking/difficulty: 🏵🏵🏵

Category: Lungs

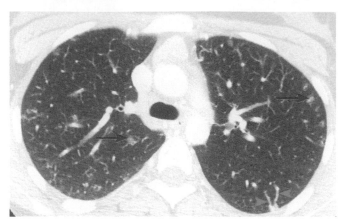

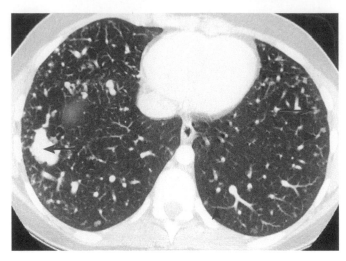

There are bilateral irregular and nodular opacities (*arrows*). Note that a larger lesion in the superior segment of the left lower lobe is associated with two vascular structures (*arrowheads*), denoting feeding and draining pulmonary vessels.

Telangiectatic vessels are also seen bilaterally (*arrowheads*), in addition to the variably sized and diffusely scattered nodular lung lesions (*arrows*).

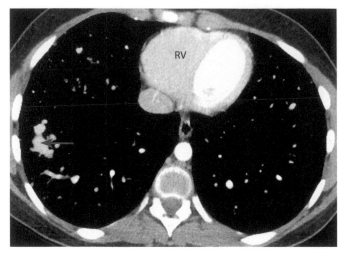

This contrast-enhanced CT image shows that the large right lower lobe lesion enhances (*arrow*) with an attenuation that is equal to that of the right ventricle (RV).

4. Brain abscesses and strokes are the major complications of a pulmonary AVM, but hemorrhage into an airway or the pleural cavity may rarely occur as well.

5. HHT is an autosomal dominant disease with variable penetrance.

Pearls

- Fifteen percent of HHT patients have pulmonary AVMs, whereas 60% of pulmonary AVM patients have HHT.
- "Simple" AVMs have a single feeding segmental vessel, whereas "complex" AVMs have more than one feeding segmental vessel.
- The major complications of pulmonary AVMs are strokes and brain abscesses.

Answers

1. There are bilateral irregular, variably sized, enhancing, nodular opacities, which are associated with feeding and draining pulmonary vessels. Scattered telangiectatic vessels are also noted bilaterally.

2. The diagnosis is that of multiple pulmonary arteriovenous malformations (AVM) in the context of hereditary hemorrhagic telangiectasia (HHT).

3. "Simple" AVMs have feeding vessel(s) arising from a single segmental pulmonary artery, whereas "complex" AVMs have feeding vessels arising from more than one segmental pulmonary artery.

Suggested Readings

Carter BW, Lichtenberger JP, Wu CC. Acquired abnormalities of the pulmonary arteries. *AJR Am J Roentgenol.* May 2014;202(5):W415-W421.

Jaskolka J, Wu L, Chan RP, Faughnan ME. Imaging of hereditary hemorrhagic telangiectasia. *AJR Am J Roentgenol.* August 2004;183(2):307-314.

Martinez-Jimenez S, Heyneman LE, McAdams HP, et al. Nonsurgical extracardiac vascular shunts in the thorax: clinical and imaging characteristics. *Radiographics.* September 2010;30(5):e41.

CT performed to exclude pulmonary embolism in a thalassemic patient

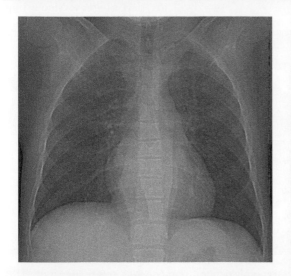

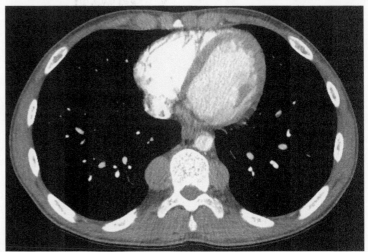

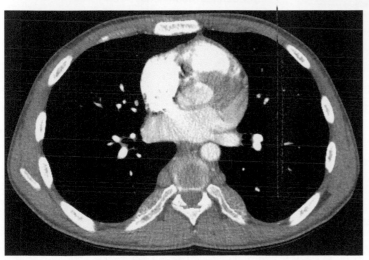

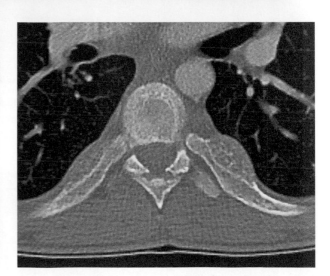

1. What abnormality is seen on the scout image?

2. What is the differential diagnosis based on the scout image?

3. What are the CT findings?

4. What causes extramedullary hematopoiesis (EMH)?

5. What is the most common location of EMH?

Case ranking/difficulty:

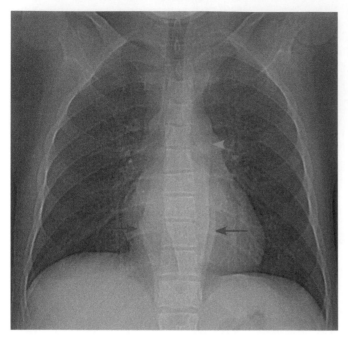

Bilateral near-symmetric, smoothly defined, convex, paravertebral opacities involve the lower two-thirds of the thoracic spine (*arrows*). A normal descending aortic contour is noted (*arrowheads*).

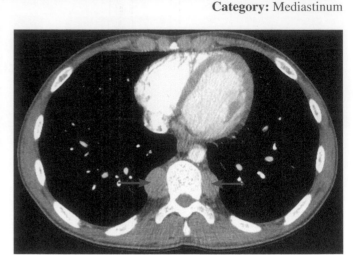

Bilateral smoothly defined, homogenous, soft tissue, paravertebral masses are seen (*arrows*).

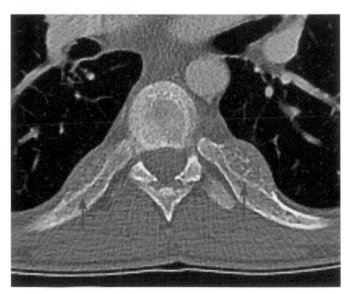

Bone remodelling is noted (*arrows*).

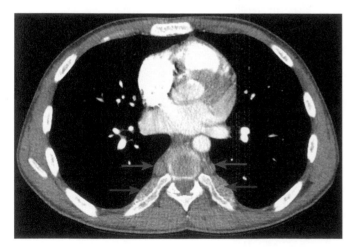

Paravertebral masses are also seen at another transverse level (*red arrows*). In addition, similar lesions are also based on the medial posterior ribs (*blue arrows*).

Answers

1. Bilateral convex paravertebral opacities are seen, in keeping with a posterior mediastinal abnormality.

2. The differential diagnosis based on the radiographic appearance includes extramedullary hematopoiesis, neurogenic tumors, lymphoma, metastases, paravertebral hematoma, and paravertebral abscesses.

3. Bilateral smoothly defined, homogenous, soft tissue, paravertebral masses are seen. In addition, similar lesions are also based on the posterior ribs. Bone remodeling is noted.

4. Transfusion-dependent thalassemia is a major cause of extramedullary hematopoiesis (EMH). However, EMH can be seen in other conditions resulting in chronic anemia, such as sickle cell anemia, myelofibrosis, and myeloproliferative disorders. EMH may be also seen in cases of bone marrow replacement, such as lymphoma or after bone irradiation.

5. The most common intrathoracic location of EMH is the posterior mediastinum, but the commonest site of EMH in general is liver and spleen.

Pearls

- EMH can have various tissue compositions, resulting in variable CT and MRI appearance.
- Bone expansion and coarse trabeculations on CT may be a hint to the patient's chronic anemic status.
- Signal intensity changes of the liver, spleen, or bone marrow on MRI may be hints to the patient's chronic anemic status.

Suggested Readings

Haidar R, Mhaidli H, Taher AT. Paraspinal extramedullary hematopoiesis in patients with thalassemia intermedia. *Eur Spine J.* June 2010;19(6):871-878.

Molinari F, Bankier AA, Eisenberg RL. Fat-containing lesions in adult thoracic imaging. *AJR Am J Roentgenol.* November 2011;197(5):W795-W813.

Trow TK, Argento AC, Rubinowitz AN, Decker R. A 71-year-old woman with myelofibrosis, hypoxemia, and pulmonary hypertension. *Chest.* December 2010;138(6):1506-1510.

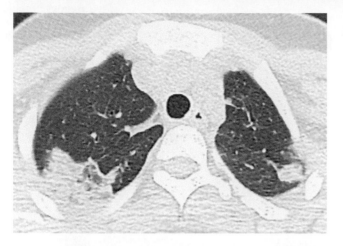
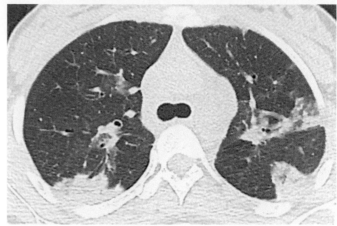
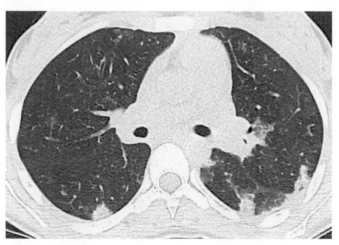
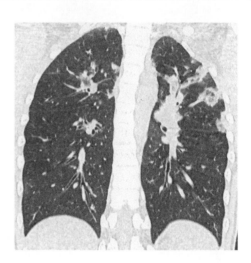

1. What are the CT findings?

2. What is the differential diagnosis in the context of the patient's chronic presentation?

3. What would the diagnosis be if the patient had peripheral eosinophilia?

4. What are the causes of pulmonary eosinophilia?

5. How is acute eosinophilic pneumonia (AEP) different from chronic eosinophilic pneumonia (CEP)?

Case ranking/difficulty: | **Category:** Lungs

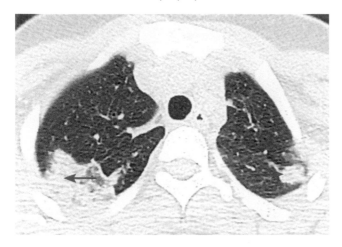

Bilateral parenchymal consolidations are seen (*arrows*).

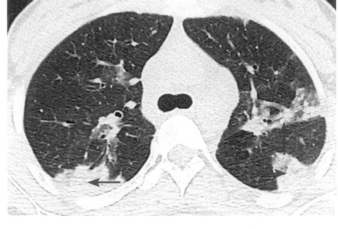

All abnormalities are peripheral (*arrows*).

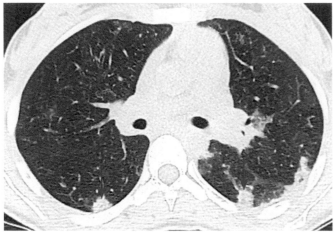

Fewer opacities are noted in the lower lung (*arrows*).

Answers

1. Bilateral peripheral airspace opacities are seen, with upper lung predominance. The lesions are predominantly consolidative, but areas of ground-glass attenuation are seen. In addition, a "reversed halo sign" is seen in the left upper lobe.

2. The differential diagnosis of chronic multifocal peripheral airspace opacities mainly includes organizing pneumonia and eosinophilic pneumonia. Note that septic embolism is not a chronic condition.

3. The diagnosis would be eosinophilic lung disease.

4. Eosinophilic lung diseases of unknown etiology are Loeffler syndrome, acute eosinophilic pneumonia, chronic eosinophilic pneumonia, Churg-Strauss syndrome, and idiopathic hypereosinophilic syndrome. Eosinophilic lung diseases caused by a known etiology are usually related to drugs and infections.

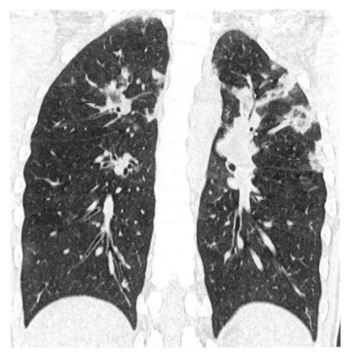

The distribution is clearly upper lung predominant on this coronal image (*arrows*). A lesion shows central ground-glass attenuation surrounded by consolidation, representing a "reversed halo sign" (*arrowhead*).

5. CEP is more common in females and may present at any age, but peaks in the fourth decade of life. Many patients with CEP are asthmatic. CEP is not associated with smoking. CEP is a chronic illness that commonly relapses after steroid therapy discontinuation. CEP mostly presents with airspace opacities and is not typically associated with pleural effusions. In contrast, AEP is more common in males and may present at

any age, but peaks in the third decade of life. Most patients with AEP are nonasthmatics and the disease is commonly associated with new-onset smoking. AEP is an acute life-threatening febrile illness that rarely relapses after steroid therapy discontinuation. AEP presents with interstitial and/or alveolar opacities and is commonly associated with pleural effusions.

Pearls

- When faced with pulmonary eosinophilia, always exclude known causes (such as drugs and infections) before embarking on differential diagnosis of idiopathic eosinophilic lung diseases.
- Different eosinophilic lung diseases have overlapping imaging findings. Acuity of the clinical presentation and the presence of multisystemic involvement can aid in their differentiation.
- Organizing pneumonia and eosinophilic lung diseases are the two main causes of chronic peripheral multifocal airspace opacities.

Suggested Readings

Jeong YJ, Kim KI, Seo IJ, Lee CH, Lee KN, Kim KN, Kim JS, Kwon WJ. Eosinophilic lung diseases: a clinical, radiologic, and pathologic overview. *Radiographics*. May-June 2007;27(3):617-637; discussion 637-639.

Kim SJ, Lee KS, Ryu YH, et al. Reversed halo sign on high-resolution CT of cryptogenic organizing pneumonia: diagnostic implications. *AJR Am J Roentgenol*. May 2003;180(5):1251-1254.

Saukkonen JJ. Pulmonary eosinophilia. Emedicine website. http://emedicine.edscape.om/article/301070-overview. Updated November 20, 2009.

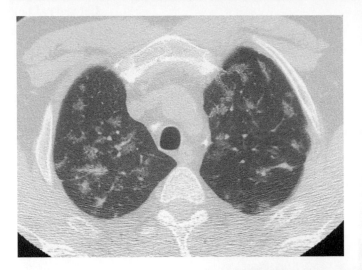

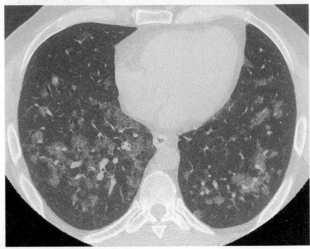

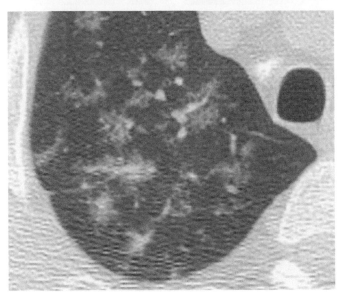

1. What are the imaging findings?

2. What is the "galaxy sign?"

3. What is the diagnosis in this case?

4. Can the featured lung finding regress with
   appropriate steroid treatment?

5. What is the percentage of pulmonary
   sarcoidosis cases that progress to fibrosis?

Case ranking/difficulty:

Category: Lungs

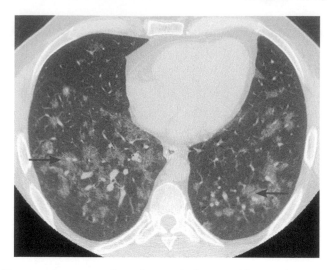

There are bilateral, predominantly central, patchy lung parenchymal ground-glass opacities (*arrows*).

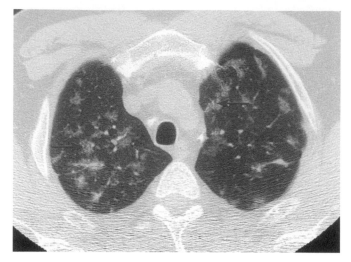

The same lung parenchymal ground-glass opacities are also seen in the lower lungs (*arrows*).

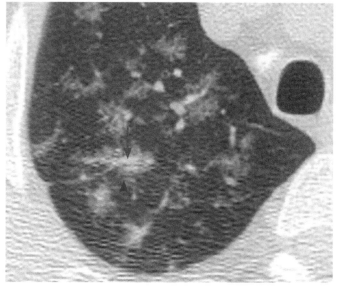

A magnified view of one of the lung parenchymal lesions shows that this opacity has a dense center (*arrow*) and an ill-defined margin demonstrating some separate nodularity (*arrowhead*), in an appearance denoting coalescent micronodules.

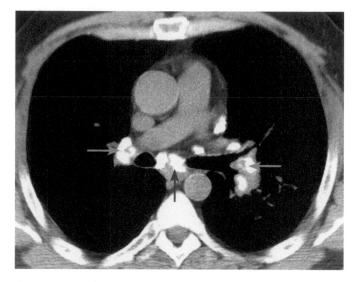

There are densely calcified bilateral hilar (*green arrows*) and mediastinal (*blue arrow*) lymph nodes.

Answers

1. There are bilateral, predominantly central, patchy lung parenchymal ground-glass opacities. The lung parenchymal lesions have a dense center and an ill-defined margin that is composed of coalescent micronodules.

2. The "galaxy sign" is seen when micronodules coalesce to form larger nodular opacities that have dense centers

and less defined peripheral borders (due to the presence of more dispersed peripheral nodularity).

3. The "galaxy sign" is seen in cases of pulmonary sarcoidosis.

4. Nodules, ground-glass opacities, and consolidation in pulmonary sarcoidosis may regress or disappear when the appropriate treatment is administrated. In contrast, treated fibrotic sarcoidosis shows features that remain stable or even progress.

5. About 20% of pulmonary sarcoidosis patients progress to fibrosis.

Pearls

- Lung parenchymal sarcoidosis may manifest in the form of the "galaxy sign."
- The "galaxy sign" is seen when micronodules coalesce to form larger nodular opacities that have dense centers and less defined peripheral borders (due to the presence of more dispersed peripheral nodularity).
- Lymph node calcifications may be secondary to remote granulomatous infections, pneumoconiosis, sarcoidosis, treated lymphoma, and amyloidosis.

Suggested Readings

Criado E, Sánchez M, Ramírez J, et al. Pulmonary sarcoidosis: typical and atypical manifestations at high-resolution CT with pathologic correlation. *Radiographics.* October 2010;30(6):1567-1586.

Kanne JP, Yandow DR, Haemel AK, Meyer CA. Beyond skin deep: thoracic manifestations of systemic disorders affecting the skin. *Radiographics.* October 2011;31(6):1651-1668.

Park HJ, Jung JI, Chung MH, Song SW, Kim HL, Baik JH, Han DH, Kim KJ, Lee KY. Typical and atypical manifestations of intrathoracic sarcoidosis. *Korean J Radiol.* November-December 2009;10(6):623-631.

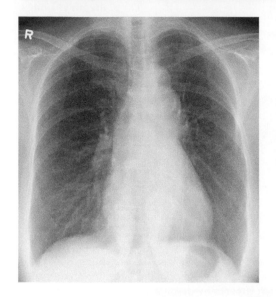

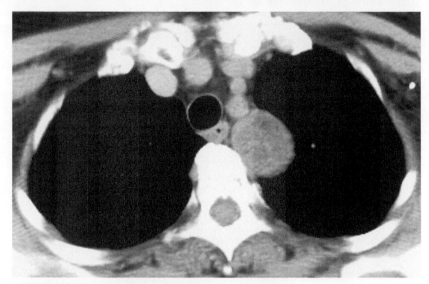

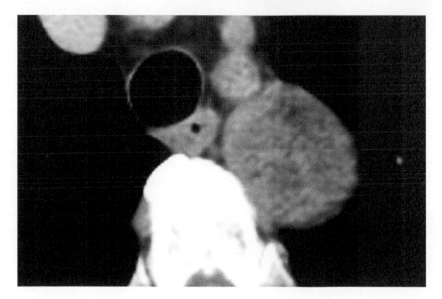

1. What are the radiographic findings?

2. What is the differential diagnosis based on the radiographic findings?

3. What are the CT findings?

4. What is the differential diagnosis based on the CT findings?

5. What pattern of calcification is most characteristic of a hamartoma?

Case ranking/difficulty: 🌰🌰🌰

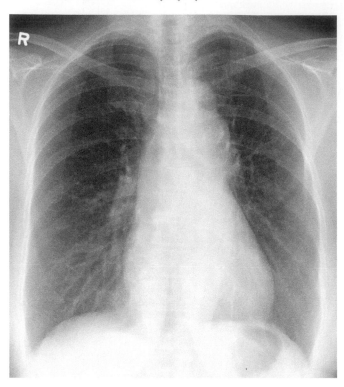

There is a left superior mediastinal contour abnormality, seen as a well-defined homogeneous bulge above the aortic arch (*arrow*). There are atherosclerotic calcifications of the aortic arch and unrelated changes of the left fifth rib due to remote surgical intervention.

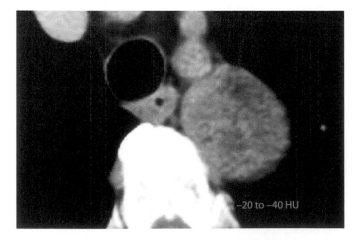

Measurement of the attenuation of the low-density areas within the lesion on this magnified view yields −20 to −40 HU, suggesting intralesional fat.

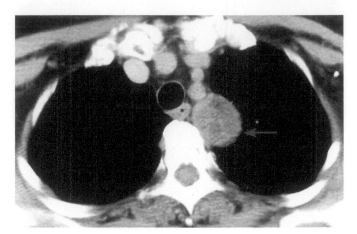

The supra-aortic lesion is a well-defined heterogeneous soft tissue mass (*arrow*) that is distinct from the aorta. The abnormality is based on the left superior mediastinal pleura, but could be mediastinal or parenchymal. The lesion has no obvious cystic or calcific components, but has internal areas of low attenuation suggesting fat (*arrowhead*).

Answers

1. There is a well-defined left superior mediastinal contour abnormality, located above the aortic arch.

2. It is most important to exclude a vascular abnormality based on the radiographic appearance, such an aneurysm or an aortic coarctation. Other entities to consider include lymphadenopathy (ie, from metastasis, lymphoma, or infection) and foregut duplication cyst (ie, bronchogenic, esophageal, or neurenteric). Rarely, paragangliomas or ectopic thymic lesions can occur in this location.

3. There is a well-defined supra-aortic lesion of heterogeneous soft tissue density. Intralesional fat is suggested, as denoted by the attenuation of −20 to −40 HU. The lesion is distinct from the aorta, but could be mediastinal or parenchymal.

4. Since intralesional fat is identified, fat-containing lesions should be included in the differential diagnosis. If the lesion is mediastinal, the following entities could be included: germ cell neoplasm, lipoma, liposarcoma, thymolipoma, transdiaphragmatic abdominal fat herniation, and epipericardial fat necrosis. If the lesion is parenchymal, the following entities could be included: hamartoma, metastatic liposarcoma, and lipoid pneumonia. It is important to ensure that the low attenuation is indeed due to fat and not an artifact. If no fat is confidently identified, other entities such as lung cancer and neurogenic tumors should be considered.

5. A "popcorn" pattern of calcification is very characteristic of a hamartoma, but is only seen in about half of the cases.

Pearls

- The radiographic abnormality of this case emphasizes the need to routinely evaluate the mediastinal contours on every chest radiograph.
- The presence of fat or popcorn calcifications in a lung nodule is highly suggestive of the diagnosis of hamartoma.
- Hamartoma can be symptomatic if it is endobronchial.
- Hamartoma may occasionally demonstrate slow growth over time or appear metabolically active on PET, features that may lead to an erroneous diagnosis of malignancy.

Suggested Readings

Brandman S, Ko JP. Pulmonary nodule detection, characterization, and management with multidetector computed tomography. *J Thorac Imaging*. May 2011;26(2):90-105.

Meyer CA, White CS. Cartilaginous disorders of the chest. *Radiographics*. September-October 1998;18(5):1109-1123; quiz 1241-1242.

Molinari F, Bankier AA, Eisenberg RL. Fat-containing lesions in adult thoracic imaging. *AJR Am J Roentgenol*. November 2011;197(5):W795-W813.

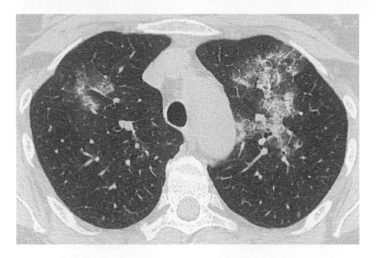
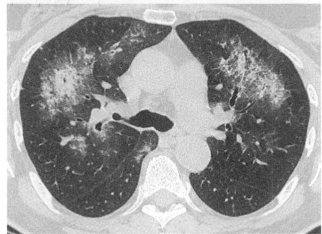
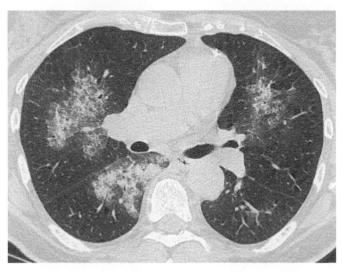
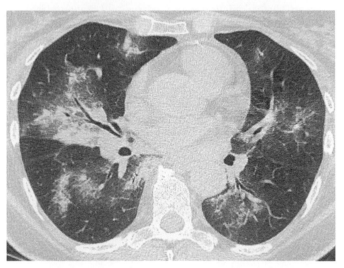

1. What are the CT findings?

2. What is the differential diagnosis based on the CT findings?

3. What would be the working diagnosis given the patient's clinical presentation?

4. What is the most common imaging pattern seen in Wegener granulomatosis (WG)?

5. What percentage of WG patients present with diffuse alveolar hemorrhage?

Wegener granulomatosis (hemorrhagic pattern)

 Case 134 (728)

Case ranking/difficulty: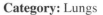

Category: Lungs

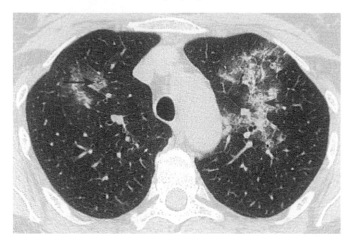

There are bilateral multifocal consolidative and ground-glass opacities (*arrows*).

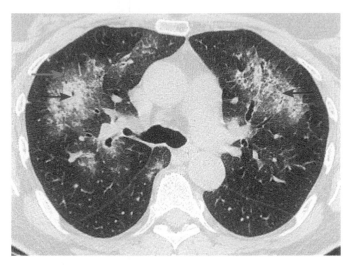

The consolidative opacities are redemonstrated (*red arrows*), with local surrounding ground-glass halo (ie, "halo sign") (*green arrow*).

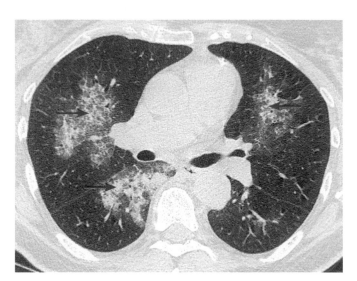

The bilateral airspace abnormalities (*arrows*) demonstrate central predominance, relatively sparing the peripheral lung zones.

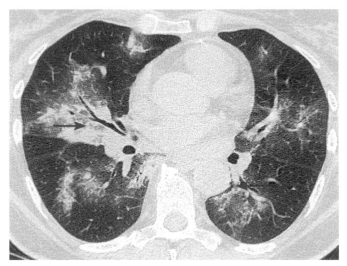

The abnormalities are intimately related to the central bronchovascular structures (*arrows*).

Answers

1. The CT images show bilateral multifocal central and peribronchovascular consolidative and ground-glass opacities, with surrounding "halo sign."

2. The major categories to consider for acute central airspace opacities are pneumonia, pulmonary edema (cardiogenic vs noncardiogenic), pulmonary hemorrhage, drug reaction, and vasculitis.

3. Diffuse alveolar hemorrhage (DAH) from any cause would be the working diagnosis in a patient with hemoptysis and a low hemoglobin level. In general, causes of DAH can be divided into pulmonary-renal syndromes and those without renal involvement.

4. The most common imaging presentation of WG is that of multiple bilateral nodules or masses, with or without cavitation.

5. About 10% of patients with WG present with DAH.

Pearls

• Pulmonary hemorrhage is a known manifestation of WG.
• New air-fluid levels or airspace opacities in the context of WG can be a manifestation of the disease, but both aforementioned appearances warrant evaluation for possible superadded infection.

462

- The "halo sign" was originally described in angioinvasive aspergillosis, but is nonspecific and occurs with a host of other pathologies.

Suggested Readings

Chung MP, Yi CA, Lee HY, Han J, Lee KS. Imaging of pulmonary vasculitis. *Radiology*. May 2010;255(2):322-341.

Marten K, Schnyder P, Schirg E, Prokop M, Rummeny EJ, Engelke C. Pattern-based differential diagnosis in pulmonary vasculitis using volumetric CT. *AJR Am J Roentgenol*. March 2005;184(3):720-733.

Mayberry JP, Primack SL, Müller NL. Thoracic manifestations of systemic autoimmune diseases: radiographic and high-resolution CT findings. *Radiographics*. November-December 2000;20(6):1623-1635.

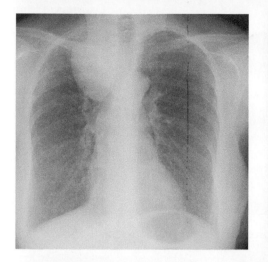
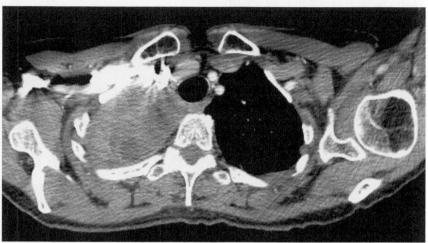
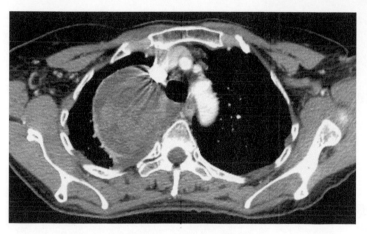
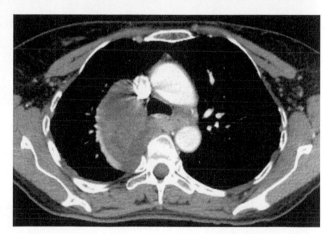

1. What are the radiographic findings?

2. What are the CT findings?

3. What does the "incomplete border sign" mean?

4. What is the most common primary pleural neoplasm?

5. What is the most common primary benign pleural neoplasm?

Case ranking/difficulty:

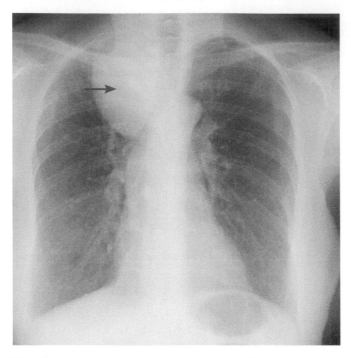

There is a large, rounded, homogenous opacity in the right medial upper hemithorax (*arrow*), with well-defined borders and no calcifications, cavitation, airway compromise, or adjacent osseous changes.

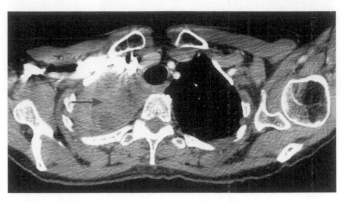

A large lesion occupies the right lung apex (*arrow*).

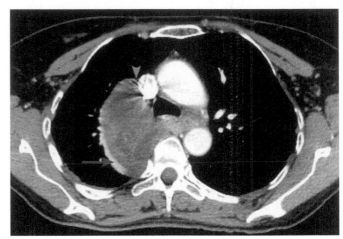

The lesion compresses the adjacent lung parenchyma (*arrow*), but shows no obvious lung invasion. This would be better assessed on dedicated lung windows. An obtuse angle with the mediastinal pleura is demonstrated (*arrowhead*).

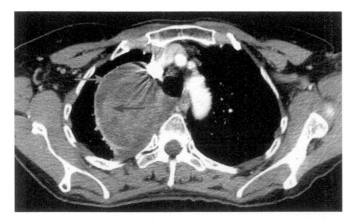

The lesion demonstrates internal areas of hypo- (*green arrow*) and hyperdensity (*red arrow*). No airway or vascular compromise is noted. Although the adjacent bones should be assessed on dedicated windows, they show no obvious abnormalities.

Answers

1. There is a large and well-defined homogenous opacity in the right medial upper hemithorax.

2. There is a large and well-defined right apical mass that is heterogeneous due to internal areas of hypo- and hyperdensity. The adjacent lung parenchyma shows compressive atelectatic changes and the trachea shows minimal anterior displacement, but no narrowing. The mass is inseparable from the right esophageal border. The vascular and osseous structures are not obviously compromised.

3. The "incomplete border sign" suggests pleural origin of a hemithoracic lesion and is seen as an abnormality with both well-defined (due to surrounding lung) and ill-defined borders (due to the pleural attachment).

4. The most common primary pleural neoplasm is a mesothelioma.

5. The most common primary benign pleural neoplasm is a fibrous pleural tumor.

Pearls

- The most common pleural neoplasm is metastasis, the most common primary pleural neoplasm is mesothelioma, and the most common primary benign pleural neoplasm is fibrous pleural tumor (FPT).
- Paraneoplastic features in the form of digital clubbing, hypertrophic osteoarthropathy (HOA), and hypoglycemia can be seen with benign or malignant FPTs.
- Although the most common tumor associated with HOA is FPT, most cases of HOA are encountered with lung cancer in daily practice.

Suggested Readings

Cardillo G, Carbone L, Carleo F, et al. Solitary fibrous tumors of the pleura: an analysis of 110 patients treated in a single institution. *Ann Thorac Surg*. November 2009;88(5):1632-1637.

Jeong YJ, Kim S, Kwak SW, et al. Neoplastic and nonneoplastic conditions of serosal membrane origin: CT findings. *Radiographics*. ;28(3):801-817; discussion 817-818; quiz 912.

Rosado-de-Christenson ML, Abbott GF, McAdams HP, Franks TJ, Galvin JR. From the archives of the AFIP: Localized fibrous tumor of the pleura. *Radiographics*. May-June 2003;23(3):759-783.

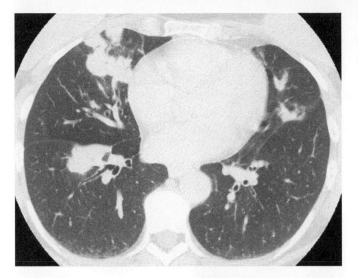 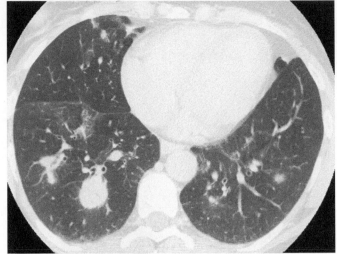

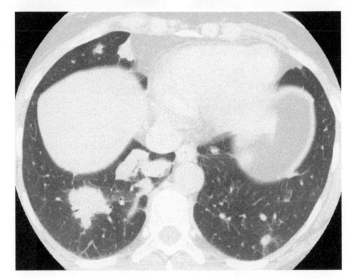

1. What are the CT findings?

2. What is the differential diagnosis based on the CT findings?

3. If sarcoidosis was the working diagnosis, would confirmation by tissue sampling be needed in this case?

4. List a few atypical described imaging features of pulmonary sarcoidosis.

5. What is the yield of endobronchial ultrasonographic tissue sampling in cases of sarcoidosis?

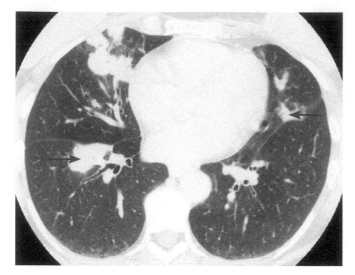

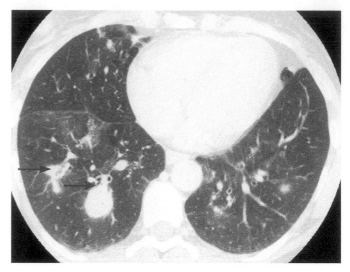

There are bilateral scattered lung parenchymal nodules and masses of variable sizes and shapes (*arrows*). The lesions are well defined with relatively smooth borders. Some lesions demonstrate an internal air bronchogram (*arrowhead*).

Some lesions demonstrate a peribronchovascular location (*arrows*).

3. Since the appearance is atypical for pulmonary sarcoidosis, other etiologies (eg, metastases and lymphoma) are possible and tissue sampling would be needed in this case.

4. Large nodules, masses, consolidations, miliary nodularity, pleural changes (ie, effusions, thickening, or calcifications), and predominant lower lung involvement may be seen in cases of sarcoidosis, but are considered atypical features.

5. Endobronchial ultrasonographic tissue sampling has a high yield for the diagnosis of sarcoidosis.

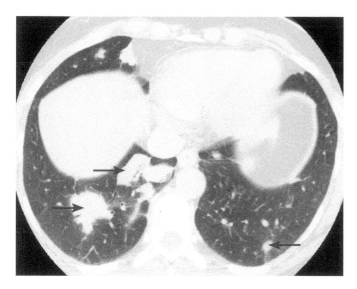

The lesions are also seen at the lung base (*arrows*).

Pearls

- Lung parenchymal large nodules or masses are well described yet atypical features of sarcoidosis.
- Endobronchial ultrasonographic tissue sampling has a high yield for the diagnosis of sarcoidosis.
- When the imaging features are typical of sarcoid and the clinical presentation is not discrepant, biopsy is not usually required for confirmation.

Answers

1. There are bilateral scattered well-defined lung parenchymal nodules and masses, with some lesions demonstrating air bronchograms and others having a peribronchovascular location.

2. When multiple lung parenchymal masses or nodules are seen, metastases, atypical infections (eg, fungal), sarcoidosis, organizing pneumonia, vasculitis, and lymphoma are possible etiologies.

Suggested Readings

Criado E, Sánchez M, Ramírez J, et al. Pulmonary sarcoidosis: typical and atypical manifestations at high-resolution CT with pathologic correlation. *Radiographics*. October 2010;30(6):1567-1586.

Kanne JP, Yandow DR, Haemel AK, Meyer CA. Beyond skin deep: thoracic manifestations of systemic disorders affecting the skin. *Radiographics*. October 2011;31(6):1651-1668.

Park HJ, Jung JI, Chung MH, et al. Typical and atypical manifestations of intrathoracic sarcoidosis. *Korean J Radiol*. Novemebr-December 2009;10(6):623-631.

Acute dyspnea after wooden tiles removal at a construction site

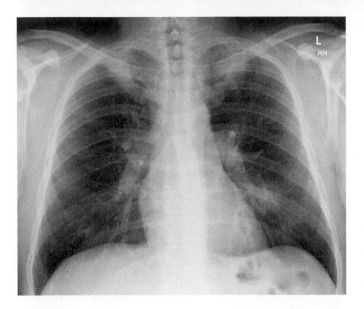
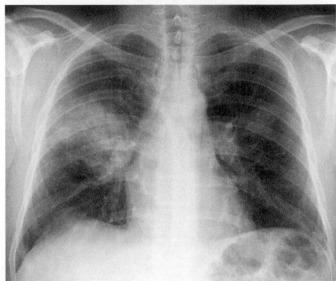
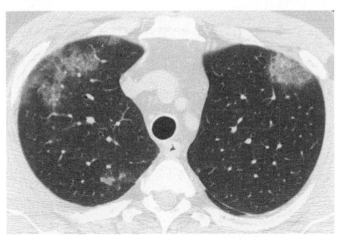
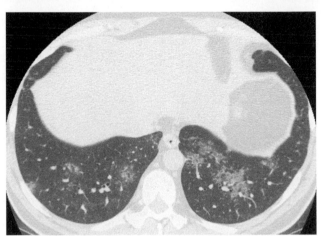

1. What are the radiographic findings (the top-right radiograph was obtained a few days after the original radiograph on the top-left)?

2. What is the differential diagnosis based on the radiographic appearance?

3. What are the CT findings?

4. Would the absence of peripheral eosinophilia exclude the diagnosis of eosinophilic pneumonia?

5. Are steroids effective in treating acute eosinophilic pneumonia (AEP)?

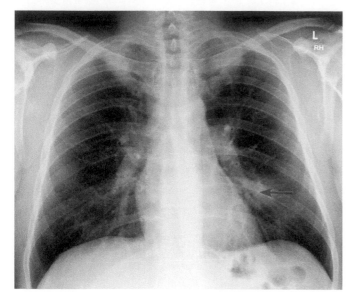

A single lower lung ill-defined opacity is seen (*arrow*).

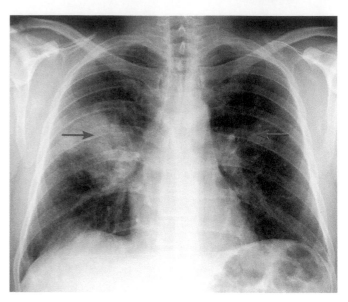

The previously noted left lower lobe opacity has resolved a few days later, but two new airspace opacities have appeared in the interval (*arrows*).

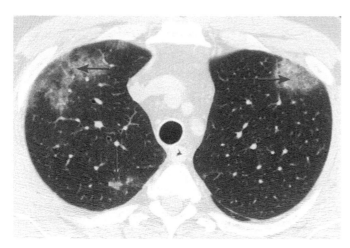

Bilateral scattered lung parenchymal ground-glass opacities are present, demonstrating a subpleural location (*arrows*).

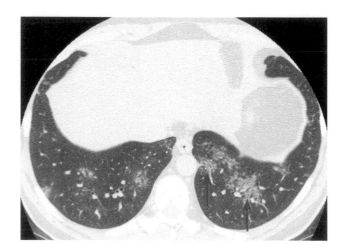

The ground-glass areas also demonstrate internal smooth septal thickening, resulting in focal crazy paving (*arrows*).

Answers

1. Multifocal parenchymal lung opacities are identified on the two presented chest radiographs. The radiographs were performed a few days apart, demonstrating a "waxing and waning" or "migratory" appearance.

2. The differential diagnosis of a "migratory" airspace pattern seen in a short interval is mainly that of organizing pneumonia, eosinophilic pneumonia, vasculitis (such as Wegener granulomatosis), aspiration pneumonitis, and allergic bronchopulmonary aspergillosis. Recurrent infection in the immunocompromised patient is also possible, but would require a longer period to resolve.

3. Bilateral scattered lung parenchymal ground-glass opacities are present, demonstrating a subpleural location and a crazy-paving pattern.

4. The absence of peripheral eosinophilia does not exclude the diagnosis of eosinophilic pneumonia, since a normal eosinophilic blood count is seen in many patients with acute eosinophilic pneumonia and proven pulmonary eosinophilia. Thus, if acute eosinophilic pneumonia is suspected and no peripheral eosinophilia is detected, proceeding to a bronchoalveolar lavage would be appropriate.

5. Steroid therapy is dramatically effective in treating AEP.

Pearls

- The absence of peripheral eosinophilia does not exclude AEP.
- AEP may cause an interstitial pattern, an airspace pattern, or both.
- Eosinophilic lung disease my cause migratory (ie, waxing and waning) lung opacities.

Suggested Readings

Jeong YJ, Kim KI, Seo IJ, et al. Eosinophilic lung diseases: a clinical, radiologic, and pathologic overview. *Radiographics*. May-June 2007;27(3):617-637; discussion 637-639.

Navaravong L, Wudhikarn K, Marini JJ. Cigarettes-induced acute eosinophilic pneumonia: a case report. *Cases J*. 2008;1(1):414.

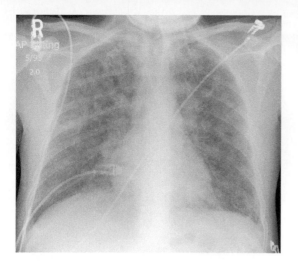
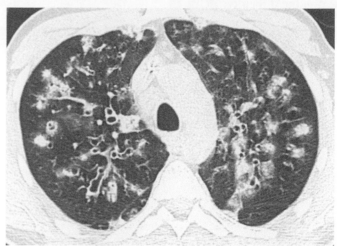

1. What are the radiographic findings?

2. What arc the CT findings?

3. What is the differential diagnosis of acute airspace lung opacities?

4. Which patient population commonly gets *Burkholderia cepacia* infection?

5. What is "cepacia syndrome?"

Case ranking/difficulty: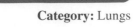

Category: Lungs

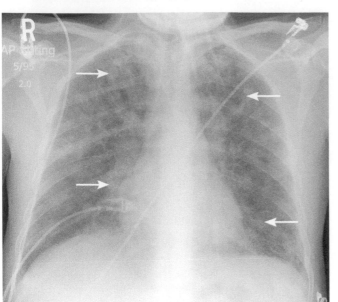

Bilateral multifocal patchy consolidations are seen (*arrows*), with preserved lung volumes and no pleural effusions.

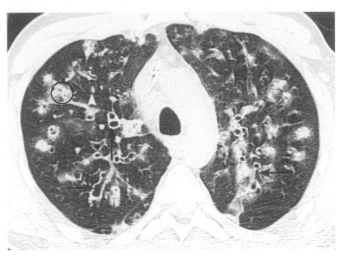

Bilateral diffuse bronchiectasis (*red arrows*), bronchial wall thickening (*blue arrow*), multiple patchy consolidations (*circle*), diffuse centrilobular nodules (*arrowhead*), and tree-in-bud pattern are noted.

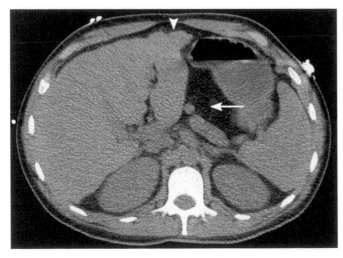

This upper abdominal image shows cirrhosis-related irregular liver border (*arrowhead*) and pancreatic lipomatosis (*arrow*), suggesting underlying cystic fibrosis.

3. The differential diagnosis of acute airspace lung opacities is bronchopneumonia, cardiogenic or noncardiogenic pulmonary edema, hemorrhage, aspiration pneumonitis, drug reactions, acute hypersensitivity pneumonitis, and acute eosinophilic lung disease.

4. Burkholderia cepacia classically infects cystic fibrosis and chronic granulomatous disease patients.

5. Cepacia syndrome is a progressive febrile illness with ensuing respiratory failure, caused by Burkholderia cepacia. The condition is often fatal.

Pearls

- Burkholderia cepacia classically infects cystic fibrosis and chronic granulomatous disease patients.
- Cepacia syndrome is difficult to treat, highly morbid, and commonly leads to death.
- Chest imaging findings in cases of cepacia syndrome are similar to any other bronchopneumonia.

Answers

1. The radiograph shows bilateral multifocal patchy consolidations. There are preserved lung volumes and no pleural effusions.

2. The CT shows bilateral diffuse bronchiectasis, bronchial wall thickening, multiple patchy consolidations, diffuse centrilobular nodules, and tree-in-bud pattern.

Suggested Readings

George RB, Cartier Y, Casson AG, Hernandez P. Suppurative mediastinitis secondary to Burkholderia cepacia in a patient with cystic fibrosis. *Can Respir J*. May-June 2006;13(4):215-218.

Jones AM, Dodd ME, Webb AK. Burkholderia cepacia: current clinical issues, environmental controversies and ethical dilemmas. *Eur Respir J*. February 2001;17(2):295-301.

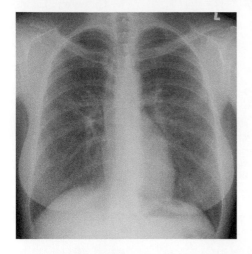
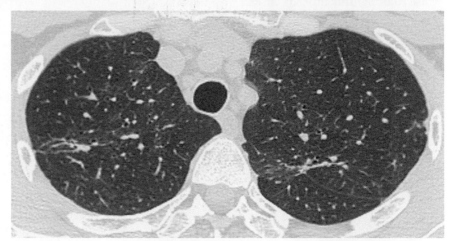
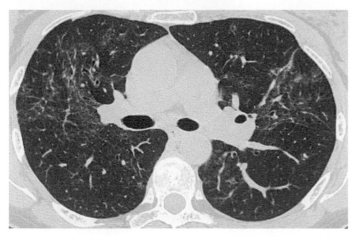
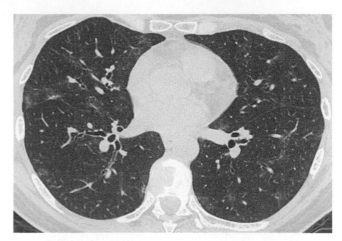

1. What are the radiographic findings?

2. What are the CT findings?

3. What should the differential diagnosis include?

4. Name a laboratory test used for diagnosing berylliosis.

5. What is the differential diagnosis for progressive massive fibrosis?

Case ranking/difficulty:

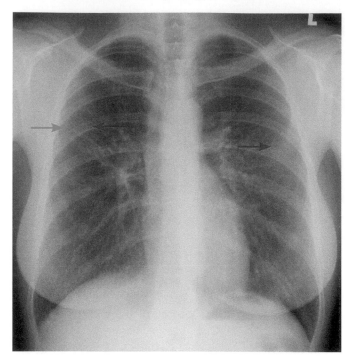

Extremely subtle, fine, linear, and irregular opacities are seen at the upper lung zones (*red arrows*). The lateral part of the minor fissure is elevated (*green arrow*).

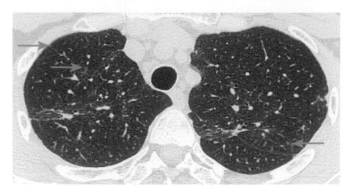

Bilateral scars are seen in the upper lung zones (*red arrows*). There are areas of questionable perilymphatic nodularity (*green arrows*).

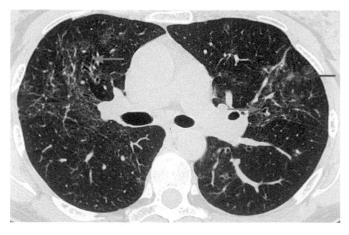

There are bilateral peribronchovascular ground-glass opacities (*red arrows*), with architectural distortion and traction bronchiectasis (*green arrows*).

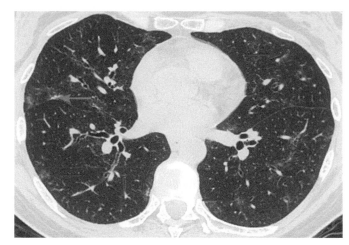

The abnormalities are less pronounced at the lower lung zones, but multiple bilateral scattered ground-glass opacities are still noted (*red arrows*). Note the focal distortion of the right major fissure (*green arrow*) due to the local fibrotic process.

Answers

1. Subtle, fine, linear, and irregular opacities are seen at the upper lung zones. The lateral part of the minor fissure is elevated.

2. The images show perilymphatic ground-glass opacities, with questionable perilymphatic tiny nodularity. A background of fibrosis is seen in the form of traction bronchiectasis and architectural distortion.

3. Given the upper lobe fibrosis and subtle perilymphatic nodularity, sarcoidosis and pneumoconiosis (such as silicosis, coal workers pneumoconiosis, and berylliosis) should be on the list.

4. Beryllium-specific lymphocyte proliferation testing of bronchoalveolar lavage or blood samples is a laboratory tool that is used to diagnose berylliosis.

5. The differential diagnosis for progressive massive fibrosis is pneumoconiosis (eg, silicosis, coal workers pneumoconiosis, hard metal exposure, and berylliosis), talcosis, and sarcoidosis.

Pearls

- Beryllium exposure may occur in workers dealing with ceramics, fluorescent lamps, metals, dental alloys, aerospace industry, and nuclear weapons.
- Acute berylliosis is a rare cause of noncardiogenic pulmonary edema.
- Chronic berylliosis is a sarcoidosis mimicker and can lead to progressive massive fibrosis.
- In contrast to sarcoidosis, lymphadenopathy in berylliosis is either absent or present only later in the course of the disease.

Suggested Readings

Sharma N, Patel J, Mohammed TL. Chronic beryllium disease: computed tomographic findings. *J Comput Assist Tomogr*. November-December 2010;34(6):945-948.

Sirajuddin A, Kanne JP. Occupational lung disease. *J Thorac Imaging*. November 2009;24(4):310-320.

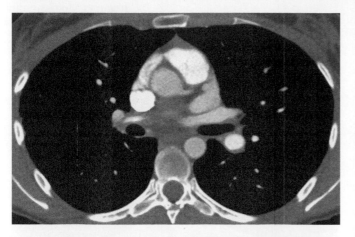
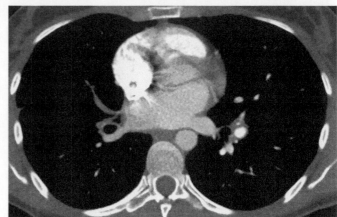
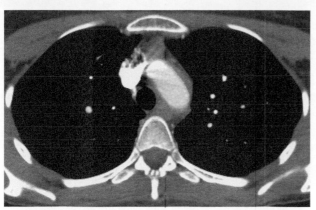
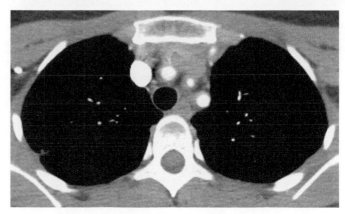

1. What are the CT findings?

2. What is the differential diagnosis?

3. List two blood tests that can be abnormal in cases of Takayasu arteritis.

4. List a few pulmonary vasculitides which can result in pulmonary arterial aneurysms or dilatation.

5. List a few points that differentiate giant cell arteritis (GCA) from Takayasu arteritis (TA).

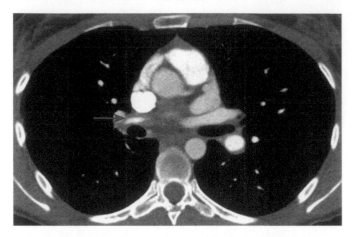

There is marked caliber attenuation of the distal right main pulmonary artery (*arrow*).

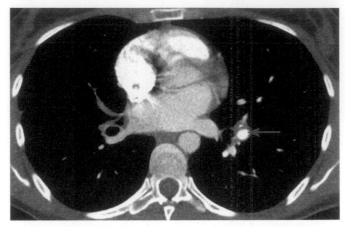

The left lower lobar pulmonary artery shows circumferential mural thickening (*arrow*). The right lung shows overall decreased vascularity compared to the left lung.

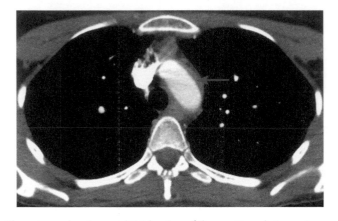

There is moderate mural thickening of the aortic arch (*arrow*).

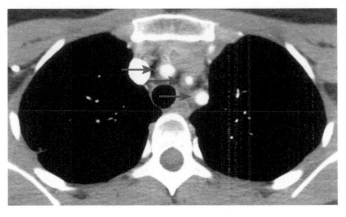

The aortic mural thickening extends to involve the origins of the major arch vessels (*arrows*).

Answers

1. The CT shows marked caliber attenuation of the distal right main pulmonary artery. The left lower lobar pulmonary artery shows circumferential mural thickening. There is moderate mural thickening of the aortic arch, which extends to involve the origins of the major arch vessels.

2. The differential diagnosis is that of large-vessel vasculitis (eg, Takayasu arteritis or giant cell arteritis) and chronic thromboembolic pulmonary arterial hypertension.

3. C-reactive protein (CRP) and erythrocyte sedimentation rate (ESR) are usually elevated in cases of Takayasu arteritis, but are nonspecific.

4. Pulmonary aneurysms are more commonly seen in Behçet disease and Hughes-Stovin syndrome, but can also be seen in giant cell arteritis. Takayasu arteritis can lead to pseudoaneurysms and poststenotic dilatation.

The central pulmonary arteries might dilate due to vasculitis-related pulmonary hypertension in the case of progressive systemic sclerosis, systemic lupus erythematosus, mixed connective tissue disease, rheumatoid arthritis, Takayasu arteritis, giant cell arteritis, and Behçet disease.

5. GCA is a large- and medium-vessel vasculitis. GCA has histological and imaging features that are identical to TA; however, GCA affects older patients (50 years and older), seen more commonly in whites, and typically affects the extracranial carotid arterial branches. Aortic arch and aortic branches involvement is less commonly encountered.

Pearls

- Takayasu arteritis commonly affects young Asian females, but is also encountered in individuals of any age, sex, or ethnicity.
- Takayasu arteritis of the pulmonary arteries can cause mural thickening and vascular dilatation, mimicking chronic pulmonary thromboembolic disease.
- Takayasu arteritis should be considered as a cause of pulmonary arterial hypertension in young females suspected to have chronic pulmonary thromboembolic disease.
- The vascular wall calcifications in Takayasu arteritis are transmural or deep within the wall, while atherosclerotic calcifications are intimal based.

Suggested Readings

Castañer E, Alguersuari A, Gallardo X, et al. When to suspect pulmonary vasculitis: radiologic and clinical clues. *Radiographics*. January 2010;30(1):33-53.

Chung MP, Yi CA, Lee HY, Han J, Lee KS. Imaging of pulmonary vasculitis. *Radiology*. May 2010;255(2):322-341.

Marten K, Schnyder P, Schirg E, Prokop M, Rummeny EJ, Engelke C. Pattern-based differential diagnosis in pulmonary vasculitis using volumetric CT. *AJR Am J Roentgenol*. March 2005;184(3):720-733.

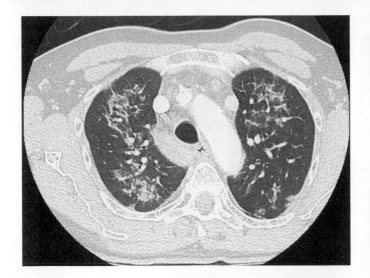
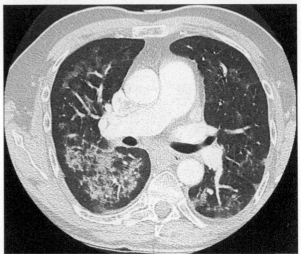
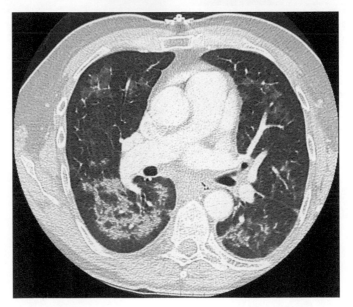

1. What are the CT findings?

2. What is the differential diagnosis?

3. What would the diagnosis be, if the analysis of the bronchoalveolar lavage (BAL) sample revealed large amounts of carbon-pigmented macrophages?

4. List a few lung abnormalities that can develop with cocaine abuse.

5. What is the likely etiology of progressive massive fibrosis (PMF) in a long-term cocaine user?

Case ranking/difficulty:

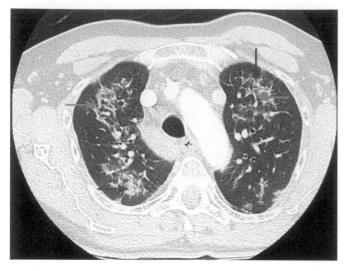

Bilateral diffuse consolidative and ground-glass lung parenchymal opacities are seen (*red arrows*), with superimposed interlobular smooth septal thickening (*green arrows*).

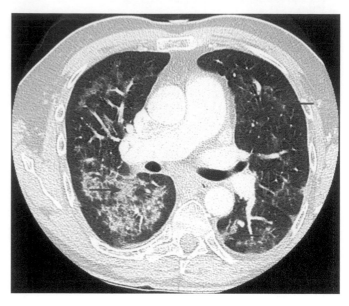

The lung parenchymal opacities are of central predominance (*arrows*), with relative peripheral sparing.

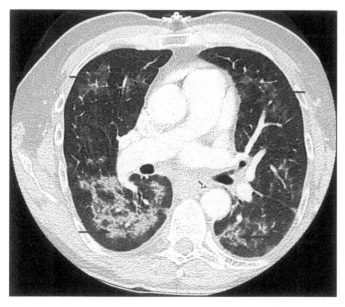

The same abnormalities are seen on this lower lung image (*arrows*), confirming the diffuse but perihilar nature of the lung parenchymal involvement.

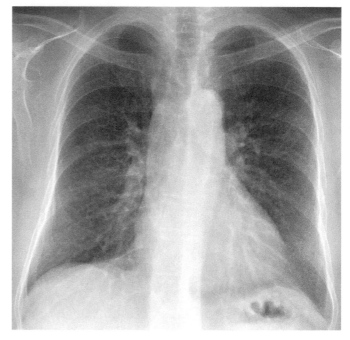

Complete resolution of the lung parenchymal abnormalities is seen on this follow-up frontal chest radiograph.

Answers

1. There are bilateral diffuse consolidations and ground-glass opacities, with central predominance and relative peripheral lung sparing. Mild smooth interlobular septal thickening is superimposed over the abnormal parenchymal areas. No features to suggest small airways involvement are seen.

2. The main diagnostic possibilities for bilateral perihilar opacities include cardiogenic and noncardiogenic pulmonary edema, alveolar hemorrhage, and infections.

3. Cocaine inhalation would be the likely diagnosis, if BAL showed large amounts of carbon-pigmented macrophages.

4. Some of the lung abnormalities that can develop with cocaine abuse are barotrauma (due to Valsalva maneuvering during drug inhalation), bronchiolitis, pulmonary edema, alveolar hemorrhage, crack lung, organizing pneumonia, eosinophilic lung disease, diffuse alveolar damage, emphysema, and superadded infection.

5. Since cocaine can be mixed with contaminants such as talc and silica, patients can develop interstitial lung diseases and PMF, if this impure form of cocaine is injected intravenously.

Pearls

- In the absence of clear history, lung imaging manifestations of illicit drug abuse may be misinterpreted, unless a high index of suspicion is maintained.
- Cocaine abuse may lead to barotrauma, airway injury and bronchiolitis, cardiogenic or noncardiogenic pulmonary edema, alveolar hemorrhage, crack lung, organizing pneumonia, eosinophilic lung disease, diffuse alveolar damage, talcosis, silicosis, fibrotic lung disease, pulmonary hypertension, emphysema, superadded infection, aspiration pneumonitis, and tumors.
- Intravenous cocaine abuse may lead to septic emboli, infective endocarditis, myocardial infarction secondary to coronary arterial spasm, or septic arthritis/spondylodiscitis.

Suggested Readings

Gotway MB, Marder SR, Hanks DK, et al. Thoracic complications of illicit drug use: an organ system approach. *Radiographics*. October 2002;22 Spec No:S119-S135.

Hagan IG, Burney K. Radiology of recreational drug abuse. *Radiographics*. July-August 2007;27(4):919-940.

Restrepo CS, Carrillo JA, Martínez S, Ojeda P, Rivera AL, Hatta A. Pulmonary complications from cocaine and cocaine-based substances: imaging manifestations. *Radiographics*. July-August 2007;27(4):941-956.

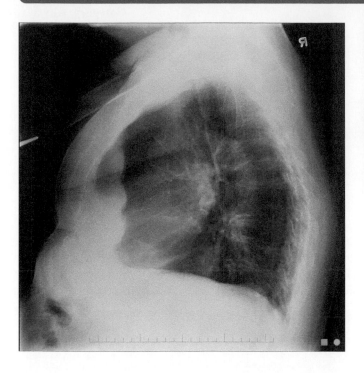

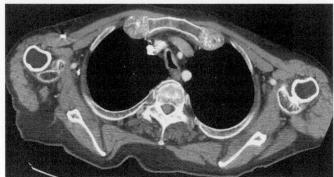

1. Which of the following clinical features do you expect this patient to have: erythema nodosum, clubbing, malar rash, auricular abnormalities, or axillary freckles?

2. What is the differential diagnosis of diffuse tracheobronchial narrowing?

3. What allows differentiation of relapsing polychondritis from other tracheobronchial pathologies?

4. What is the most common thoracic complication of relapsing polychondritis?

5. What is the treatment for relapsing polychondritis?

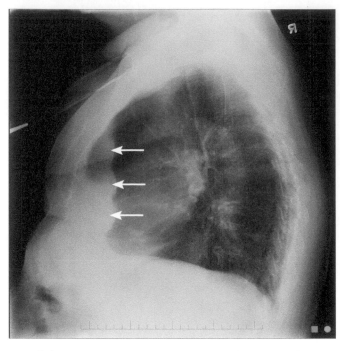

Lateral chest x-ray demonstrating an abnormal retrosternal polylobulated opacity (*arrows*).

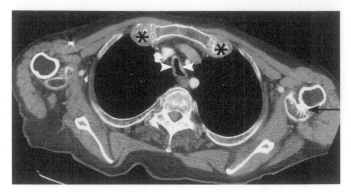

CT chest demonstrating diffuse thickening of the costal cartilage (*asterisks*), smooth thickening of the tracheal wall (*arrowheads*) sparing the posterior membrane, tracheal luminal narrowing, and left glenohumeral joint degenerative changes (*arrow*).

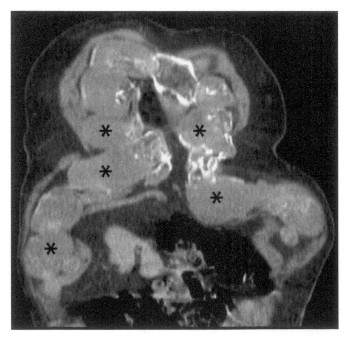

Coronal reformation image of the chest CT demonstrating diffuse thickening of the costal cartilage (*asterisks*).

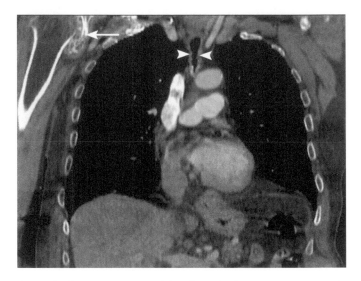

Coronal reformation image of the chest CT demonstrating smooth thickening of the tracheal wall (*arrowheads*), tracheal luminal narrowing, and right shoulder degenerative changes (*arrow*).

Answers

1. In relapsing polychondritis, recurrent inflammation of auricular cartilage leads to clinically apparent auricular swelling and redness, sparing the lobules.

2. Differential diagnosis of diffuse tracheobronchial narrowing includes amyloidosis, scleroma, Wegener granulomatosis, tracheobronchopathia osteochondroplastica, and relapsing polychondritis.

3. Relapsing polychondritis and tracheobronchopathia osteochondroplastica spare the posterior tracheal membrane, a feature that differentiates these two entities from other causes of diffuse tracheal thickening.

4. Severe pulmonary infections are the most common thoracic complication of relapsing polychondritis. Other clinical manifestations of relapsing polychondritis include vertigo, hoarseness, joint deformity, epiglottitis, uveitis, and aortic and mitral valve regurgitation.

5. Prednisone is the drug of choice for relapsing polychondritis. It is used in acute flares and for long-term suppression of inflammation. In severe cases, tracheostomy or tracheal stents might be necessary.

Pearls

- Relapsing polychondritis (RP) is a rare inflammatory condition involving cartilaginous structures throughout the body.
- Classically, RP patients have swollen and tender ears.
- RP causes smooth wall thickening of the central airway with sparing of the posterior membrane.

Suggested Readings

Im JG, Chung JW, Han SK, Han MC, Kim CW. CT manifestations of tracheobronchial involvement in relapsing polychondritis. *J Comput Assist Tomogr.* Septemebr-October 1988;12(5):792-793.

Prince JS, Duhamel DR, Levin DL, Harrell JH, Friedman PJ. Nonneoplastic lesions of the tracheobronchial wall: radiologic findings with bronchoscopic correlation. *Radiographics.* October 2002;22 Spec No:S215-S230.

SVC syndrome

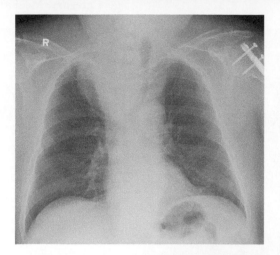
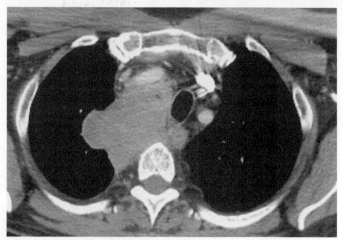
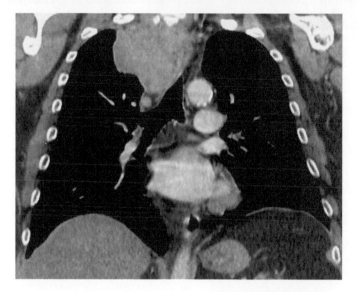

1. What are the findings?

2. What is the differential diagnosis?

3. What are the recognized forms of plasma cell dyscrasia?

4. What is the association between extramedullary plasmacytomas (EMP) and multiple myeloma (MM)?

5. What is the usual management of primary EMP?

Case ranking/difficulty:

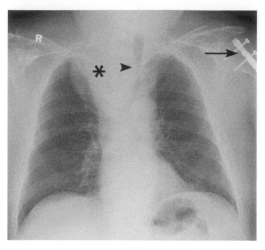

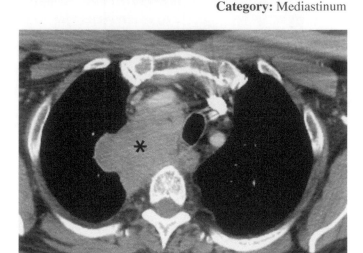

There is a large right paratracheal mass (*asterisk*) causing leftward deviation of the trachea (*arrowhead*). There is a left humeral intramedullary nail with proximal interlocking screws (*arrow*).

CT chest confirms a right superior mediastinal solid mass (*asterisk*) extending from anterior to posterior mediastinum.

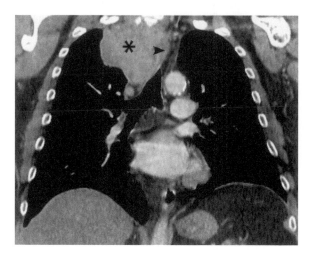

Coronal reformation again shows a superior mediastinal solid mass (*asterisk*), exerting mass effect on the trachea (*arrowhead*).

Answers

1. There is an upper mediastinal soft tissue lesion that exerts mass effect on the trachea. There is a left humeral intramedullary nail.

2. The differential diagnosis of an upper mediastinal mass includes lymphadenopathy (reactive, metastatic, or secondary to lymphoproliferative disorders or sarcoidosis), germ cell tumors (seminomas, mature and immature teratomas), thymic lesions (thymoma, thymic carcinoma, thymic cyst, thymolipoma), thyroid lesions (retrosternal goiter, thyroid neoplasms), and aneurysm of the thoracic aorta.

3. Plasma cell dyscrasias include multiple myeloma, plasmacytoma, primary amyloidosis, and monoclonal

gammopathy of unknown significance. Chloroma is an extramedullary manifestation of acute myeloid leukemia and represents a solid collection of leukemic cells outside of the bone marrow.

4. Only 5% of EMP patients will have MM.

5. The standard of care for primary EMP is surgical excision, followed by radiotherapy.

Pearls

- Plasmacytoma is a form of plasma cell dyscrasia.
- Plasmacytoma may be primary or secondary to disseminated MM.
- Plasmacytomas may be solitary or multiple.
- Plasmacytomas may be osseous or extramedullary.
- Plasmacytoma may precede MM, but most cases of EMP do not develop MM.
- The most common site for EMP is the upper aerodigestive tract.

Suggested Readings

Masood A, Hudhud KH, Hegazi A, Syed G. Mediastinal plasmacytoma with multiple myeloma presenting as a diagnostic dilemma. *Cases J*. 2008;1(1):116.

Moran CA, Suster S, Fishback NF, Koss MN. Extramedullary plasmacytomas presenting as mediastinal masses: clinicopathologic study of two cases preceding the onset of multiple myeloma. *Mod Pathol*. April 1995;8(3):257-259.

Ooi GC, Chim JC, Au WY, Khong PL. Radiologic manifestations of primary solitary extramedullary and multiple solitary plasmacytomas. *AJR Am J Roentgenol*. March 2006;186(3):821-827.

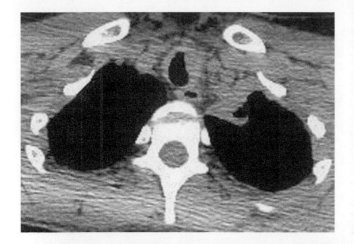
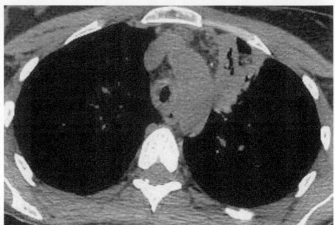
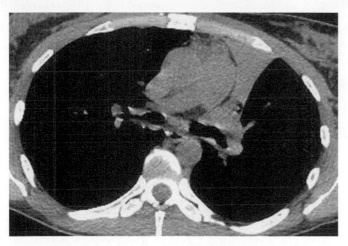
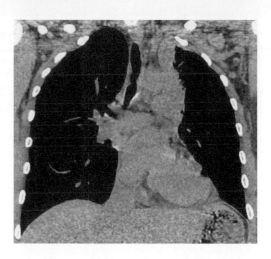

1. What are the findings?

2. What is the differential diagnosis of diffuse tracheal wall thickening?

3. What intestinal pathology can be associated with tracheal wall thickening?

4. What are common extraintestinal manifestations of inflammatory bowel disease (IBD)?

5. What are recognized pulmonary manifestations of IBD?

Case ranking/difficulty: **Category:** Airways

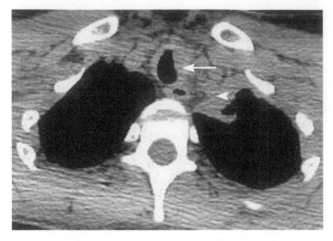

There is an asymmetrical upper tracheal wall thickening (*arrow*) and a left upper lobe subpleural opacity (*arrowhead*).

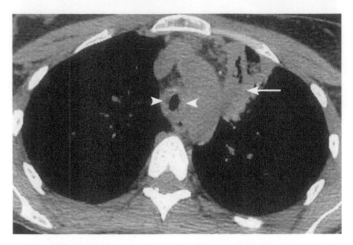

There is circumferential lower tracheal wall thickening (*arrowheads*) and luminal stenosis, and left upper lobe collapse (*arrow*).

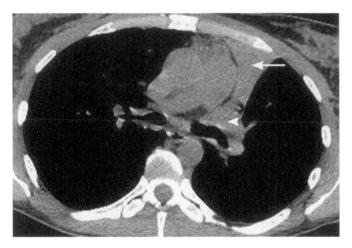

There is left upper lobe collapse (*arrow*) secondary to left upper lobar mucous plugging (*arrowhead*).

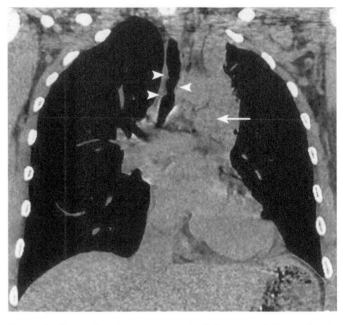

Coronal reformation demonstrates the full extent of the tracheal wall thickening (*arrowheads*) and the left upper lobe collapse (*arrow*).

Answers

1. The CT images show asymmetric upper and circumferential lower tracheal wall thickening, with mild tracheal luminal stenosis. There is left upper lobe collapse secondary to lobar mucous plugging.

2. The differential diagnosis of diffuse tracheal wall thickening includes sarcoidosis, amyloidosis, scleroma, Wegener granulomatosis, tracheobronchopathia osteochondroplastica, and relapsing polychondritis.

3. Tracheal wall thickening is one of the recognized thoracic manifestations of ulcerative colitis and Crohn disease.

4. Common extraintestinal manifestations of IBD are aphthous ulcers, pyoderma gangrenosum, iritis/uveitis, erythema nodosum, sclerosing cholangitis, arthritis, and digital clubbing.

5. Approximately 22% of IBD patients with symptomatic respiratory involvement will show bronchiectasis; 20%, chronic bronchitis; 18%, interstitial lung disease; 12%, cryptogenic organizing pneumonia; and 6%, necrobiotic nodules.

Pearls

- Thoracic involvement in IBD may include airway inflammation, predominantly affecting the intermediate-size bronchi and manifesting as bronchiectasis or chronic bronchitis, suppurative large airway disease, cryptogenic organizing pneumonia, pulmonary drug toxicity, eosinophilic pneumonia, nonspecific interstitial pneumonia, pulmonary necrobiotic nodules, serositis involving pleura and pericardium, and increased rate of pulmonary thromboembolic disease.
- Airway involvement is more common with ulcerative colitis than with Crohn disease.
- Thoracic involvement can occur even after total colectomy in IBD patients.

Suggested Reading

Betancourt SL, Palacio D, Jimenez CA, Martinez S, Marom EM. Thoracic manifestations of inflammatory bowel disease. *AJR Am J Roentgenol*. September 2011;197(3):W452-W456.

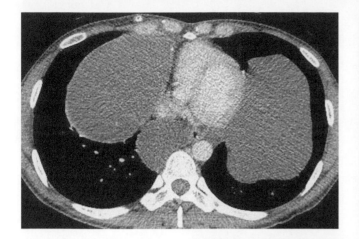
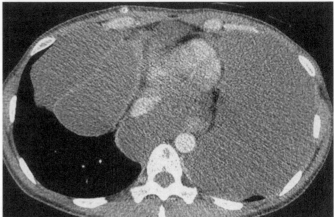

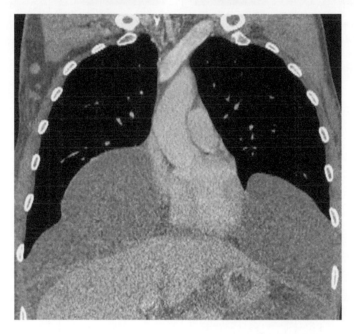

1. What are the findings?

2. What is the most likely anatomical location of the chest lesions?

3. What is the differential diagnosis?

4. What are common anatomical sites of lymphangiomatosis involvement?

5. What is the most common pattern of bone involvement by lymphangiomatosis?

Case ranking/difficulty:

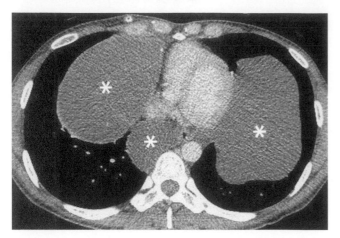

CT at the level of the lower chest demonstrates large bilateral cystic lesions with very thin, smooth walls (*asterisks*).

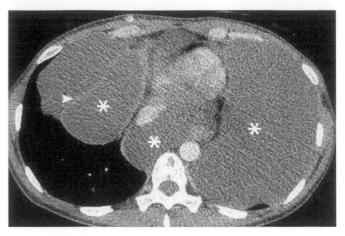

CT chest at a lower level redemonstrates the large bilateral cystic lesions (*asterisks*), one with a thin internal septation (*arrowhead*).

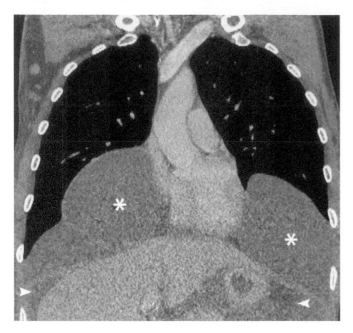

Coronal reformation image better depicts craniocaudal extent of the large bilateral cystic lesions (asterisks) and ascites (*arrowheads*).

Answers

1. CT images show multiple intrathoracic cystic lesions without calcifications or solid components, and upper abdominal ascites.

2. The lesions are most likely located in the pleural space.

3. The differential diagnosis includes loculated pleural effusions, cystic metastases, lymphangiomas, hemangiomas, and echinococcal cysts.

4. Bones, pleural and peritoneal spaces, mediastinum, and spleen are commonly involved in lymphangiomatosis.

5. Osteolytic lesions with multiple septae are the most common pattern of bone involvement by lymphangiomatosis.

Pearls

- Generalized cystic lymphangiomatosis (GCL) is a rare congenital malformation of the lymphatics.
- GCL may involve pleural space, peritoneum, spleen, and bones.
- On imaging, GCL presents as multiple cystic lesions of various size, which are pliable and usually insinuate themselves around adjacent structures.

Suggested Readings

Wong CS, Chu TY. Clinical and radiological features of generalised lymphangiomatosis. *Hong Kong Med J.* October 2008;14(5):402-404.

Wunderbaldinger P, Paya K, Partik B, et al. CT and MR imaging of generalized cystic lymphangiomatosis in pediatric patients. *AJR Am J Roentgenol.* March 2000;174(3):827-832.

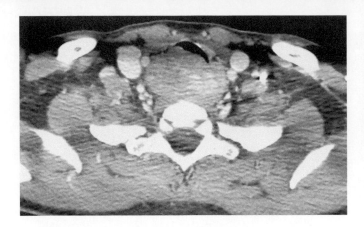 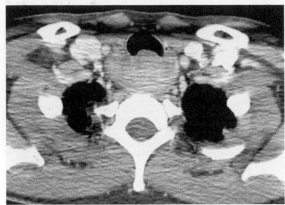

1. What is the finding?

2. What is the differential diagnosis of a central airway mass?

3. What is the most common primary tracheal neoplasm in adults?

4. What is the second most common primary tracheal neoplasm in adults?

5. What type of organ tissue/cell type does the second most common primary tracheal neoplasm in adults arise from?

Case ranking/difficulty:

Category: Airways

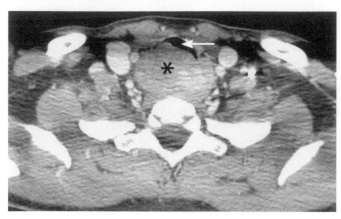

There is an enhancing mass (*asterisk*) posterior to the upper trachea, markedly narrowing the tracheal lumen (*arrow*).

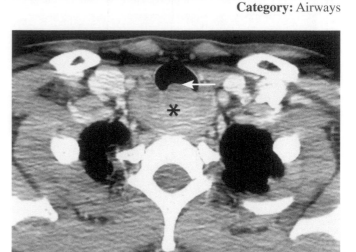

The enhancing mass (*asterisk*) is indenting the posterior tracheal wall (*arrow*).

Answers

1. There is an enhancing mass arising from the posterior wall of the upper trachea.

2. The differential diagnosis of a central airway mass includes squamous cell carcinoma, adenoid cystic carcinoma, mucoepidermoid carcinoma, carcinoid, and hamartoma.

3. Squamous cell carcinoma is the most common primary tracheal neoplasm in adults.

4. Adenoid cystic carcinoma (ACC) is the second most common primary tracheal neoplasm in adults.

5. ACC arises from the minor salivary glands.

Pearls

- ACC is the second most common tracheal tumor in adults, preceded by squamous cell carcinoma.
- ACC is considered a low-grade malignancy.
- ACC is not related to smoking.
- ACC usually arises in the lower trachea.
- Since ACC is infiltrative and may have various degree of longitudinal tracheal wall extension, assessing the trachea in coronal and sagittal planes is important.

Suggested Reading

Kwak SH, Lee KS, Chung MJ, Jeong YJ, Kim GY, Kwon OJ. Adenoid cystic carcinoma of the airways: helical CT and histopathologic correlation. *AJR Am J Roentgenol.* August 2004;183(2):277-281.

Suspected nodular sarcoidosis

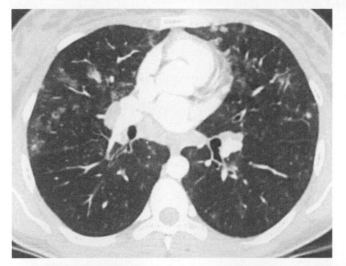
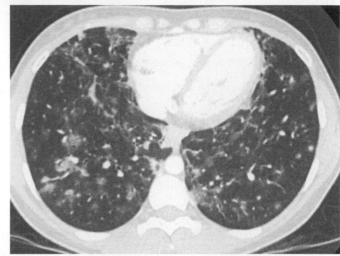
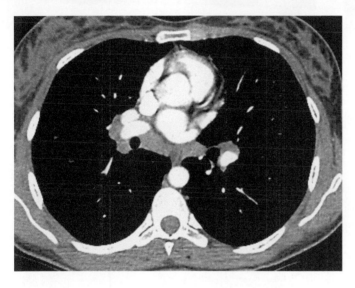
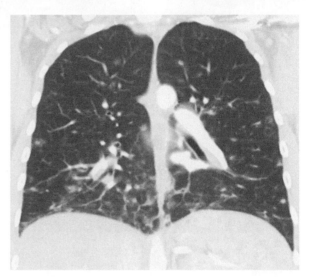

1. What is the dominant pattern of nodular distribution in this case?

2. What lung pathologies can be associated with this pattern?

3. What underlying immunological disease is associated with this pulmonary condition?

4. What is the etiologic agent of this pulmonary condition?

5. What are possible extrapulmonary findings of the underlying immunological disease?

Case ranking/difficulty:

Category: Lungs

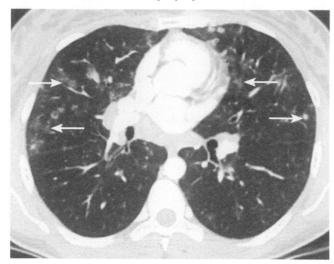

CT chest in lung windows demonstrating bilateral peribronchovascular ground-glass and mixed density nodules (*arrows*).

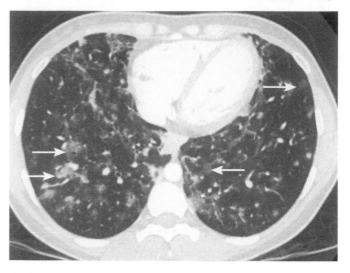

CT chest in lung windows shows that the nodules (*arrows*) predominate at the lung bases.

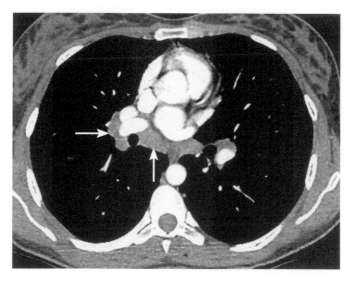

CT chest in mediastinal windows demonstrating subcarinal and hilar lymphadenopathy (*arrows*).

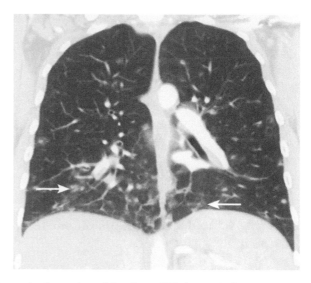

Coronal reformation of the chest CT in lung windows demonstrating apicobasilar gradient of nodular distribution (*arrows*), with relative sparing of the apices.

Answers

1. All the nodules are adjacent to the bronchovascular bundles. There is sparing of pleural surfaces and fissures. No tree-in-bud centrilobular nodules clearly identified. This is in keeping with peribronchovascular distribution.

2. Sarcoidosis, pulmonary lymphoma, Kaposi sarcoma, metastases and cryptogenic organizing pneumonia (COP) can give rise to peribronchovascular nodules.

3. Granulomatous-lymphocytic interstitial lung disease (GLILD) is a recognized noninfectious complication of common variable immunodeficiency (CVID).

4. The etiology of GLILD is unknown.

5. Extrapulmonary manisfestations of CVID may include abdominal lymphadenopathy, hepatomegaly, splenomegaly, nonspecific hypoattenuating splenic lesions, and nonspecific hypoattenuating renal lesions.

Pearls

- GLILD is a known complication of CVID.
- On imaging, GLILD could be confused with sarcoidosis.
- Basilar predominance of the lung nodules is characteristic of GLILD.

Suggested Readings

Bates CA, Ellison MC, Lynch DA, Cool CD, Brown KK, Routes JM. Granulomatous-lymphocytic lung disease shortens survival in common variable immunodeficiency. *J Allergy Clin Immunol*. August 2004;114(2):415-421.

Park JS, Brown KK, Tuder RM, Hale VA, King TE Jr, Lynch DA. Respiratory bronchiolitis-associated interstitial lung disease: radiologic features with clinical and pathologic correlation. *J Comput Assist Tomogr*. July 2005;26(1):13-20.

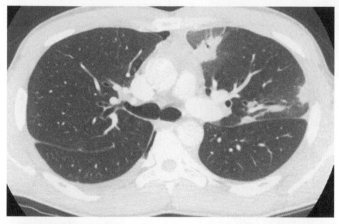

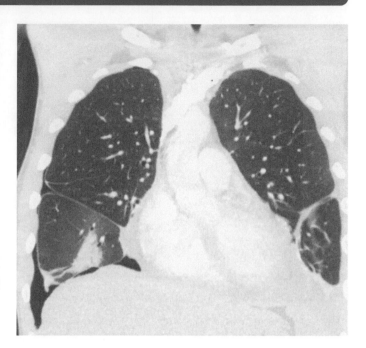

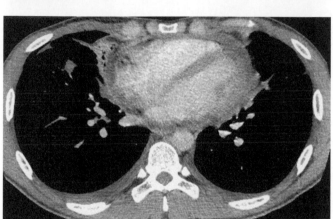

1. What are the findings?

2. What is the differential diagnosis of secondary spontaneous pneumothorax?

3. What is the differential diagnosis of multiple, subpleural poorly marginated pulmonary nodules?

4. What is the most likely diagnosis for this patient?

5. What is the risk factor for contracting this disease?

Case ranking/difficulty:

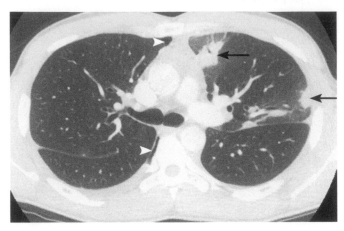

CT chest demonstrates a small right loculated pneumothorax (*arrowheads*) and left upper lobe subpleural nodular opacities (*arrows*).

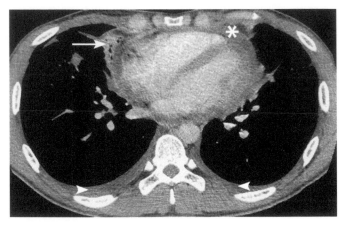

CT in mediastinal windows shows small bilateral pleural effusions (*white arrowheads*), a small pericardial effusion (*asterisk*), and right middle lobe atelectasis (*arrow*).

Answers

1. There are small bilateral pleural effusions, small right loculated pneumothorax, and bilateral subpleural nodular opacities.

2. Differential diagnosis of secondary spontaneous pneumothorax should include cystic lung diseases (eg, bullae, emphysema, *Pneumocystis jiroveci* pneumonia, lymphangioleiomyomatosis, Langerhans cell histiocytosis, cystic fibrosis), asthma, pulmonary necrosis (eg, necrotizing pneumonia, tuberculosis), cavitating neoplasms (eg, squamous cell carcinoma), metastatic osteosarcoma, and pleural endometriosis.

3. Common differential diagnostic considerations of multiple, subpleural poorly marginated pulmonary

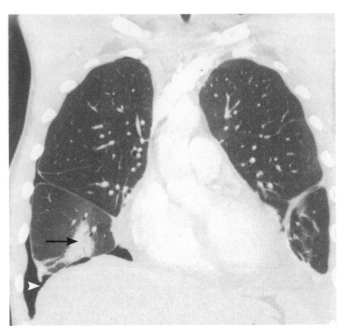

Coronal reformation redemonstrates a small right loculated pneumothorax (*arrowhead*) and shows a right lower lobe subpleural nodular opacity (*arrow*).

nodules are pulmonary contusions, pulmonary infarcts, cryptogenic organizing pneumonia, chronic eosinophilic pneumonia, vasculitis, and multifocal adenocarcinoma spectrum (previously known as bronchioloalveolar carcinoma).

4. The classical CT findings of subpleural poorly marginated nodules, pleural effusions, and spontaneous pneumothorax, together with history of recent travel to Southeast Asia, make paragonimiasis the most likely diagnosis.

5. Pleuropulmonary paragonimiasis is a parasitic disease caused by the lung fluke *Paragonimus*. Human infection starts with ingestion of raw or inadequately cooked freshwater crab or crayfish infested with the metacercariae.

Pearls

- Pleuropulmonary paragonimiasis is a parasitic disease caused by the lung fluke *Paragonimus*, endemic to Southeast Asia, Far East, Africa, and South America.
- Infection follows consumption of contaminated raw or undercooked fresh water crab or crayfish.
- Classical CT presentation is that of focal pleural thickening and subpleural linear opacity leading to a necrotic, peripheral pulmonary nodule, together with pleural effusion and pneumothorax.
- Clinically, paragonimiasis is often misdiagnosed as tuberculosis.

Suggested Readings

Haswell-Elkins MR, Elkins DB. Lung and liver flukes. In: Collier L, Balows A, Sussman M, eds. *Topley and Wilson's Microbiology and Microbial Infections.* 9th ed. New York: Oxford University Press; 1998:507-520.

Kim TS, Han J, Shim SS, et al. Pleuropulmonary paragonimiasis: CT findings in 31 patients. *AJR Am J Roentgenol.* September 2005;185(3):616-621.

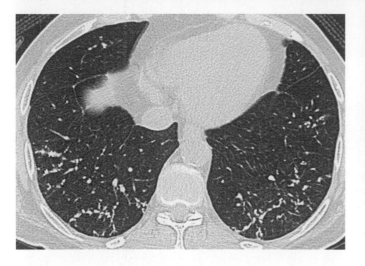 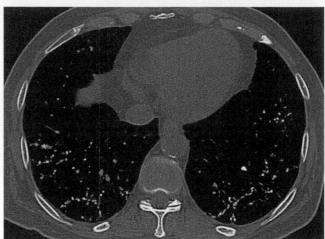

1. What are the imaging findings?

2. What is the differential diagnosis?

3. What is the diagnosis in this patient?

4. What are some secondary causes of pulmonary ossification?

5. What is the most common cause of small calcific lung nodules?

Case ranking/difficulty:

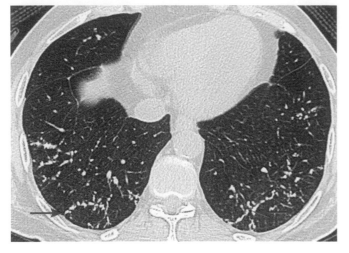

There are bilateral, basal, tiny, high-density nodular opacities, demonstrating linear and branching arrangement (*arrows*).

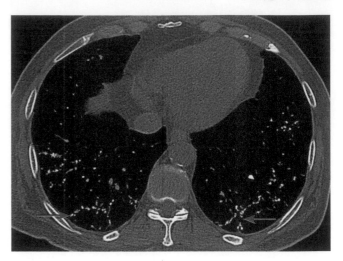

The bone window shows that the nodules have calcific density (*arrows*).

Answers

1. There are bilateral, basal, tiny, high-density nodular opacities, demonstrating a linear and branching arrangement.

2. The differential diagnosis of multiple bilateral small calcified nodular opacities: idiopathic pulmonary ossification, infection (eg, tuberculosis, histoplasmosis, and remote varicella pneumonia), pneumoconiosis (eg, silicosis, coal worker pneumoconiosis, and berylliosis), sarcoidosis, alveolar microlithiasis, injected or embolized material (eg, talcosis, mercury injection, and cement embolization), and metastases from bone-forming sarcomas (eg, osteosarcoma and chondrosarcoma) or adenocarcinomas.

3. The diagnosis in this patient is idiopathic pulmonary ossification (IPO).

4. Lung fibrosis (eg, idiopathic pulmonary fibrosis) and chronic pulmonary venous congestion (eg, longstanding mitral valve disease or chronic pulmonary edema) have been associated with pulmonary ossification.

5. Infectious granulomatous disease (eg, tuberculosis or histoplasmosis) is the most common cause of small calcific lung nodules.

Pearls

- Pulmonary ossification is a process of metaplastic mature bone formation.
- Pulmonary ossification can be an isolated idiopathic finding, or may be seen in cases of long-standing insults (ie, fibrosis or chronic pulmonary venous congestion).
- Pulmonary ossification is classified into *noduar* and *dendriform* types.
- Pulmonary ossification should not be confused with granulomatous or fibrotic lung disease.

Suggested Readings

Brown K, Mund DF, Aberle DR, Batra P, Young DA. Intrathoracic calcifications: radiographic features and differential diagnoses. *Radiographics*. November 1994;14(6):1247-1261.

Marchiori E, Souza AS, Franquet T, Müller NL. Diffuse high-attenuation pulmonary abnormalities: a pattern-oriented diagnostic approach on high-resolution CT. *AJR Am J Roentgenol*. January 2005;184(1):273-282.

Reddy TL, von der Thüsen J, Walsh SL. Idiopathic dendriform pulmonary ossification. *J Thorac Imaging*. September 2012;27(5):W108-W110.

Follow-up in patient with long-standing upper airway disease

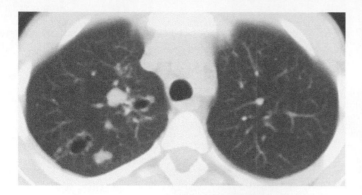
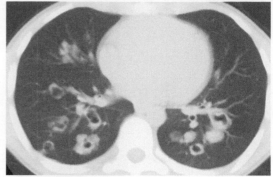
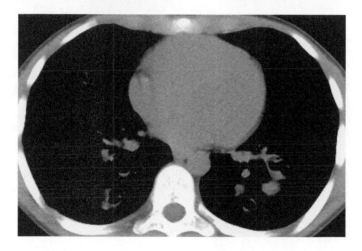

1. What are the findings?

2. What is the differential diagnosis based on the CT findings?

3. What is the causative agent of this disease?

4. What is the most feared complication of this condition?

5. What is the standard treatment for this condition?

Case ranking/difficulty: 🐾🐾🐾   **Category:** Lungs

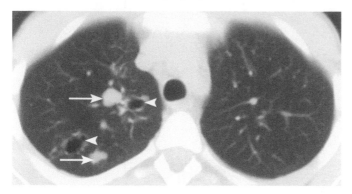

There are right upper lobe nodules (*arrows*) and thick-walled gas-filled cysts (*arrowheads*).

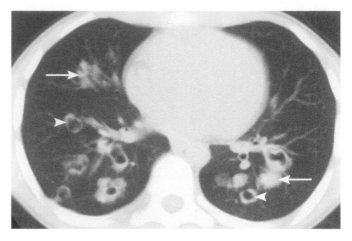

There are numerous bilateral nodules (*arrows*) and thick-walled cysts (*arrowheads*) at the lung bases.

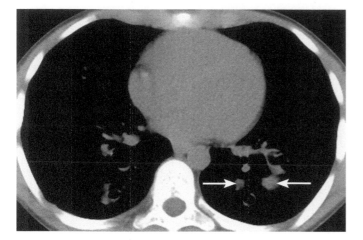

The mediastinal windows show that some nodules are solid (*arrows*).

Answers

1. There are numerous bilateral solid pulmonary nodules, cavitary nodules, and lobulated cysts with thick walls.

2. The differential diagnosis of multiple cavitary pulmonary nodules should include metastases, septic emboli, tuberculosis, fungal pneumonia, respiratory papillomatosis, Wegener granulomatosis, and necrobiotic nodules.

3. Recurrent respiratory papillomatosis is caused by human papillomavirus types 6 and 11.

4. Transformation of the pulmonary papillomas into squamous cell carcinoma is a rare, but ominous complication of respiratory papillomatosis.

5. The current standard of care is surgical therapy with a goal of complete removal of papillomas and preservation of normal structures. When surgical therapy is needed

more frequently than four times in 12 months or there is extralaryngeal disease, adjuvant medical therapy should be considered. Adjuvant therapies that have been investigated include dietary supplements, control of gastroesophageal reflux disease, potent antiviral and chemotherapeutic agents, and photodynamic therapies.

Pearls

- Recurrent respiratory papillomatosis is caused by human papillomavirus types 6 and 11.
- It is characterized by the proliferation of benign squamous papillomas within the aerodigestive tract.
- Larynx is most commonly affected.
- Pulmonary involvement is characterized by centrilobular cavitary nodules, which grow over time.
- Malignant transformation to squamous cell carcinoma is a rare complication.

Suggested Readings

Derkay CS, Wiatrak B. Recurrent respiratory papillomatosis: a review. *Laryngoscope*. July 2008;118(7):1236-1247.doi: 10.097/MLG.b013e31816a7135. Review.

Harman EM. Recurrent respiratory papillomatosis. http://emedicine.edscape.om/article/302648-overview. Updated November 20, 2013.

Chapter Index

Note: Numbers in parentheses refer to Case IDs.

Subchapter Index

Note: Numbers in parentheses refer to Case IDs.

Alphabetical Subject Index

Note: Numbers in parentheses refer to Case IDs.

Difficulty Level Index

Note: Numbers in parentheses refer to Case IDs.

Author Index

Note: Numbers in parentheses refer to Case IDs.